Breaking Down Barriers

Pat Langdon · Jonathan Lazar
Ann Heylighen · Hua Dong
Editors

Breaking Down Barriers

Usability, Accessibility and Inclusive Design

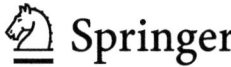 Springer

Editors
Pat Langdon
Department of Engineering
University of Cambridge
Cambridge, Cambridgeshire
UK

Jonathan Lazar
Department of Computer
　and Information Sciences
Towson University
Towson, MD
USA

Ann Heylighen
Department of Architecture, Research[x]
　Design
University of Leuven
Leuven
Belgium

Hua Dong
College of Design
　and Innovation
Tongji University
Shanghai
China

ISBN 978-3-319-75027-9   ISBN 978-3-319-75028-6 (eBook)
https://doi.org/10.1007/978-3-319-75028-6

Library of Congress Control Number: 2018930141

© Springer International Publishing AG, part of Springer Nature 2018
This work is subject to copyright. All rights are reserved by the Publisher, whether the whole or part of the material is concerned, specifically the rights of translation, reprinting, reuse of illustrations, recitation, broadcasting, reproduction on microfilms or in any other physical way, and transmission or information storage and retrieval, electronic adaptation, computer software, or by similar or dissimilar methodology now known or hereafter developed.
The use of general descriptive names, registered names, trademarks, service marks, etc. in this publication does not imply, even in the absence of a specific statement, that such names are exempt from the relevant protective laws and regulations and therefore free for general use.
The publisher, the authors and the editors are safe to assume that the advice and information in this book are believed to be true and accurate at the date of publication. Neither the publisher nor the authors or the editors give a warranty, express or implied, with respect to the material contained herein or for any errors or omissions that may have been made. The publisher remains neutral with regard to jurisdictional claims in published maps and institutional affiliations.

Printed on acid-free paper

This Springer imprint is published by the registered company Springer International Publishing AG part of Springer Nature
The registered company address is: Gewerbestrasse 11, 6330 Cham, Switzerland

Preface

The Cambridge Workshops on Universal Access and Assistive Technology (CWUAAT) are a series of workshops, which is held every 2 years at Fitzwilliam College in Cambridge University. This volume, *Breaking Down Barriers*, comes from the 9th workshop in this series held in April 2018.

In the context of developing demographic changes leading to greater numbers of older people and people living with impairments, the general field of inclusive design research strives to relate the capabilities of the population to the design of products, services and spaces. CWUAAT has always had a successful multidisciplinary focus, but if genuine transdisciplinary fields are to evolve from this, the final barriers to integrated research must be identified and characterised. Only then will benefits be realised in an inclusive society. Barriers do not arise from impairments themselves but, instead, are erected by humans, who often have not considered a greater variation in sensory, cognitive and physical user capabilities. Barriers are not only technical or architectural but they also exist between different communities of professionals. Our continual goal with the CWUAAT workshop series is to break down barriers in technical, physical and architectural design, as well as barriers between different professional communities.

The main sections of this book reflect the themes that we have identified in the emerging field of design for inclusion:

I Breaking Down Barriers Between Disciplines: Different disciplines, such as Engineering design, Assistive Technology, and Architecture and Medical design, are poor at communicating to each other on the basis of their approach to inclusive design and their criteria for good research in inclusive design;

II Breaking Down Barriers Between Users, Designers and Developers: A specific problem has been identified as the relationship between designers and the likely end users of their products or services;

III Removing Barriers to Usability, Accessibility and Inclusive Design: These different sub-disciplines of human computer interaction and user centred design actually evolved from similar roots. Nevertheless, despite some consideration of ageing and impairment in each field, they do not share a common theoretical or practical framework as a basis for progress;

IV Breaking Down Barriers Between People with Impairments and Those Without: It is an important consideration during the design or development of inclusive products. In particular, new ways of working together with disability have to be found if we are to realise the potential of this area. This includes collaborative, participative and user-centred design but also addresses each designer and user at the social–cultural level;

V Breaking Down Barriers Between Research and Policymaking: Here, important deficiencies have been identified in the translation of inclusive understanding into policy and practice. Hence, despite the existence of inclusive laws and guidelines based on inclusive research and the presence of websites, services and products that are predicated on them, considerable barriers have emerged in the access, use and construction of these offerings. Very often this affects the very population they were intended to serve.

The greatly appreciated aspect of these workshops is that they are a single session running over 3 days in pleasant surroundings with many delegates from home and abroad staying on site. CWUAAT allows speakers longer presentation times and question sessions, carrying discussion on through the day into plenaries. The shared social, temporal and leisure spaces generate an enjoyable academic environment that is both creative and innovative. CWUAAT is one of the few gatherings where people interested in inclusive design, across different fields, including **designers, computer scientists, engineers, architects, ergonomists, ethnographers, policymakers and user communities, meet, discuss and collaborate**. CWUAAT has also become an international workshop, representing diverse cultures including Portugal, Germany, Trinidad and Tobago, Canada, Australia, China, Norway, USA, Belgium, UK and many more.

This book contains the reviewed papers from CWUAAT 2018 that were invited for oral presentation. The papers that have been included were selected by peer review carried out by an international panel of currently active researchers. The chapters forming the book represent an edited sample of current national and international research in the fields of inclusive and architectural design, universal access, engineering design, HMI, and assistive and rehabilitative technology.

We would like to thank all those authors and researchers who have contributed to CWUAAT 2018 and to the preparation of this book. We would also like to thank the external reviewers who took part in the review process. Many thanks are also due to the reviewing members of the Programme Committee who have renewed their intention to support the workshop series. We are grateful to the staff at Fitzwilliam College for their patience and help. We must also thank the contributors of images for the cover and these are acknowledged as follows:

The wheelchair in the snow—Megan Strickfaden, University of Alberta
The wall—Natalia Pérez Liebergesell, KU Leuven
The map—Jo-Anne Bichard, 'Our Future Foyle', www.futurefoyle.org
The car—Miles Garner, RDM, UK Autodrive

Cambridge, UK
April 2018

Pat Langdon
The CWUAAT Editorial Committee

Contents

Part I Breaking Down Barriers Between Disciplines

Creating an Inclusive Architectural Intervention as a Research Space to Explore Community Well-being 3
J. Bichard, R. Alwani, E. Raby, J. West and J. Spencer

The Effect of Age and Gender on Task Performance in the Automobile 17
L. Skrypchuk, A. Mouzakitis, P. M. Langdon and P. J. Clarkson

Introducing Assistive Technology and Universal Design Theory, Applications in Design Education 29
Y. M. Choi

Exploring User Capability Data with Topological Data Analysis 41
U. Persad, J. Goodman-Deane, P. M. Langdon and P. J. Clarkson

Enhancing the Fashion and Textile Design Process and Wearer Experiences 51
W. Moody, P. M. Langdon and M. Karam

Part II Breaking Down Barriers Between Users, Designers and Developers

Using Inclusive Design to Drive Usability Improvements Through to Implementation 65
J. Goodman-Deane, S. D. Waller, M. Bradley, P. J. Clarkson and O. Bradley

Improving Pool Design: Interviewing Physically Impaired Architects 77
C. M. Pereira, T. V. Heitor and A. Heylighen

Intelligent Support Technologies for Older People: An Analysis of Characteristics and Roles 89
H. Petrie, J. S. Darzentas and S. Carmien

Participatory Design Resulting in a 'Do-It-Yourself Home Modification' Smartphone App 101
C. Bridge

Identifying Barriers to Usability: Smart Speaker Testing by Military Veterans with Mild Brain Injury and PTSD 113
T. Wallace and J. Morris

Part III Removing Barriers to Usability, Accessibility and Inclusive Design

Breaking Down Barriers: Promoting a New Look at Dementia-Friendly Design 125
J. Kirch, G. Marquardt and K. Bueter

Usability of Indoor Network Navigation Solutions for Persons with Visual Impairments 135
G. A. Giannoumis, M. Ferati, U. Pandya, D. Krivonos and T. Pey

Physical Barriers to Mobility of Stroke Patients in Rehabilitation Clinics 147
M. Kevdzija and G. Marquardt

A Practical Tool for the Evaluation of Contrast 159
S. Danschutter and B. Deroisy

Part IV Breaking Down Barriers Between People with Impairments and Those Without

Breaking Down Barriers Between Undergraduate Computing Students and Users with Disabilities 171
Jonathan Lazar

Improving Design Understanding of Inclusivity in Autonomous Vehicles: A Driver and Passenger *Taskscape* Approach 181
M. Strickfaden and P. M. Langdon

The Role of Inclusive Design in Improving People's Access to Treatment for Back Pain 195
Y. Liu, T. Dickerson, S. D. Waller, P. Waddingham and P. J. Clarkson

Inclusivity Considerations for Fully Autonomous Vehicle User Interfaces 207
T. Amanatidis, P. M. Langdon and P. J. Clarkson

**At Home in the Hospital and Hospitalised at Home: Exploring
Experiences of Cancer Care Environments** 215
P. Jellema, M. Annemans and A. Heylighen

**Do Exergames Motivate Seniors to Exercise? Computer Graphics
Impact** 227
R. Alyami and H. Wei

**Part V Breaking Down Barriers Between Research and
Policy-making**

**On Becoming a Cyborg: A Reflection on Articulation Work,
Embodiment, Agency and Ableism** 239
Jennifer Ann Rode

**Breaking Well-Formed Opinions and Mindsets by Designing with
People Living with Dementia** 251
Paul A. Rodgers and E. Winton

**The Effect of Simulation in Large-Scale Data Collection—An Example
of Password Policy Development** 263
J. Chakraborty and N. Nguyen

**Education and Existing Knowledge of Architects in Germany About
Accessibility and Building for the Older Generation** 275
E. Rudolph and S. Kreiser

Author Index 285

Contributors

R. Alwani Royal College of Art Helen Hamlyn Centre for Design, London, UK

R. Alyami Department of Computer Science, University of Reading, Reading, UK

T. Amanatidis Department of Engineering, Cambridge Engineering Design Centre, University of Cambridge, Cambridge, UK

M. Annemans Department of Architecture, Research[x]Design, KU Leuven, Leuven, Belgium

J. Bichard Royal College of Art Helen Hamlyn Centre for Design, London, UK

M. Bradley Cambridge Engineering Design Centre, University of Cambridge, Cambridge, UK

O. Bradley Unilever, Leatherhead, England, UK

C. Bridge UNSW, Sydney, Australia

K. Bueter Faculty of Architecture, Technische Universitaet Dresden, Dresden, Germany

S. Carmien Human Computer Interaction Research Group, Department of Computer Science, University of York, York, UK

J. Chakraborty Towson University, Towson, MD, USA

Y. M. Choi Georgia Institute of Technology, Atlanta, GA, USA

P. J. Clarkson Department of Engineering, Cambridge Engineering Design Centre, University of Cambridge, Cambridge, UK

S. Danschutter Belgian Building Research Insitute, Limelette, Belgium

J. S. Darzentas Human Computer Interaction Research Group, Department of Computer Science, University of York, York, UK

B. Deroisy Belgian Building Research Insitute, Limelette, Belgium

T. Dickerson Department of Engineering, Cambridge Engineering Design Centre, University of Cambridge, Cambridge, UK

M. Ferati Oslo and Akershus University College of Applied Sciences, Oslo, Norway

G. A. Giannoumis Oslo and Akershus University College of Applied Sciences, Oslo, Norway

J. Goodman-Deane Cambridge Engineering Design Centre, the University of Cambridge, Cambridge, UK

T. V. Heitor University of Lisbon, Lisbon, Portugal

A. Heylighen Department of Architecture, Research[x]Design, KU Leuven, Leuven, Belgium

P. Jellema Department of Architecture, Research[x]Design, KU Leuven, Leuven, Belgium

M. Karam Kings College London, London, UK

M. Kevdzija Technische Universität Dresden, Dresden, Germany

J. Kirch Network Aging Research, Heidelberg University, Heidelberg, Germany

S. Kreiser Faculty of Architecture, TU Dresden, Dresden, Germany

D. Krivonos Oslo and Akershus University College of Applied Sciences, Oslo, Norway

P. M. Langdon Department of Engineering, Cambridge Engineering Design Centre, University of Cambridge, Cambridge, UK

Jonathan Lazar Department of Computer and Information Sciences, Towson University, Towson, MD, USA; University of Pennsylvania Law School, Philadelphia, PA, USA

Y. Liu Department of Engineering, Cambridge Engineering Design Centre, University of Cambridge, Cambridge, UK

G. Marquardt Faculty of Architecture, Technische Universität Dresden, Dresden, Germany

W. Moody Cambridge School of Art, Anglia Ruskin University, Cambridge, UK

J. Morris Shepherd Center, Atlanta, GA, USA

A. Mouzakitis Jaguar Land Rover Research, Coventry, UK

N. Nguyen Towson University, Towson, MD, USA

U. Pandya Wayfindr, London, UK

C. M. Pereira University of Lisbon, Lisbon, Portugal

Contributors

U. Persad The University of Trinidad and Tobago, Arima, Trinidad and Tobago

H. Petrie Human Computer Interaction Research Group, Department of Computer Science, University of York, York, UK

T. Pey Royal Society for Blind Children, London, UK

E. Raby Royal College of Art Helen Hamlyn Centre for Design, London, UK

Jennifer Ann Rode University College London, London, UK

Paul A. Rodgers Imagination, Lancaster University, Lancaster, UK

E. Rudolph Faculty of Architecture, TU Dresden, Dresden, Germany

L. Skrypchuk Jaguar Land Rover Research, Coventry, UK

J. Spencer Royal College of Art Helen Hamlyn Centre for Design, London, UK

M. Strickfaden Department of Human Ecology, University of Alberta, Edmonton, AB, Canada

P. Waddingham Cambridgeshire Community Services NHS Trust, Cambridge, UK

T. Wallace Shepherd Center, Atlanta, GA, USA

S. D. Waller Department of Engineering, Cambridge Engineering Design Centre, University of Cambridge, Cambridge, UK

H. Wei Department of Computer Science, University of Reading, Reading, UK

J. West Royal College of Art Helen Hamlyn Centre for Design, London, UK

E. Winton Imagination, Lancaster University, Lancaster, UK

Part I
Breaking Down Barriers Between Disciplines

Creating an Inclusive Architectural Intervention as a Research Space to Explore Community Well-being

J. Bichard, R. Alwani, E. Raby, J. West and J. Spencer

Abstract This paper outlines a 2-year active design research project coordinated in collaboration with Public Health Northern Ireland and set in the city of Derry/Londonderry to explore how inclusive design methodologies can produce interventions to improve community well-being. The research focuses on the waterfront of the River Foyle and how an inclusive architectural intervention challenged the areas' negative associations. In the last decade, the waterfront has become synonymous with mental health crisis and suicide. This has led to the phrase 'I'm ready for the Foyle' becoming embedded within the communities' language as a colloquial term for stress. This project seeks to extend inclusive design within the community, creating well-being spaces around the bridges and banks of the river, with outcomes focused on drawing people to the area as a place of celebration and life-affirming activities. The project has helped to develop Inclusive Design as a means of engaging a whole city in the redesign of public spaces for improved well-being.

1 Introduction

Historically, the city of Derry/Londonderry has a turbulent past in which the river has acted as a 'natural' divide between opposing communities. In a region where peace is relatively new, tensions remain regarding access to shared resources.

J. Bichard (✉) · R. Alwani · E. Raby · J. West · J. Spencer
Royal College of Art Helen Hamlyn Centre for Design, London, UK
e-mail: jo-anne.bichard@rca.ac.uk

R. Alwani
e-mail: ralf.alwani@network.rca.ac.uk

E. Raby
e-mail: elizabeth.raby@network.rca.ac.uk

J. West
e-mail: jonathan.west@network.rca.ac.uk

J. Spencer
e-mail: jak.spencer@rca.ac.uk

© Springer International Publishing AG, part of Springer Nature 2018
P. Langdon et al. (eds.), *Breaking Down Barriers*,
https://doi.org/10.1007/978-3-319-75028-6_1

This division required careful organisation to avoid separate research enquiries with each community but to also draw on the neutrality of the river as a symbol of the shared home of the city.

Inclusive Design is a way of designing products, services and environments that include the needs of the widest number of people as possible. It is often used to understand marginalised, overlooked or vulnerable populations to help innovation for the good of society. This project seeks to understand how inclusively designed interventions can improve community well-being.

Through our initial engagements with community representatives, mental health professionals, police and rescue services, a story emerged around the river that told of an Orca's visit to the city at the height of 'the Troubles' in the 1970s. The whale was seen in the river for nearly a week, was reported in the press and given the name 'Dopey Dick'. Many people visited the River Foyle to witness their unusual guest and for many children, it was their first experience of meeting others from across the river. This historical encounter was a shared community memory that conjured a positive recollection of a period that has previously been linked to destruction and violence. With the need to develop a neutral space in which to extend inclusive design with the larger community, the tale of 'Dopey Dick' provided the impetus for the design of an architectural intervention as shared research space.

Created in collaboration with community activists and creatives within Derry/Londonderry, the structure of a whale was designed and built as a space for the communities to come together. Within this space, the research team was able to organise inclusive and interactive activities to begin the process of exploring how well-being is perceived and how suicide prevention might be understood and tackled. The structure was subsequently featured in news reports and was a major attraction at two city events drawing crowds of up to 80,000 people. This paper reflects on the creation of this research space and how this shared history opened a space of design-led navigation of the city's and communities' response to well-being, the design initiatives and briefs that have emerged from these engagements and how this might offer key learnings for understanding how the design of the built environment may afford positive mental health opportunities.

2 Addressing Suicide in Derry/Londonderry

The World Health Organisation (WHO 2014) report *Preventing suicide: A global imperative* found that suicide is a major public health concern and estimated that globally, every 40 s a person will die by suicide. Northern Ireland has the highest suicide rate of the UK nations, which has increased dramatically over the last 30 years (Samaritans 2017) with Derry/Londonderry identified as the city with the highest rate of suicide in Northern Ireland (MHFI 2013). Instances of young male suicide, noted by *The Atlantic* as 'the ceasefire babies', are at 'crisis' level (McKee 2016). Within the locality of Derry/Londonderry, the term 'I'm ready for the Foyle' has become embedded within the city as a saying associated with feelings of despair, distress or desperation, and is associated with suicide by jumping, notably from one of the three bridges that crosses the city's river.

Knapp et al. (2011) estimate that each instance of suicide in the UK has a cost equivalence of £1.7 million. Their calculations include direct costs, i.e. the services used by the individual leading up to and immediately following the suicide; GP visits, prescribed medication, counselling, funeral costs, court costs, use of emergency services, insurance claims and medical services. Indirect costs encompass the costs to society of each suicide including time lost from work, lost production from an exit or absence from the workforce. Consideration is also noted towards the human cost such as lost years of disability-free life in addition to the pain and grief experienced by family and friends.

The Public Health Agency (Northern Ireland) have looked at traditional approaches to addressing suicide prevention involving rivers and bridges but often found possible resolutions ineffective or failing to address the core reasons why people choose to die by suicide. The Agency also acknowledges that the Foyle area is a very unique situation; it is not just about the river itself, but why people are attracted to it as a means of suicide.

The River Foyle is a natural formation within the urban area of Derry/Londonderry Northern Ireland (Fig. 1). The riverfront is a six-mile loop with three bridges connecting the areas known as city-side and waterside. The largest bridge in Ireland spanning 866 m is the Foyle Bridge. To the south of the city is the Craigavon Bridge, one of the few double-decker road bridges in Europe. Between these two iconic structures is the newest bridge, the Peace Bridge a pedestrian-only walkway. The east bank of the river has a railway line (towards/from Belfast) that runs along its edge, and acts as a boundary between the water and pedestrian walkways. The river's east banks include large areas of park and wetland with residential clusters. The west bank is more urban and includes a hardscape riverfront. There are some commercial and residential blocks in the centre, whereas the south-west of the riverfront is disconnected to the city centre by a busy road. The north-west of the site emerges into a retail park and then industrial land connected along the water's edge to a nature reserve which encompasses the Foyle Bridge.

In the context of the River Foyle, individuals have lost their lives to suicide which, as Knapp et al. suggest, has an associated economic cost. However, this cost does not include unreported cases and individuals that have not lost their life but that have been intervened with at the river's edge. The cost of such attempts is undetermined.

The more intangible but central impact of suicide is how it affects the mental health and well-being of friends, family, the community and a place. Suicide in a public place can lead to further instances and spaces can become stigmatised. San Francisco's Golden Gate Bridge holds the reputation as the world's leading suicide destination, whilst England's Beachy Head holds a similar reputation in Europe. Suicides that occur in public places have far-reaching consequences for the health of others and thereby contribute to the overall burden of mental illness and

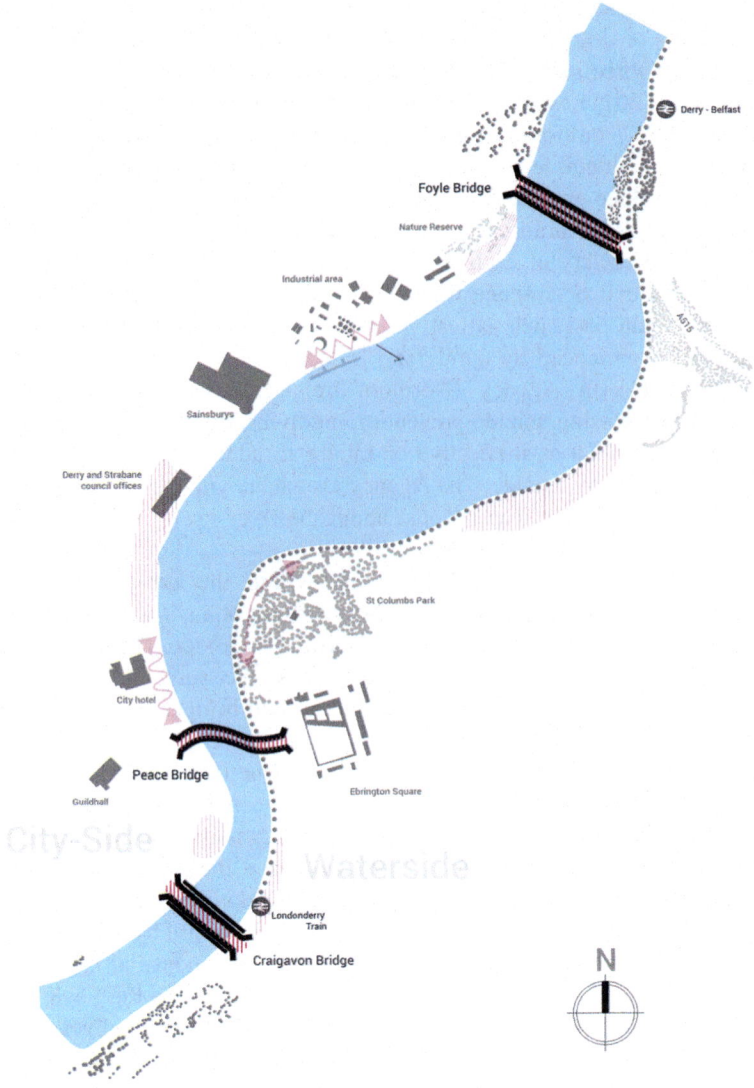

Fig. 1 Map of River Foyle showing the three city bridges

psychological distress. Such identification can potentially influence others to take their own lives at that location (Reisch and Michel 2005).

The River Foyle and its banks currently have a critical reputation for suicidal behaviour. With area associations evolving over generations, it is recognised that it will take time to shift public and community perceptions and as with many other public health initiatives will involve a complex and broad approach that empowers people and communities to collaborate as agents of change. Inclusive innovation will contribute to creating the right conditions, offering avenues for people-centred engagement in the cities design. A current innovative initiative is the partnership between Public Health Northern Ireland and The Royal College of Art Helen Hamlyn Centre for Design (2016–2019) who have created 'Our Future Foyle' as a research and design initiative that seeks to develop, through community facing inclusive design, social and cultural interventions around arts and leisure that impact the banks and bridges of the River Foyle. This multidisciplinary collaboration brings together; an architect, an information experience designer, an industrial designer with expertise in healthcare, a design anthropologist and public health experts as well as the residents, businesses and community groups within the Derry/Londonderry locality.

3 Our Future Foyle

The team established 'Our Future Foyle' (PHA & HHCD) in early 2016 as the public face for the project with a wider vision of community health and well-being. The brief highlighted how arts, leisure and technology could play a part in interventions with a wider vision of improving well-being and community use of the space for the people of the city.

Establishing the organisation has centred the project as a neutral and empowering voice within the community, allowing the public to have their say on how to improve their riverfront through urban regeneration without reinforcing the stigma of mental health crisis in the area. Public feedback on future public art, disjointed areas and community spaces through to better amenities such as public toilets, cycle lanes and retail spaces have been combined with more in-depth research and engagement with stakeholders. Such public engagement activities have been further informed by focused interviews with experts and individuals about suicidal behaviour. These research insights have informed an iterative design process based on both community and contextual responses and developed towards solutions that are inclusive, enjoyable and that benefit the whole community whilst also acting as a suicide prevention measure.

Our Future Foyle has also had to consider the communities' historical context. Derry/Londonderry caught the world's attention from the late 1960s and through the end of the twentieth century as a city divided by conflict, known as 'the Troubles'. This period resulted in community segregation and divisions that despite considerable progress since the 'Good Friday Agreement' of 1999 still exist today. The legacy of this period continues to impact Northern Ireland's well-being. The World Mental Health Survey Initiative covering 28 countries noted Northern to have the highest rate of post-traumatic disorder amongst those who were not born during this period (the ceasefire babies) (McLafferty et al. 2016). Such trauma is now considered to be intergenerational and has been identified from Holocaust survivors.

Many of the risk factors for suicide, including history of trauma, unemployment, drugs and alcohol misuse, social isolation and deprivation (O'Reilly et al. 2008), are all prevalent in the city of Derry/Londonderry and it is thought that the higher levels of suicide are also due to post-traumatic stress of the troubles (McLafferty et al. 2016).

Further consideration needs to address the premeditation of suicide, which has been noted to fall into two categories: planned and impulsive. Planned suicides maybe considered over a period of months, weeks or days. In contrast, impulsive suicides may have been considered for less than five minutes (Anderson 2008). Considering incidents on the River Foyle, it is noted that those who have planned their suicide are most likely to have entered the water from the Foyle Bridge, the highest point to the river (Fig. 2). Indications of such planning include its car accessibility as well as relatively quiet periods where visits can be undisturbed. The Foyle Bridge's height also contributes to a high 'completion' rate and to date, only two people are known to have survived a fall from this bridge. In contrast, impulsive suicides are more likely to have entered the river from the banks or lower Peace and Craigavon bridges. The accessibility of the lower bridges and riverbanks from the town centre, coupled with the close proximity to venues selling alcohol, presents a greater opportunity for impulsive suicides.

Combined consideration of these geographical, social and historical factors have been crucial in building co-design relationships with Derry/Londonderry communities and addressing how the project is presented to the community and how consultation will engage.

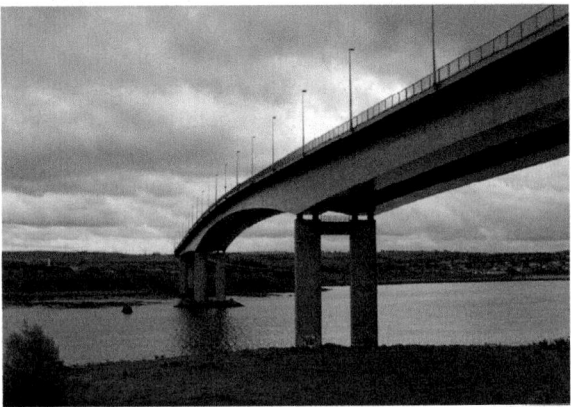

Fig. 2 The Foyle bridge (Our Future Foyle 2016)

4 The Tale of the Whale

In November 1977, the front page of *The Derry Journal* announced 'Huge whale in the Foyle' and reported that to the bafflement of marine experts an orca (killer whale) had swum up the River Foyle. The whale was given the name 'Dopey Dick', and crowds congregated around the river to see the visitor. Dopey would subsequently enter into Derry/Londonderry folklore. The timing of the whale's visit at the height of 'the Troubles' meant that many children were taken down to the river to witness this event, and Dopey became a neutral visitor in the predominantly divided community.

Prior to the research starting, Dopey Dick had again made the front pages of both *Derry Journal* and the *Guardian* with a report that he (although rumour had it he was really a she) was still alive and living off the coast of Scotland—although the 1 April news date might prove difficult to verify. The research team saw the power of this story, especially its occurrence during this specific period of the city's history, as well as its possible transgenerational appeal and opportunities for engagement with older people who remembered Dopey's visit, and younger people, especially children who might enjoy the story of the whale in their river. During a stakeholder workshop, it became apparent that the team's planned community consultation may have to take place 'over here and over there' due to each community's preference for specific spaces of the city. This would effectively double the resourcing of the engagement process. On reviewing the activities and information gathered at the workshop, the team's architect suggested building a specific 'neutral' structure in which to hold engagement activities, and that this structure could take the form of a whale (Fig. 3).

Construction of the whale was to be wholly community focused. The whale's bones were cut by community FabLab, whilst the whale's skin would draw from the cities historical industry of shirt making and was created by material donated by *Smyth & Gibson*—the last shirt makers in the city. Through its toy-like design, the space aimed to attract both children and adults, into inclusive research activities.

During the construction of the whale, the researchers carried out further consultations within the community through a series of workshops that involved 50 people. By annotating scale maps of the area around the river, the participants recorded spaces they thought were negative and positive, as well as putting forward ideas and hopes for the future of the river. The information gathered in these workshops was then assessed and cross-referenced to see if the identified areas reflected wider findings from previous community consultations. It was found that information correlated to wider consultations and pinpointed areas of concern that were shared across ages and cultural heritage. Predominantly, negative areas were the area of the riverside path to the south of the river; the Craigavon and Foyle

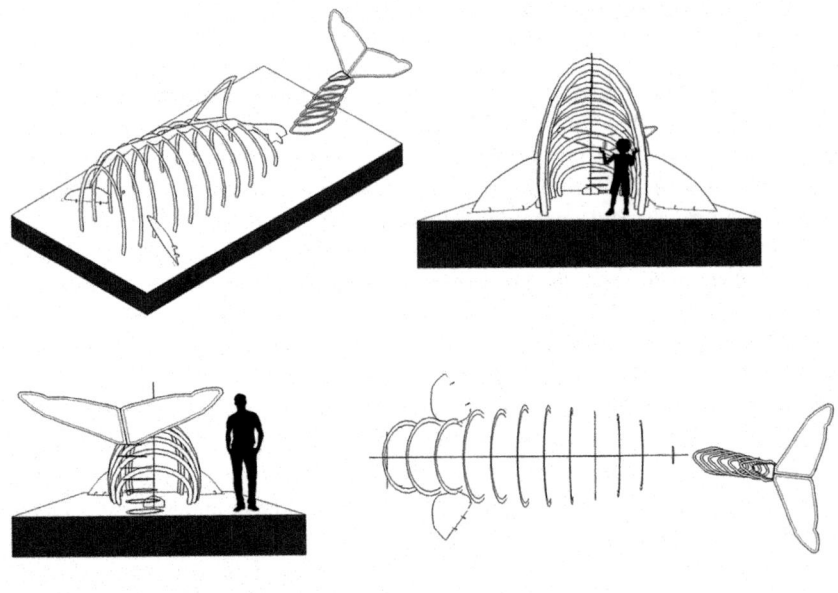

Fig. 3 Outline of whale structure (Alwani; Our Future Foyle 2016)

bridges were also highlighted as negative areas with concerns raised on low lighting, high incidences of anti-social behaviour and less human activity/flow. Positive areas identified included the Peace Bridge and the cafes that had been located close to the river.

5 Extending Inclusive Consultations Through Events

The design and construction of the whale structure presented an opportunity to create a community built neutral space for public engagement and consultation in Our Future Foyle project. Further consultation with research partners identified that a key place for the whale structure would be on the bank of the River Foyle for the cities Maritime Festival. This key event in Derry/Londonderry's calendar has the city as host port for the Clipper round the world race. The Clipper 9-day festival drew an estimated 163,000 people. The whale structure—now formally called Dopey—was on site for 2 days and became the Our Future Foyle research space open to the public. Approximately, 1250 people came to the space and one in five engaged with the consultation through commenting on postcards that were then displayed inside Dopey. Sticker boards were also used for people to vote on various ideas and hopes previously emerging from the workshops. Children and young people were encouraged to decorate Dopey's skin with pictures and comments highlighting their hopes and aspirations for the River Foyle.

Derry/Londonderry is also known locally as 'LegenDerry' and this status is reflected in the cities world-renowned status for hosting Halloween celebrations. Dopey would return this time as the 'Ghost of Dopey Dick' and set up in the city centre for 4 days over the Halloween weekend. During this event, an estimated 3,000 people visited the research space, and consultations were extended to include video interviews and recorded 'voxpops' of people's thoughts about the river and the opportunities it may present. During the Halloween event, the space also became a central point for community activities and performances including a choir, poetry recitals (Fig. 4) and a music performance.

In the evening, Dopey's interior became a pop-up cinema showing clips from number of water-themed horror films. The weekend's events around and inside Dopey culminated in the taking down and reconstruction of the structure onto a barge. Working in collaboration with Loughs and River's Agencies Dopey was floated down the river during the cities Halloween costume parade and closing firework display (Fig. 5), drawing an estimated crowd of 30,000 people, and featured on local BBC news.

It should be noted that the consultations and activities did not directly discuss the issue of suicide. Participants did comment on incidents and the area's association with suicide behaviour but it was decided that this would not directly be addressed during these public engagements, so that the tone of the event remained positive

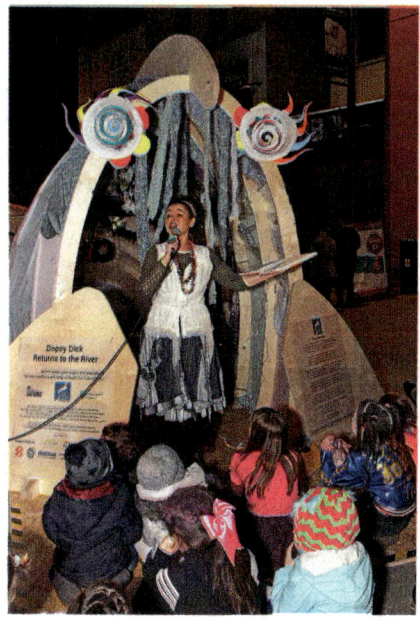

Fig. 4 Dopey as community performance space (Our Future Foyle 2016)

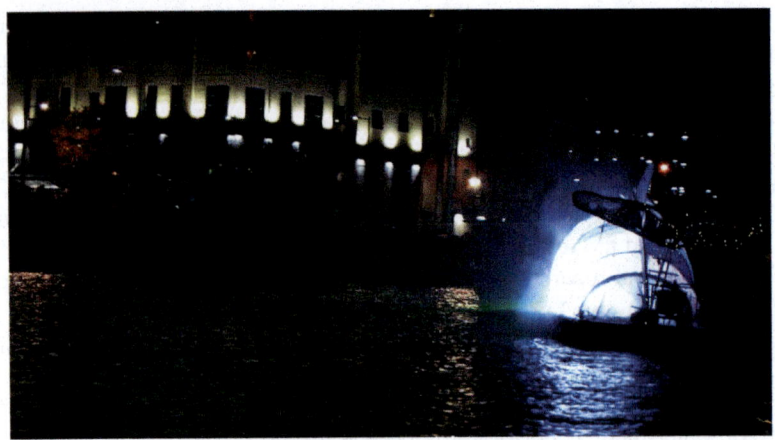

Fig. 5 'Dopey Dick' on the river for Halloween celebrations (Gavin Patton 2016)

and highlighted opportunities for future development around the River Foyle. The key question asked at these events was 'what do you want your riverfront to become?'

By focusing on key events in the cities' calendar, the research engaged over 4000 individuals using a variety of inclusive methods. Participation of the research and the Our Future Foyle initiative at these events was designed to engage with ideas formulated at earlier workshops, gather new ideas, gain feedback and increase the presence of the project.

Our Future Foyle events have continued with a pop-up cinema. The research team continues to plan future events as a key method to engage with the community and gather citywide insights from those who attend. These events also help to showcase the design work to as wider audience as possible. Centred around and on the river, the events contribute to tackling the stigma of the area and suggest innovative uses for the space extending inclusive engagement with communities that may not visit the riverfront.

6 Design Proposals

From the extensive engagement with the community, it was clear that a holistic approach to designing interventions for improved well-being would be required, rather than a single physical intervention. The engagement showed the best way to achieve a positive, lasting impact would be to incorporate physical, behavioural, environmental, social and digital interventions. As a result, five design proposals are currently being developed as direct outcomes from these event-based public engagements and design research activities. These social and cultural interventions address suicidal behaviour on the Foyle whilst positively impacting on wider physical health, well-being, education, tourism and community-specific agenda. As with all Inclusive Design projects, they are created through co-design, with the Derry/Londonderry community regularly consulted throughout the design process. They comprise the following:

- *Foyle Reeds*: a non-imprisoning prevention barrier over the Foyle Bridge and comprising the largest public art sculpture in Northern Ireland. Its aim is to act as an effective suicide prevention installation whilst changing the perception of the bridge to a positive icon with a sense of community ownership (Fig. 6).
- *Foyle Bubbles*: a series of portable satellite spaces set along the river bank, reconnecting disjointed spaces and providing navigational points, to be facilitated by existing organisations and individuals from community, arts and commercial sectors. Hosts of the bubbles will undertake mental health training and offer educational alternatives acting as a community response to the river without clinical stigma.
- *Foyle Experience*: reducing suicides through sensory means. These 'soft' interventions focus on reducing suicide attempts from the Craigavon and Peace bridges. This intervention explores deploying a series of sensory objects that influence how design can affect social perception and cognitive behaviours in a place.
- *Foyle Connect*: a media campaign looking at suicide prevention. By improving public awareness of identifying suicidal behaviour within the home, workplace and community, individuals may feel supported to discuss suicide with potentially vulnerable individuals. This intervention aims to support people before a potential point of crisis at the riverfront.
- *Foyle Digital*: Digital Platform. The creation of a digital platform that promotes community and tourism use along the riverfront; through publicising events, information and facts along the river, the platform acts as a way finding aid with elements of gamification and a discussion platform.

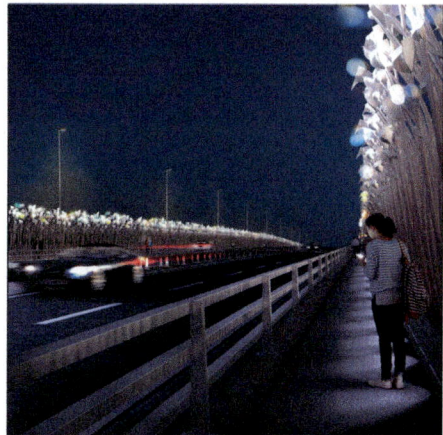 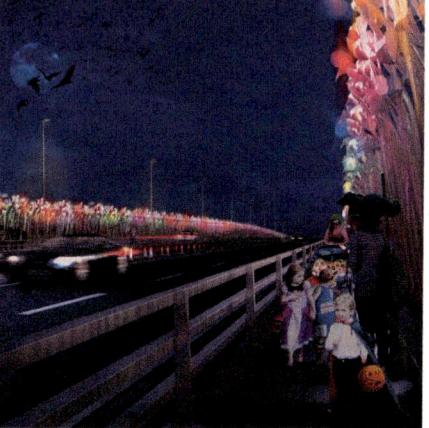

Fig. 6 Proposed 'Foyle Reeds' light installation on the Foyle Bridge showing daily and special event adaptation (Our Future Foyle 2017)

All five of these design proposals directly involve the communities of Derry/Londonderry in their development, and as much as feasibly possible, the building and delivery of the proposals, ensuring a community-led initiative that can proudly announce that it was conceived, built and delivered in the city for the city.

7 Conclusions

Our Future Foyle incorporates elements of inclusive architectural, information, health service and experience design to explore how a key area of a city may develop new opportunities, whilst tackling negative associations with a specific public space. The project's principle aim is to address the issue of suicide in public, but its focus explores how a space may be reconceptualised as an area associated with life-affirming activities and well-being. The design of the whale structure based on a historical occurrence and local memory generated a neutral space in which a still divided community could visit and participate in the project.

A crucial element of this design work has been to engage with the community and understand the issues of the space and city. Both design researchers Alwani and Raby have attended and completed initial and advanced suicide awareness training. As the research has developed and the realisation of design briefs materialises, it has become necessary in both time and budget for one of the researchers to spend extended periods in the city. This gives the design researcher time to build on community and stakeholder networks and immerse themselves in the day-to-day happenings of the communities creating a deeper understanding of what may or may not be accepted by this specific UK population. Such in-depth design ethnography can be seen to be essential to understand a space, a place and the people who inhabit it, and therefore begin to address directly the issue of suicide in public space and contribute to creating improved health and well-being within the city.

The design of the whale pushed the boundaries of design provocations as an Inclusive Design tool to engage participants, to an architectural scale, enabling the participation of the entire city in the redesign of its public space. The findings from this develop Inclusive Design as a tool, from one that has traditionally worked with small, typically excluded groups to open the potential of working with entire populations. The design proposals are specifically focused on social and cultural outcomes that aim to reach all members of the community. The research space of the whale generated cross-community and transgenerational outreach, enabling the design team to focus on well-being outcomes that may benefit the whole community. The design proposals focus on greater sensitivity and improved place making that also acts, in this specific case, as suicide prevention measures.

References

Anderson S (2008) The urge to end it all. New York Times Magazine, July 6. www.nytimes.com/2008/07/06/magazine/06suicide-t.html?mcubz=1. Accessed 28 Sept 2017

Derry Journal (2011) Whale of a tale that had the city hooked for a week. Derry Journal, Sunday 06 November 2011. www.derryjournal.com/lifestyle/nostalgia/whale-of-a-tale-that-had-the-city-hooked-for-a-week-1-3215091. Accessed 28 Sept 2017

Derry Journal (2016) Dopey Dick has retired to Scotland. Derry Journal, Friday 01 April 2016. www.derryjournal.com/news/dopey-dick-has-retired-to-scotland-1-7307581. Accessed on 28 Sept 2017

Foyle Search and Rescue (2017) Internal communication

Knapp M, McDaid D, Parsonage M (eds) (2011) Mental health promotion and mental illness prevention: the economic case. Personal Social Service Research Unit, London School of Economics and Political Science. www.lse.ac.uk/businessAndConsultancy/LSEEnterprise/pdf/PSSRUfeb2011.pdf. Accessed 28 Sept 2017

McKee L (2016) Suicide among the ceasefire babies. The Atlantic, 6 January 2016. www.theatlantic.com/health/archive/2016/01/conflict-mental-health-northern-ireland-suicide/424683/. Accessed 28 Sept 2017

McLafferty M, Armour C, O'Neill S, Murphy S, Ferry F, Bunting B (2016) Suicidality and profiles of childhood adversities, conflict related trauma and psychopathology in the Northern Ireland population. J Affect Disord 200:97–102

MHFI (2013) Young men and suicide project. A report on all-Ireland young men and suicide project. Men's Health Forum Ireland. www.mhfi.org/ymspfullreport.pdf. Accessed 28 Sept 2017

O'Reilly D, Rosato M, Connolly S, Cardwell C (2008) Area factors and suicide: 5-year follow-up of the Northern Ireland population. Br J Psychiatry 192(2):106–111

Reisch T, Michel K (2005) Securing a suicide hotspot: Effects of a safety net at the Bern Muenster Terrace. Suicide Life Threat Behav 35(4):460–467

Samaritans (2017) Suicide statistics report. Samaritans. www.samaritans.org/sites/default/files/kcfinder/files/Suicide_statistics_report_2017_Final.pdf. Accessed 30 Sept 2017

The Guardian (2016) Dopey Dick, killer whale that swam into Derry in 1977, still alive and well. The Guardian, Friday 01 April 2016. www.theguardian.com/environment/2016/apr/01/dopey-dick-killer-whale-derry-1977-west-coast-scotland. Accessed 28 Sept 2017

WHO (2014) Preventing suicide: a global imperative. World Health Organisation, Geneva

The Effect of Age and Gender on Task Performance in the Automobile

L. Skrypchuk, A. Mouzakitis, P. M. Langdon and P. J. Clarkson

Abstract The automobile is becoming more complex as vehicle technologies advance. As a result, driver awareness of internal and external aspects of the environment will influence performance for a range of activities. Inclusivity is an important aspect of vehicle design, especially as autonomous driving functionality increases. This paper examines how users of differing gender and age perform within the vehicle. A simulator study was carried out to assess performance on a range of tasks, whilst driving under different driving conditions. The results show that differences exist between males and females, and older and younger operators for a range of driving and non-driving measures. Older operators generated higher steering wheel variation than younger drivers in driving-only conditions, whilst older and female operators require more button presses and glances away from the road than younger and male operators. The implications relating to in-vehicle interface design are discussed.

1 Introduction

There are many aspects of the automobile that are changing rapidly, such as alternative power sources (Zapata and Nieuwenhuis 2010) and autonomous driving (Luettel et al. 2012). These are aimed at reducing the impact of large global issues such as CO_2 emissions and vehicle safety. As such, rapid changes are also being

---

L. Skrypchuk (✉) · A. Mouzakitis
Jaguar Land Rover Research, Coventry, UK
e-mail: LSKRYPCH@jaguarlandrover.com

A. Mouzakitis
e-mail: AMOUZAK1@jaguarlandrover.com

P. M. Langdon · P. J. Clarkson
Cambridge Engineering Design Centre, University of Cambridge, Cambridge, UK
e-mail: pml24@eng.cam.ac.uk

P. J. Clarkson
e-mail: pjc10@eng.cam.ac.uk

made on the interior of the vehicle. The number of features and technologies offered to consumers is increasing (Abelein et al. 2012). Thus, whilst drivers are in manual control, another factor associated with vehicle safety is the impact these alternative tasks have when attempted in parallel with driving. Whether built-in onboard or through brought in devices (such as mobile phones), the user has access to more functionality than ever. Many of these cause the driver to shift attention away from the road. This combined with human desire to access information, increasingly fuelled by a fear of missing out, increases the likelihood of multitasking in the car (Przybylski et al. 2013).

Multitasking in the vehicle can be classified in a number of ways. The first relates to the driving act itself. The driver has to navigate, manoeuvre, check speed and avoid hazards, all of which have to be carried out successfully to complete a journey. The second type is when the driver attempts to carry out a Non-Driving Related Activity (NDRA) whilst the Driving Related Activity (DRA) is active, achieving this either in serial or parallel mode (Salvucci et al. 2009). It is this second type of multitasking that will be the focus of this paper.

One aspect of this challenge is the effect of natural variation within the user group and to what extent differences are evident that may impact how the vehicle systems are designed. Two prevalent differences are gender and age. Figure 1 shows the profile of active drivers in the United States of America. The first observation of note is the equal split of gender between male and female drivers, whilst the second is the wide age range. This diverse profile potentially makes designing and testing interface systems more challenging, especially when combined with the increasing complexity found within the driving environment. The question therefore being considered here is what is the effect of gender or age on performance in an automotive multitasking situation? This question will be examined using a driving simulator study along with a discussion about the implications for interface systems.

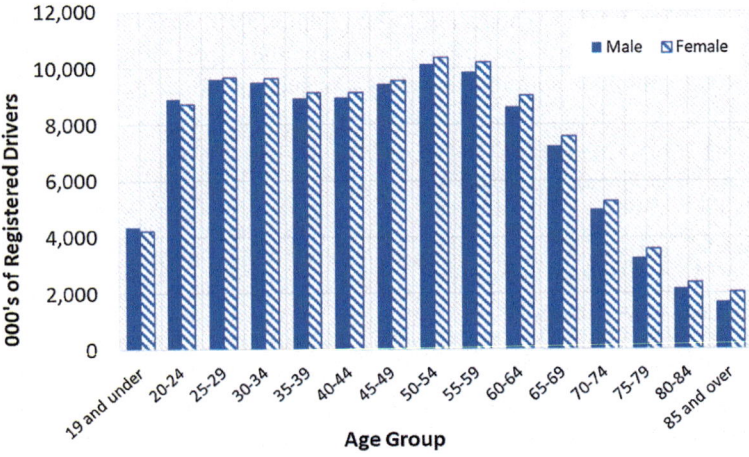

Fig. 1 Age profile of drivers in the United States of America, accurate as of 2015 (FHWA 2015)

1.1 Age and Gender Differences

Previous research has shown effects of both gender and age on human performance. Age appears more frequently in the literature. A number of the age-related findings are associated with reduced performance with old age, such as eyesight (Guirao et al. 1999), psychomotor response (Smith et al. 1999) and cognitive function (Hasher and Zacks 1988) amongst others (Charness and Bosman 1994, Reimers and Maylor 2005). Higher level functions, such as anticipation of hazards, gained through many years of experience, however, are sometimes lacking in the young (Borowsky et al. 2010).

There has been a large amount of age-related driving research focussing on different aspects of driving control through to the effects of multitasking. A number of simulator and real-world studies have been carried out to assess how age affects driving behaviour. Borowsky et al. (2010) found that older adults are more able to recognise hazards than younger adults when presented with videos of hazardous situations. Another study looked at age-related decline in cognitive ability and found differences in driving behaviour for older adults, such as adopting a larger headway to a leading vehicle. They also found that older drivers with high cognitive ability showed a greater ability to anticipate hazards, whilst the converse was true for younger drivers (Andrews and Westerman 2012). Crook et al. (1993) found a decline in performance relating to cognitive rather than psychomotor factors when testing reaction time in a simulator study. Kline et al. (1992) established that there are a number of factors caused by visual difficulties. Visual processing speed, light sensitivity, dynamic vision, near vision and visual search are areas where older drivers struggle. Related to this, Wood and Troutbeck (1994) found driving performance reductions for elderly drivers with cataracts when compared to elderly and younger drivers with normal vision. Cantin et al. (2009) found that driving led to a greater perceived mental workload for older drivers, an effect that heightened under complex driving environments.

A number of age-related studies have focussed on distraction. Shinar et al. (2005) looked at how younger and older adults dealt with phone conversations whilst driving. They found diminishing interference with practice across all age groups, especially in the young, as a result of learning. Older groups showed greater interference and a slower learning effect than younger adults. Horberry et al. (2006) found stable effects, regardless of age, with different environment complexities and in-vehicle tasks. This pointed towards no major differences as a function age. Hakamies-Blomqvist et al. (1999) used an instrumented vehicle to establish that older drivers were less able to multitask than younger driver. They found that younger drivers were able to use more concurrent controls than older drivers. This pointed towards a serial mode of operation for older drivers. Ponds et al. (1988) used a driving simulator and three age groups to examine performance under divided attention. The older group performed significantly worse than the middle-aged and younger groups who performed similar. Thompson et al. (2012) found that distraction caused reduced driving performance when comparing middle-aged and elderly drivers. The middle-aged drivers show the greatest variation.

When it comes to gender, there are clear physiological differences. The same is true for attitudes towards driving risk, including distraction, that may lead to performance differences. The result could be that males and females differ in how they handle the operational aspects of driving, such as acceleration, braking, car following distance, lane keeping and manoeuvring. If these basic driving behaviours differ, the same may be true for multitasking. In gender research to date, DeJoy (1992) found, when using a subjective questionnaire, that female drivers took driving incidents more seriously than males but both had similar perceptions of the frequency and likelihood of accidents. Similarly, Yagil (1998) found that males had a lower perception of the importance of traffic laws compared to female drivers. In an empirical study, Mäntylä (2013) found that in a multitasking situation, where one of the tasks was monitoring, that males outperformed females. This was explained by differences in spatial awareness. Rhodes and Pivik (2011) carried out a survey of teen and adult drivers to establish a relationship between risk perception, positive affect and risky driving. They found that risky driving behaviour was more likely to be found in teen males than in adult females. Simon and Corbett (1996) found that females offended on the road less often than males but experienced more stress as a result of an incident.

Despite a large amount of research on gender and age, there does not appear to be any distinction of the effect of performance on in-vehicle activities. In terms of gender-related driving research, there is a lack of reported empirical data regarding the relative performance of males and females and particularly for multitasking. Therefore, the key question relating to this paper is what effect does gender and/or age have on task performance in a multitasking driving situation. To answer this question empirically, an experimental study was carried out.

2 An Experimental Study

2.1 Study Design and Procedure

A low fidelity driving simulator was used to carry out the experiment at the research labs of Jaguar Land Rover, UK. Participants of varying age (groups of over and under 40 years of age) and gender were recruited against a specified profile. Sixty participants volunteered, were pre-screened for simulator sickness and asked to arrive for a specified time slot. The recruitment campaign resulted in a 56% male and 44% female split. The mean age of the over 40 group was 49.93 (± 7 years) and 29.6 (± 5.7 years) for the under 40 group. The experimental design was a repeated measures design with two factors, each with two levels: Age (under 40 years and over 40 years) and gender (male and female). The dependant variables collected were a range of performance measures relating to both the DRA and the NDRA. These were steering wheel position variation, speed, NDRA task time, button presses, mean number of glances per task and mean glance time. There were two main hypotheses. In Hypothesis 1 [H1], there will be a significant effect of age group on task performance measures and in Hypothesis 2 [H2], there will be a significant effect of gender on task performance measures.

The setup contained a half-vehicle cabin with integrated steering wheel and pedals (Logitech G27), a digital instrument cluster and centre console touchscreen. The roadway environment was represented in front of the driver on an 85 LCD TV containing a digital rear-view mirror. Side mirror displays presented wing mirror views. The driving environment was programmed using STISIM (v3) and consisted of a 10 min drive along a three-lane UK highway with typical lane width and curvature. Light to moderate traffic was programmed into the scenario whereby the driver had to periodically overtake slow moving traffic. During the drive, the participants were asked to maintain 70 mph and stay in the left-hand lane as frequently as possible. If they came upon a slower vehicle, they were asked to safely overtake the vehicle before moving back to the left-hand lane as soon as was safe to do so. This remained consistent between runs.

The in-vehicle tasks were all carried out using the centre console-mounted touchscreen, programmed using Qt (v5.7). Five tasks were used, all of which represented typical tasks available on a modern day automotive touchscreen. The tasks included were list scrolling, typing, option selection, menu navigation and setting adjustment. The simulator software reported several driving parameters (steering, lane position and speed) which were logged onto a PC. Moment-to-moment eye glance data was recorded from a SmartEye remote eye tracker (v6.1) mounted on the dashboard. Task performance data (button pushes, errors) was also recorded onto the same PC. All data was synchronised using a UNIX timestamp.

When participants arrived, they were asked to read an information sheet before signing a consent form. They were then asked to make themselves comfortable in the simulator by adjusting the seat and steering wheel. They were all given an opportunity to get used to the driving simulator setup during a brief familiarisation period which included them attempting to carry out the NDRA whilst driving. Following this, the participant was trained to some specific criteria on the NDRA interface to improve their awareness of how to successfully complete the tasks. The criteria consisted of observing the instructor complete the task before successfully completing the task five consecutive times themselves. Following this, they completed three further experimental runs. Each experimental run consisted of 1 min baseline driving periods interlaced with task epochs (counterbalanced in order). This and all subsequent runs lasted 10 min.

2.2 Results and Analysis

The data was coded and tested using a repeated measures ANOVA. The factors used were gender (male and female) and age group (Under 40 and over 40). No significant results were found for speed, NDRA task time or mean glance time ($p > 0.05$) and these are not included below.

2.2.1 Standard Wheel Position Variation

For baseline driving, the ANOVA of steering wheel position variation (Fig. 2; Table 1) found a significant effect of age group [$F(1, 152) = 8.18$, $p = 0.005$] with the over 40 s having a significantly higher steering variation than the younger group. There was no effect of gender and no interaction of gender by age group ($p > 0.05$). For multitasking, the ANOVA of steering wheel position variation (Fig. 2; Table 1) found no significant effect of gender, age group or gender by age group ($p > 0.05$).

2.2.2 Mean Number of Button Presses and Glances Per Task

For mean number of button presses (Fig. 3; Table 2), the ANOVA found a significant main effect of gender [$F(1, 143) = 6.14$, $p = 0.014$] and also for age group [$F(1, 143) = 12.72$, $p = 0.000$]. The female and over 40 groups requiring significantly more button presses to complete a task than the male and under 40 groups. There was no effect of gender by age group ($p > 0.05$). For mean number of glances per task (Fig. 3; Table 2), the ANOVA found a significant main effect of gender

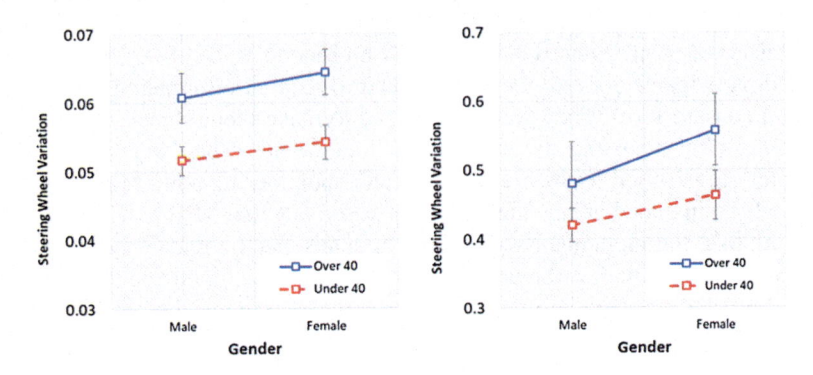

Fig. 2 Steering variation during baseline (left) and multitasking conditions (right)

Table 1 Steering variation for baseline and multitasking grouped by gender and age group, with the values in brackets indicating the standard error of the mean

Steering wheel position variation mean (standard error)		Baseline conditions		Multitasking conditions	
		Age group			
		Over 40	Under 40	Over 40	Under 40
Gender	Male	0.06078 (0.00359)	0.05165 (0.00213)	0.4804 (0.0609)	0.4199 (0.0245)
	Female	0.06439 (0.00329)	0.05424 (0.00254)	0.4199 (0.0245)	0.4629 (0.0355)

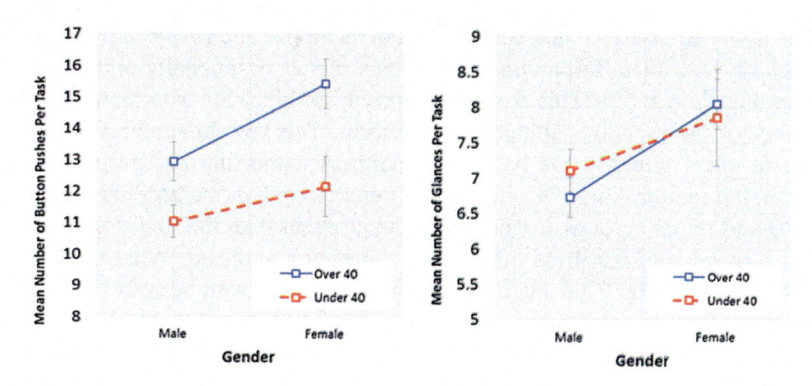

Fig. 3 Mean number of button pushes (left) and mean number of glance (right) per task

Table 2 Mean number of button pushes and mean number of glances per task grouped by gender and age group, values in brackets are the standard error of the mean

Mean (standard error)		Mean button pushes		Mean number of glances	
		Age group			
		Over 40	Under 40	Over 40	Under 40
Gender	Male	12.937 (0.613)	11.039 (0.519)	6.727 (0.285)	7.106 (0.303)
	Female	15.412 (0.795)	12.15 (0.958)	8.053 (0.353)	7.859 (0.688)

$[F(1, 151) = 6.86, p = 0.010]$ with the female group needing significantly more glances per task than males. There was no effect of age group or gender by age group ($p > 0.05$).

3 Discussion and Design Implications

When looking at DRA performance, the baseline driving condition showed an effect of age group on general lane-keeping ability. The scenario used was consistent with typical highway driving, but even so, the effects of age group on steering wheel variation were evident in this simulator study. There was no effect of gender on baseline driving and so the male and female groups performed equally as well as each other. Figure 2 shows that the male participants mean steering variation value was marginally lower than the female participants mean steering variation. This was consistent between age groups with a high standard error seen with the over 40 s. This is as expected, the driving-only conditions were well within the capability of the operators. The scenario used was familiar and thus the only observation was that over 40 s were not as good at maintaining lane position as the under 40 s. This could be explained by any of the aspects described earlier (such as visual, cognitive or psychomotor).

This result in itself is not surprising but is important in the context of the multitasking data. First, the multitasking data were all significantly higher than the baseline data ($p < 0.05$). This was as expected, multitasking puts extra strain on the ability of the user to maintain lane position. The key difference was that the significant effect found in the baseline conditions within the age groups was not present in the multitasking data. The same trend as seen in the baseline data exists (over 40 and female groups producing a higher mean than the under 40 and male groups, respectively) but these differences were not significant. What is evident is that the variance (Fig. 2 standard error bars) is greater with respect to the mean values meaning a much greater variation in individual ability to maintain lane position. This is again not surprising considering that the NDRA takes focus away from driving and so deviations in lane are more likely. This makes corrective actions more likely and thus increases the amount of variation in wheel position.

For the NDRA performance, the number of button presses shows effects of both gender and age. For female participants, the over 40 s take two to three more button presses than under 40 s. The same distinction exists for the males where the difference is about one button press. Male participants took two to three fewer button presses than females to successfully carry out the same activities. This could be evidence of females making more errors or being less accurate with the touchscreen than the males. This points to consideration of button sizes and accuracy with this difference in mind. The differences in age are likely down to similar reasons, with under 40 s requiring fewer touches than over 40 s by around two to three pushes. Errors caused by physical or cognitive limitations are likely causes for the need to make more button pushes. There is also a potential exposure issue. Despite these participants being well trained in how to carry out these activities, younger members of society have more exposure to touchscreen devices and so could, in general, be more proficient.

For glance performance, effects were found for gender but not for age. The males required on average one fewer glances than females per task, indicating a difference in glance behaviour. Glance performance gives us indication of how drivers balance their visual resource between DRA and NDRA. More glances to a task could equally indicate more attention required to complete a task or a driver more conscious of the risk associated with the driving environment. The differences found here could be down to a number of reasons. One explanation could be linked to button presses. The greater number of button presses by female drivers could have led to the need for more glances. Another explanation could be the time required to find and locate a button. Longer visual search time leads to the need for more glances because of unsuccessful glance instances. This could also be explained by an increase in the number of glances back at the road for females influenced by risk aversion, as described in prior literature (DeJoy 1992).

In summary, there appears to be performance differences in baseline driving between age groups, but not between genders. There is also a general reduction in DRA performance between baseline and multitasking periods. What are the implications of these findings in terms of interface design? The first implication relates to the type of support on offer to the occupant. Interfaces that can help the user to maintain lane would certainly help to support the older individuals in this study. Equally, this functionality would offer support to all drivers during multitasking. The aim would be to reduce the amount of lane deviation during these multitasking situations and, therefore, could be activated when the user is identified as being multitasking.

This study demonstrates a general difference in steering performance between males and females. Although not significant, this could lead to making sure that there is a good balance of both in any testing campaign. This would help ensure that differences are accounted for in the evaluation process and assist in identifying issues that can be improved through an iterative design process. The gender difference may also offer insight into how interfaces could be more empathic. If females are more conscious of the effect of distraction, extra thought can be given to how an interface could be designed to be more conservative in this sense.

Consideration for the effects of age is required. Recent trends for minimalist graphics and modern design strategies that can make interpreting what a button is more difficult. This could increase the number of button presses (i.e. attempting to press something that is not a button) and glances (locating a button). In general, understanding the capability range of individuals with reduction in vision, psychomotor or cognitive performance, can help to develop better interfaces. Varying button sizes and greater clarity of touch areas could be applied dynamically, dependent upon age, to assist when multitasking (Biswas et al. 2014).

4 Conclusions

The act of multitasking in vehicle is very challenging. What is more, the design of interface systems that can take into account variation in the users attempting to use them is also complex. In this simulator study, there were significant differences found for a range of driving and non-driving tasks. For driving, there were no significant effects of gender but significant effects of age were found in relation to the variation in steering wheel movements. The over 40 age group produces a greater variation than the under 40 age group. Whereas for non-driving, significant effects for both age and gender were present with the male and under 40 age group producing fewer glances and button presses than the female and over 40 age group, respectively. This offers fresh insight into refining requirements for in-vehicle interface systems to account for differences that can influence performance for large numbers of people.

Acknowledgements This work is funded by Jaguar Land Rover Research through the Centre for Advanced Photonics and Electronics at Cambridge University.

References

Abelein U, Lochner H, Hahn D, Straube S (2012) Complexity, quality and robustness—the challenges of tomorrow's automotive electronics. Des Autom Test Eur Conf Exhib 870–871

Andrews EC, Westerman SJ (2012) Age differences in simulated driving performance: compensatory processes. Accid Anal Prev 45:660–668

Biswas P, Langdon P, Umadikar J, Kittusami S, Prashant S (2014) How interface adaptation for physical impairment can help able bodied users in situational impairment. In: Langdon PM, Lazar J, Heylighen A, Dong H (eds) Inclusive designing. Joining usability, accessibility and inclusion, pp 49–67, Springer

Borowsky A, Shinar D, Oron-Gilad T (2010) Age, skill, and hazard perception in driving. Accid Anal Prev 42:1240–1249

Cantin V, Lavallière M, Simoneau M, Teasdale N (2009) Mental workload when driving in a simulator: effects of age and driving complexity. Accid Anal Prev 41:763–771

Charness N, Bosman E (1994) Age-related changes in perceptual and psychomotor performance: implications for engineering design. Exp Aging Res 20:45–59

Crook TH, West RL, Larrabee GJ (1993) The driving-reaction time test: assessing age declines in dual-task performance. Develop Neuropsychol 9:31–39

DeJoy DM (1992) An examination of gender differences in traffic accident risk perception. Accid Anal Prev 24:237–246

FHWA (2015) Highway statistics 2015. US Department of Transportation, Federal Highway Administration. https://www.fhwa.dot.gov/policyinformation/statistics/2015/pdf/dl20.pdf. Accessed 5 Dec 2017

Guirao A, Gonzalez C, Redondo M, Geraghty E, Norrby S, Artal P (1999) Average optical performance of the human eye as a function of age in a normal population. Invest Ophthalmol Visual Sci 40(I):203–213

Hakamies-Blomqvist L, Mynttinen S, Backman M, Mikkonen V (1999) Age-related differences in driving: are older drivers more serial? Int J Behav Develop 23:575–589

Hasher L, Zacks RT (1988) Working memory, comprehension, and aging: a review and a new biew. Psychol Learn Motiv 22:193–225

Horberry T, Anderson J, Regan M, Brown J (2006) Driver distraction: the effects of concurrent in-vehicle tasks, road environment complexity and age on driving performance. Accid Anal Prev 38:185–191

Kline DW, Kline TJB, Fozard JL, Kosnik W, Schieber F, Sekuler R (1992) Vision, aging, and driving: the problems of older drivers. J Gerontol 47:27–34

Luettel T, Himmelsbach M, Wuensche H-J (2012) Autonomous ground vehicles—concepts and a path to the future. Proc IEEE 100:1831–1839

Mäntylä T (2013) Gender differences in multitasking reflect spatial ability. Psychol Sci 24:514–520

Ponds RWHM, Brouwer WH, Van Wolffelaar PC (1988) Age differences in divided attention in a simulated driving task. J Gerontol 43:151–156

Przybylski AK, Murayama K, Dehaan CR, Gladwell V (2013) Motivational, emotional, and behavioral correlates of fear of missing out. Comput Hum Behav 29:1841–1848

Reimers S, Maylor EA (2005) Task switching across the life span: Effects of age on general and specific switch costs. Dev Psychol 41:661–671

Rhodes N, Pivik K (2011) Age and gender differences in risky driving: the roles of positive affect and risk perception. Accid Anal Prev 43:923–931

Salvucci DD, Taatgen NA, Borst J (2009) Toward a unified theory of the multitasking continuum: From concurrent performance to task switching, interruption, and resumption. In: Proceedings of the 27th international conference on human factors in computing systems, CHI'09, Boston, MA, USA, 4–9 Apr 2009

Shinar D, Tractinsky N, Compton R (2005) Effects of practice, age, and task demands, on interference from a phone task while driving. Accid Anal Prev 37:315–326

Simon F, Corbett C (1996) Road traffic offending, stress, age, and accident history among male and female drivers. Ergonomics 39:757–780
Smith MW, Sharit J, Czaja SJ (1999) Aging, motor control, and the performance of computer mouse tasks. Hum Factors 41:389–396
Thompson KR, Johnson AM, Emerson JL, Dawson JD, Boer ER, Rizzo M (2012) Distracted driving in elderly and middle-aged drivers. Accid Anal Prev 45:711–717
Wood MJ, Troutbeck JR (1994) Effect of age and visual impairment on driving and vision performance. Transp Res Rec 84–90
Yagil D (1998) Gender and age-related differences in attitudes toward traffic laws and traffic violations. Transp Res Part F: Traffic Psychol Behav 1F(2):123–135
Zapata C, Nieuwenhuis P (2010) Exploring innovation in the automotive industry: New technologies for cleaner cars. J Clean Prod 18:14–20

Introducing Assistive Technology and Universal Design Theory, Applications in Design Education

Y. M. Choi

Abstract The aim of this study was to better understand student assumptions related to the challenges of developing a universally designed device compared to designing a dedicated assistive device. Two projects were conducted in a sophomore industrial design studio class. Data was collected from students via surveys. Results of the projects and suggestions for conducting similar projects are presented.

1 Introduction

The aim of this paper is to examine methods for introducing undergraduate design students to the concepts of Universal Design (UD) and to the design of Assistive Technology (AT) devices. UD here is defined as the design of environments and products to be usable by all people to the greatest extent possible so that adaptations without the need for adaptation or specialised design (CUD 1997). In practice, universal design helps to ensure that more people with varying abilities will have a better chance to be able to effectively use and benefit from a product. Design schools in the United States have been slow to adopt universal design, even as the number of individuals who will experience some level of limited ability is forecast to increase in the future (Fletcher et al. 2015). This makes it more important that designers are trained to consider a wider range of abilities when designing future products.

It is similarly important to introduce students to the design of assistive products. Assistive technology here is defined as any item, piece of equipment or product system, whether acquired commercially off the shelf, modified or customised, that is used to increase, maintain or improve the functional capabilities of people with disabilities. AT is distinct from UD in that the objective is to improve a specific functional ability rather than to achieve broad, general usability.

Y. M. Choi (✉)
Georgia Institute of Technology, Atlanta, GA, USA
e-mail: christina.choi@gatech.edu

A key element of this learning is enabling students to interface with potential users, particularly, those with disabilities (Burgstahler 2007). This is an important component to allow students to develop confidence in their ability to interface with people who may have very different needs and perspectives. Without it students may not have a way to solicit feedback on their designs (or may not take the initiative to seek feedback) and test/challenge their own assumptions.

It is arguably important to educate design students early about both Universal Design and Assistive Design and provide the opportunity to gain practical experience with both. With an early introduction to these concepts, students will have the opportunity to apply their experience to both future projects during the course of their training and into their professional careers (whether product design or other fields).

2 Method

This study was performed in a university industrial design class. All students were sophomores taking a foundational project-based studio course which is focused on teaching foundational product design skills and methodologies. Many user engagement techniques are introduced in the second semester. The aim of this study was to better understand student assumptions related to the challenges of developing a universally designed device compared to designing a dedicated assistive device.

The students completed two projects: the first (UD) focused on a universally designed device followed by a second (AT) to design an assistive focused device. Students were given surveys at two points during these projects. The first survey was given at the end of the UD project. It included questions asking students to provide their opinions about various aspects of the UD project and what they learned. It also included questions about their assumptions of assistive design. The second survey was given at the end of the AT project. It asked students to provide their opinion about various aspects of the AT project and what they learned. It also included several questions asking them about their general perceptions (after completing both projects) of universal design, assistive design and the differences between them.

A total of 34 students between two class sections completed the surveys. Participation was voluntary and the surveys were administered by a neutral party (not the instructor) and held until after grades were finalised for the semester. Since the project was conducted within a class, the process was outlined in the informed consent provided to the students to make clear that their participation, and any opinion provided about the projects, would have no impact on their course grade.

The primary feature of both of these projects was the recruitment of real, potential end users of products the students would be designing and scheduling their participation in the class. The projects were organised so that students prepared for user visits by formulating interview questions, preparing surveys or planning tests to gather data about their prototypes/designs. This allowed students the opportunity to realistically exercise their user engagement skills.

The universal design project was assigned first. It was a team project performed by students in teams of 3–4 students. The assigned goal of the project was to create a universally designed carry-on travel bag which included mobile-enabled features. This bag had to meet the needs of the general travelling public (business/leisure travellers, flight attendants, etc.) and also the needs of users with limited mobility. Some of the specific project requirements were as follows:

- The specific use environment for this exercise was air travel, with other types of travel (train, bus, car, etc.) being considered as secondary uses.
- The luggage had to be of a carry-on size (such as a carry-on roller bag). Bags of a size that require them to be checked were not to be considered).
- The luggage had to include mobile/wireless-enabled features intended specifically to meet the needs of users in the air travel environment.

Students were provided with the opportunity to interact with mobility limited users during class time at several points during the project. This was arranged to ensure that all students undertaking the project had equal opportunity to meet with this user group, since many students may not have the resources/connections to be able to connect with them on their own. It also provided a consistent and controlled environment.

The first meeting, consisting of manual wheelchair users, was arranged during the second week of the project at the Shepherd Center, a spinal cord and brain injury rehabilitation centre. The goal of this meeting was to allow students to interview users and to learn about their travel related needs. Students spent the first week conducting research, preparing questions and engaging with other users on their own. After the class user meeting, students completed development of personas for mobility limited users as well as for other users met on their own. Students then developed and tested initial design concepts in order to fabricate a study model to use to conduct formative testing with users.

In the third week of the project, another meeting with mobility limited users was arranged. This meeting was used to test their study models with users and to obtain feedback on their chosen design direction and features. Students used the results of this testing, along with testing performed on their own with other users, to refine their design and fabricate a final mock-up for testing.

A final meeting with mobility limited users was provided in the fifth week of the project. This allowed students to perform summative testing of their design and obtain final feedback on what changes/additions worked well (or not) between the initial and final design concepts.

The assistive design project was assigned next. This project was not performed as a team, and each student developed his/her own design. Each student was responsible for researching/investigating an assigned task scenario to identify a potential design problem, success criteria for the design and then to design a solution to the identified problem.

Students were assigned to one of two possible scenarios focusing on users with low vision:

- Travelling from the studio building to a bookstore across campus via the campus shuttle, making a purchase and then returning to the studio via the shuttle.
- Travelling from the studio building to the student centre and ordering food at the cafeteria, selecting food, paying for it, eating the food and then returning to the studio.

Within these scenarios, each student was required to identify a problem/barrier and then to design and fabricate a working product prototype to reduce/overcome it. It is important to note that this was NOT a re-design project. One of the boundary conditions was that the new product had to work within the existing environment, not re-design the environment itself. For example, a student would not design a new tray for the cafeteria but could instead design a product that worked with the current trays in order to solve a problem/barrier. This was a necessary condition to limit the scope of the problem space to something more appropriate for a relatively short project and help the students focus on more manageable problems.

For this project, groups of low vision users were scheduled to visit class in order to provide input and feedback. Students spent the first week of the project researching and defining the problem they would design for. As they began developing design concepts, initial testing was performed via simulation. Students were provided with Zimmerman Low Vision Simulation Kits. These allowed simulation of visual acuity conditions (20/70, 20/200, 20/500 and 20/800), peripheral field of view loss conditions (3°, 7° and 10°) as well as conditions including macular degeneration (near and far), cataract, scotoma and hemianopsia.

The first meeting with users was arranged during the second week of the project. During this visit, students interacted with the users to discuss their solutions and to solicit feedback. Most importantly, each student personally walked through the scenario with three different users. This gave them the opportunity to both perform observation as well as to discuss issues with the users within the actual scenario environment. Students were challenged to think about how their simulation approach compared to the experience of users who actually have the disability and find out possible approaches directly from the users to allow them to more accurately recreate the user experience. Ultimately, students were encouraged to reflect on what insights they were able to discover about the user's experience in going through the task with them that they could not discover through simulation (Fig. 1).

The gathered input was used to update the designs and to fabricate a final, testable prototype. Low vision users again visited class at the end of the third week in order to test the design concepts and to engage the users in a participatory fashion to identify potential improvements. Students again worked with users to test their concepts within the actual scenario environment. Students then used this input to fabricate a final prototype. The final designs were evaluated by a panel of external reviewers, which included visually impaired academics and assistive technology design professionals.

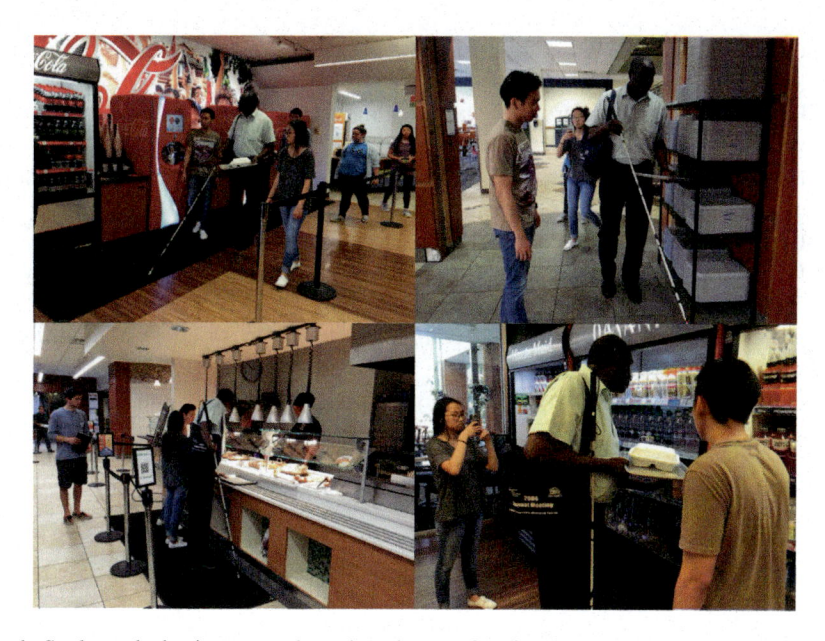

Fig. 1 Students shadowing a user through each step of performing a task in an assigned scenario

3 Results

The following tables show the results of the two surveys. The questions in the first survey, and responses presented below and in Table 1, included

(1) Have you ever temporarily lost your vision (such as from an injury)?
(2) Have you ever temporarily lost the use of your arm (such as a broken arm or other injury)?
(3) Have you ever known a close friend or family member who has permanently lost their vision?

Table 1 Student answers to the first survey

Question	Yes	No	a.	b.	c.	d.
1	7	27				
2	7	27				
3	4	30				
4	7	26				
5	2	32				
6	2	32				
7	18	16				
8	10	9				
9	0	34				
10			0	1	20	12
11			0	7	24	2
12			0	28	6	

(4) Have you ever known a close friend or family member who has permanently lost the use of one or both of their arms?
(5) Have you ever had to provide care for someone who has permanently lost their vision?
(6) Have you ever had to provide care for someone who has permanently lost the use of one or both of their arms?
(7) Have you ever used a device to simulate a condition or situation?
(8) If yes, did you find that the simulation was an accurate representation of the condition or situation?
(9) Have you ever tried to design or build a device to simulate a condition or situation?
(10) How easy do you think it would be to build an accurate simulation tool?

   a. Very easy,
   b. Somewhat easy,
   c. Somewhat difficult or
   d. Very difficult.

(11) Do you think a simulation tool will be able to allow you to experience *everything* in *exactly* the same way as an end user?

   a. Yes, I think it is possible to make a simulation tool that allows me to have the *same* experience as an end user.
   b. I think it is possible to make a simulation tool that allows me to experience *mostly* the same experience as an end user.
   c. I think it is possible to make a simulation tool that allows me to experience *some specific aspect* as an end user.
   d. No, I don't think a simulation tool can provide me with the same experience as an end user.

(12) Do you think a simulation tool would provide you with the ability to test a product in the absence of an end user?

   a. I think a simulation tool would provide a fully accurate way to test a product.
   b. I think a simulation tool would provide an accurate way to test for specific scenarios.
   c. I don't think a simulation tool would provide an accurate way to test a product.

The questions in the second survey and responses are presented below and in Table 2. The questions on the second survey included

(1) How easy was it to build an accurate simulation tool for the situation in this project?

Introducing Assistive Technology and Universal ...

Table 2 Student answers to the second survey

Question	Yes	No	a.	b.	c.	d.	e.
1			2	8	12	3	
2			0	9	9	7	1
3	11	10					
4			0	6	7	4	0
5	3	17					
6	12	8					
7			7	17	2		
8			21	2	2		
9	4	17					

   a. Very easy,
   b. Somewhat easy,
   c. Somewhat difficult or
   d. Very difficult.

(2) Was your simulation tool able to accurately replicate your problem condition?

   a. Yes, it was the same as the problem condition in every way.
   b. Yes, it was the same in most ways, but not perfect.
   c. It was the same in some ways but not the same in others.
   d. No, it was only the same in a few ways, but mostly different.
   e. No, it was different from the problem condition in every way.

(3) Did you validate your simulation tool with actual users?
(4) If yes, how closely did the users say that the simulation tool was able to match their own experience?

   a. It was the same as the problem condition in every way.
   b. It was the same in most ways, but not perfect.
   c. It was the same in some ways but not the same in others.
   d. It was only the same in a few ways, but mostly different.
   e. It was different from the problem condition in every way.

(5) If your simulation was not accurate in some way, were you able to correct it?
(6) Did product testing with your simulation tool give the same results as when you tested your product with end users?
(7) What did you learn about the design of your product based on the simulation tool?

   a. A lot. I was able to find many design problems that I wouldn't have known without simulation.
   b. Some. I was able to find some useful design problems that I wouldn't have known otherwise.
   c. Nothing. The simulation tool did not help me identify any new design problems.

(8) What did you learn about the design of your product based on feedback from users?

   a. A lot. I was able to find many design problems that I wouldn't have known otherwise.
   b. Some. I was able to find some useful design problems that I wouldn't have known otherwise.
   c. Nothing. I did not learn about any new design problems from the users.

(9) Based on your experience from this project (project 3) do you think that it is possible to design a universally designed product that will always work for all people with different abilities?

   - Yes, I think a universally designed product is always possible.
   - No, I think a specifically designed product that works best for particular people is sometimes needed.

The second survey included several free-form questions. These are presented below along with some select responses.

(10) What was the biggest challenge related to assistive design that you encountered during project 3? Were you able to solve it?

   - Some users found the device unuseful because they didn't think their vision was as bad as others and therefore did not need the device.
   - The biggest challenge was finding unique ways to relay information to the users with limited vision. I solved it by finding creative ways that use the other senses (hearing, though, etc.).
   - Not over thinking the design. I kept trying to do too much when the solution was very simple.
   - The sheer variety of different users and different impairments.
   - Because my initial exposure and preconceived ideas about 'visually impairment' was very little to none. I thought that it would be very difficult adapting to a brand new perspective, possibly even changing them as well. But I found that research into specific diagnosis helped. The user interviews and simulations helped the most.

(11) Was there anything that you expected would be a big challenge before starting project 3 but turned out to be easier than you thought?

   - No, I expected that everything would be hard and they were.
   - No, everything was challenging.
   - I thought making a product for a limited vision users functional would be the most difficult. This required me to think outside the box for building and simulation tools.

(12) Comparing project 2 (universal design) and project 3 (assistive design), what do you feel is the biggest difference between them?

- Project 2 included so many other considerations because it included a wide range of target users. But project 3 was easier because it focused on a specific group.
- You have a smaller audience and can focus on working to solve some of their problems and not focusing on trying to accommodate the majority.
- Specifically making a product for a target demographic, or users, is something I prefer. Project 3 allowed me to focus all efforts onto solving a single issue rather than project 3.
- The bigger challenge of project 3 was the open-ended scenario.
- Project 3 was probably more difficult because simulating (and testing) it was more challenging and visual impairment is even more difficult to understand if you don't live with it.

4 Discussion

One of the main aims of both projects is to get students to think outside of the box and learn to identify design opportunities. For many students, this aspect (identifying design opportunities) was one of the most difficult tasks. To this point, most students' experiences are that assignments/projects generally give a very specified problem with particular boundaries, and consequently a limited number of solutions. That was not the case with either project as students were simply given a defined scenario/environment and were tasked with identifying a design problem along with the performance and success requirements for a viable solution. This is a difficult skill to learn and requires practice (and room to fail) but it is critical for a designer as it relates directly to innovation.

The vast majority of the students in the class were non-disabled. A small percentage of them reported personal experience with temporary disability or have known/cared for a close friend or family member with a disability. Most students began the AT project with mixed expectations on the effectiveness of simulation. Most did not expect that it would be perfectly representative or completely useless. Most had moderate expectations that it would be somewhat to very useful. At the end of the project, their experiences seemed to match initial expectations. They found simulation provided some insight, but that it was not perfect. By walking through the assigned scenarios and directly discussing their simulated experiences to users' own experience with the scenario, students found that their product testing results through simulation and testing results with actual users were almost always different. Students reported that they were able to improve their simulations in some ways after comparing their experiences with users, but that it was not a substitute.

Simulation under any circumstance is not perfect. There are advantages and limitations. Students were able to experience and learn from this first hand through the assignment. The best way to begin to know this is through experience, but students need to have some real understanding that there actually are limitations that could lead them to bad assumptions and poor design decisions. Many students often assume that their first ideas of a simulation are perfect without realising that they have not considered many factors. Through this project, they were able to experience this first hand and become aware of the possible issues to consider in their future design work.

The broader lessons in both projects, beyond the actual design solutions, were the most important: practice engaging actual users and directly tackling unexpected issues; building empathy through direct interaction; learning about the advantages, disadvantages and appropriate use of simulation; challenging assumptions of personal views of the designed world; and understanding the differences between universal and assistive design. The engagement of actual users, while logistically difficult to coordinate in a class/project setting, is critical for allowing these to be learned, and are a powerful experience for most students.

5 Future Suggestions

The short time frames of both projects presented challenges to addressing user's problems in a meaningful manner. This limited the level of finish achievable in testable prototypes and left little time to refine designs based on feedback or results from usability testing.

Working with users unfamiliar with the design process was sometimes problematic as end user participants in both projects were often enamoured with what the students accomplished and tended not to be particularly objective or critical of the solutions offered by the students. The subjective nature of their feedback was not universally helpful. It is suggested that users, as a group, be briefed on the design process before interaction with students in order to set their expectations and help them to provide more relevant feedback.

Acknowledgements The contents of this report were developed under a grant from the National Institute on Disability, Independent Living, and Rehabilitation Research (NIDILRR grant number 90RE5007-01-00). NIDILRR is a Center within the Administration for Community Living (ACL), Department of Health and Human Services (HHS). The contents of report do not necessarily represent the policy of NIDILRR, ACL, HHS, and you should not assume endorsement by the Federal Government.

The contents of this report were also supported under an AccessEngineering minigrant which support engineering activities, training and experiential learning opportunities. The AccessEngineering project is funded by the National Science Foundation (grant number EEC-1444961).

References

Burgstahler S (2007) Universal design: process, principles, and applications. DO-IT: University of Washington, Seattle
CUD (1997) The principles of universal design. The Center for Universal Design, North Carolina State University, NC, US
Fletcher V, Bonome-Sims G, Knecht B, Ostroff E, Otitigbe J, Parente M et al (2015) The challenge of inclusive design in the US context. Appl Ergonom 46:267–273

Exploring User Capability Data with Topological Data Analysis

U. Persad, J. Goodman-Deane, P. M. Langdon and P. J. Clarkson

Abstract This paper presents an analysis of user capability data using Topological Data Analysis (TDA) (unsupervised machine learning) to extract insight. The aim was to explore the global shape and sub-groupings (clusters of profiles) of people using data collected from the Cambridge Better Design Pilot Study of 362 people from across England and Wales. The resulting topological network demonstrated the global shape of the sample and distribution of sensory, cognitive and motor capability across the sample. The TDA network was automatically grouped into 14 distinct clusters, and distinguishing features of each cluster was extracted. The results demonstrate the value of applying TDA to analyse and visualise user capability data, and it is proposed that the cluster descriptions could be used for developing empirically based design tools such as personas for Inclusive Design.

1 Introduction

Inclusive Design is becoming more important with the ageing of the world's population and improvements in medical care. Designers are required to respond to this population shift by executing an Inclusive Design process to produce practical inclusive consumer products across a range of sectors. To enact this approach, design and manufacturing business practices are required to become more people

---

U. Persad (✉)
The University of Trinidad and Tobago, Arima, Trinidad and Tobago
e-mail: umesh.persad@utt.edu.tt

J. Goodman-Deane · P. M. Langdon · P. J. Clarkson
Cambridge Engineering Design Centre, the University of Cambridge, Cambridge, UK
e-mail: jag76@cam.ac.uk

P. M. Langdon
e-mail: pml24@eng.cam.ac.uk

P. J. Clarkson
e-mail: pjc10@eng.cam.ac.uk

© Springer International Publishing AG, part of Springer Nature 2018
P. Langdon et al. (eds.), *Breaking Down Barriers*,
https://doi.org/10.1007/978-3-319-75028-6_4

and population aware to accommodate the mainstream approach that Inclusive Design advocates.

However, there remains a need for a better understanding of how data on human capability variation across populations can support the inclusive approach (Johnson et al. 2010). Current user data is fragmented and lacking (Johnson et al. 2010), and though designers and researchers have made the best use of such data for product evaluation (Waller et al. 2010), the lack of integrated data with proven predictive value continues to plague the field (Persad et al. 2011; Tenneti et al. 2013). In addition, the databases on user capability require transformation into visual representations that are easy to understand and use. To this end, this paper presents an exploratory study using a relatively new unsupervised machine learning technique termed Topological Data Analysis (TDA) on a recent pilot study of user capabilities across the UK population (Tenneti et al. 2013).

2 Background

Previous work in this area explored the underlying structure of disability data via hierarchical cluster analysis (Langdon et al. 2006). By using numerical methods of classification, it is possible to extract the underlying structure in data without any prior assumptions. However, the resulting clusters and interpretations were found to be difficult for practitioners to understand (Langdon et al. 2006). Given recent progress in machine learning and big data analytics, a new method has emerged to understand the global structure in datasets. This method combines the mathematical field of Topology with Machine Learning and Visualisation resulting in TDA (Carlsson 2009; Lum et al. 2013).

In essence, the TDA method is built on the principle that data has a multidimensional shape, and this shape conveys meaning. Fundamentally, TDA is a geometric method to detect patterns and shapes within the data. By recognising these shapes and patterns in the data, important features and groupings could be identified. Lum et al. (2013) describe three key ideas of topology that make extracting of patterns via shape possible. First, TDA defines a metric space between all multidimensional points in a dataset, i.e. the 'distance' between any pair of points. Since this is a coordinate-free way of defining the data, the TDA depends only on the distance function that specifies the shape. Second, TDA shapes and representation are invariant under small deformations. Third, TDA generates a compressed representation of the shape of the data using a simplicial complex or network. Shapes, such as circular segments (loops) and linear segments (flares), appear in the data visualisation leading to new insight.

The advantage of TDA is that it can detect patterns missed by traditional multidimensional methods, such as PCA, MDS and cluster analysis. Specifically, clustering methods produce several distinct and unrelated groups without clearly showing how these groups relate to each other. Therefore, TDA provides a new tool in the data science toolbox for understanding multidimensional datasets as found in the field of ergonomics/human factors. The study presented in this paper uses TDA to explore the Better Design pilot survey data of 362 people from across England and Wales (Tenneti et al. 2013).

3 Methodology

The dataset of 362 people contained capability variables describing the age, gender, vision, hearing, cognition and motor function of participants. Thirty nine (39) variables were selected for inclusion fulfilling the assumption that the measures were ratio or interval level data in order to be compatible with the TDA analysis. Apart from age and gender, the other variables selected were as follows:

Sensory Variables: Near-vision comfort (high contrast): majority of the day setup; near-vision comfort (low contrast): majority of the day setup; distance vision, distance vision comfort: majority of the day setup; distance vision comfort: general setup (distance aid if participants did the distance aid test, majority setup otherwise), hearing at different volumes (no background noise) and hearing at medium volume at different levels of background noise.

Motor Variables: Moberg test results: right hand, Moberg test results: left hand, grip strength: comfort non-dominant hand, grip strength: comfort dominant hand, grip strength: threshold non-dominant hand, grip strength: threshold dominant hand, getting out of a chair (with arms), getting out of a chair (without arms), reaching floor level, out in front (Left arm), out in front (Right arm), above head (Left arm) and above head (Right arm).

Cognitive Variables: Immediate recall memory, delayed recall memory, number of letters scanned and search efficiency (executive function measures), literacy: number of correct answers, numeracy: number of correct answers, perseverance when things go wrong, ability to find a solution when confronted with a problem, confidence in learning to use technology products, anxiety about new technology products, experience with the following—make calls on a mobile phone, send text message on a mobile phone, take pictures with a digital camera or phone, use a remote control for digital TV, use the Internet, listen to MP3 tracks on a portable device, use a gaming console, such as XBOX, playstation or Wii and use satellite navigation, like a tom-tom.

The data was imported and analysed in Ayasdi platform, a TDA software tool for analysis and visualisation (AYASDI 2017). This TDA method requires no prior assumptions allowing the data to speak for itself.

The first step in the analysis was to select an appropriate metric for the data that could account for missing values and deal with continuous variables that measure different phenomena. Only variables with interval or ratio level data were used in the analysis. A norm angle metric was selected where the procedure first normalises all capability variables in the dataset to have a mean of 0 and a variance of 1 (making the variables comparable). The norm angle distance is then calculated as the angle distance between the mean-centred, variance-normalised points.

This metric handles nulls by projecting the pair of rows to the intersection of their non-null columns.

The second step in the analysis was to select an appropriate lens for the data. A lens is a filter that converts the dataset into a vector, where each row in the original dataset contributes to a real number in the vector turning every row into a single number. Neighbourhood Lenses 1 and 2 were selected. These lenses generate an embedding of high-dimensional data into a two-dimensional plane by embedding a k-nearest neighbours graph of the data using Ayasdi's proprietary graph layout algorithm. These lenses work to emphasise the metric structure of the data. The software then used a mapping and clustering algorithm to group people into connected clusters (nodes) producing TDA network visualisations. For exploratory data analysis, the resolution and the gain of the lenses were varied to produce networks of varying levels of detail. These networks could be coloured by any variable in the dataset.

For clustering the network, the Community auto-grouping algorithm was used via the provided Python SDK. This network algorithm, based on Louvain modularity optimisation, operates on the topological model's graph structure. It tries to find the best grouping of nodes that have high intragroup connectivity and low intergroup connectivity, resulting in highly connected clusters. The clusters were compared to the rest of the dataset using comparison tests of P value and KS scores (Kolmogorov–Smirnov tests) to determine which variables differentiated each cluster (with $p < 0.05$ representing significant variables on the KS test). Cases in each of the 14 clusters were exported out of the AYASDI platform software and further analysed in MS Excel and JASP for descriptive statistics. In the next section, these results are presented.

4 Results

Figure 1 shows the TDA network produced from the Better Design data. The overall shape of the network indicates a structure similar to a neuron with a core at the left end with three small protruding 'flares' and a fourth large protruding 'flare' out to the right end with smaller flares protruding from it. Some nodes were also not included in the main structure seen as singletons above the main structure. The network is coloured by 'Rows per Node', which translates to the number of people grouped in a node. The main structure on the left contains the most people in each node shown with the red and yellow colouring. Flares (i.e. sub-groupings of interest) therefore contain fewer individuals than the inner core on the left.

Figure 2 shows 14 clusters resulting from the application of the Community Algorithm on the TDA network structure. For ease of interpretation, these clusters have been grouped into three categories with average age less than 40 years, average age 40–60 years and average age greater than 60 years. These are shown in Figs. 3, 4 and 5, respectively, with qualitative cluster descriptions.

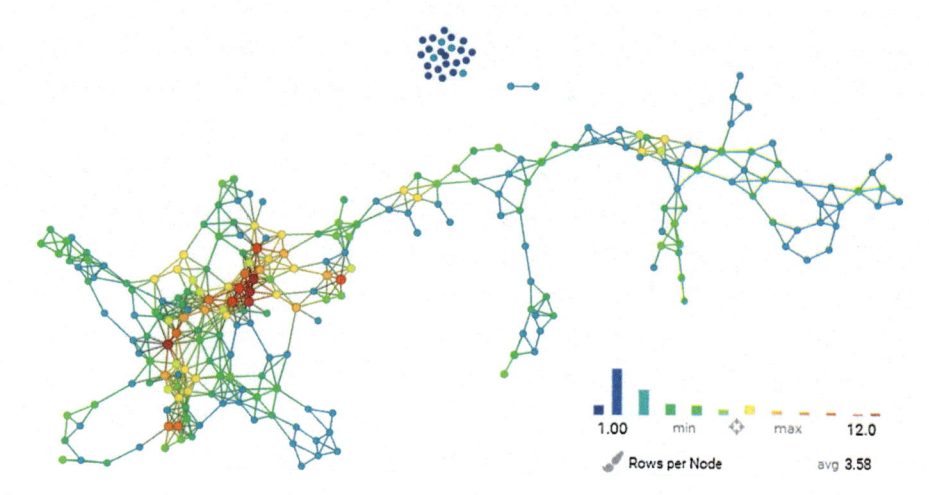

Fig. 1 TDA network coloured by rows per node. Metric: norm angle, Lens 1: neighbourhood Lens 1 (res: 30, gain: 2.5), neighbourhood Lens 2 (res: 30, gain: 2.5)

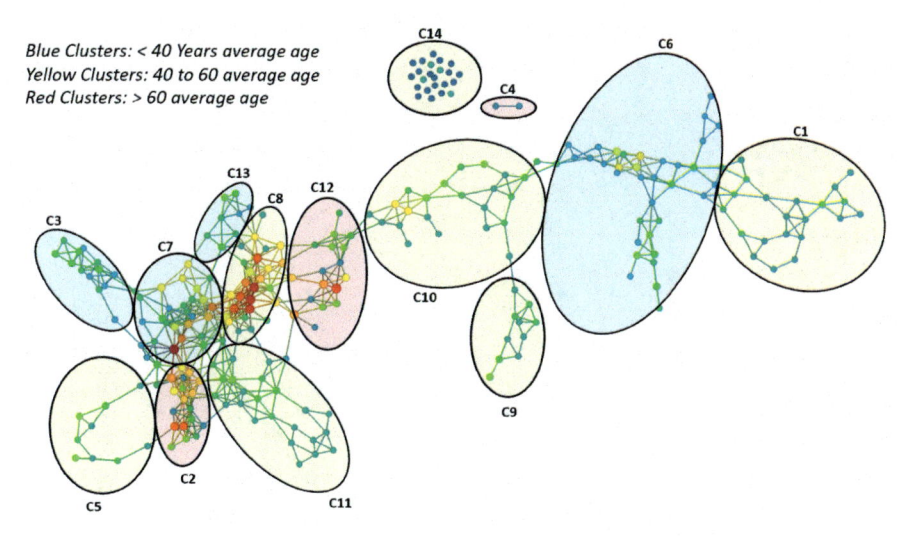

Fig. 2 TDA clustering of topological network of the Better Design data using auto-grouping (community algorithm) showing the resulting 14 distinguishing clusters in three broad age groups: <40 years, 40–60 years and >60 years

Four clusters are shown in Fig. 3 for the less than 40 years age group. In this age group, people showed sample average and above scores or experience with digital technology. However, clusters 3 and 7 show some minor capability loss in cognitive and motor capabilities. Seven clusters are shown in Fig. 4 for the 40–60 years age group. In this age group, the clusters ranged from above sample

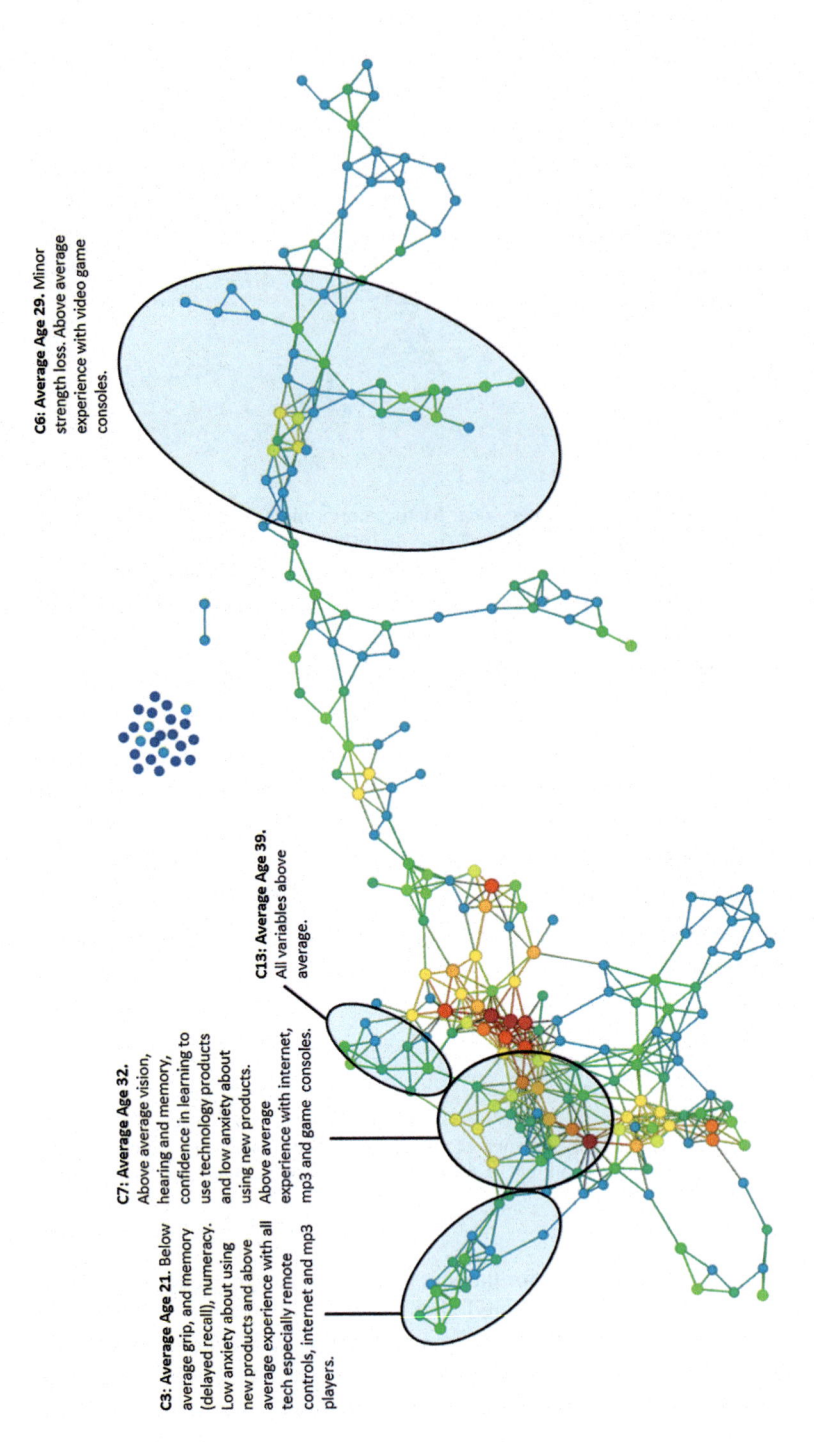

C6: Average Age 29. Minor strength loss. Above average experience with video game consoles.

C7: Average Age 32. Above average vision, hearing and memory, confidence in learning to use technology products and low anxiety about using new products. Above average experience with internet, mp3 and game consoles.

C3: Average Age 21. Below average grip, and memory (delayed recall), numeracy. Low anxiety about using new products and above average experience with all tech especially remote controls, internet and mp3 players.

C13: Average Age 39. All variables above average.

Fig. 3 Cluster descriptions for the <40 years age group

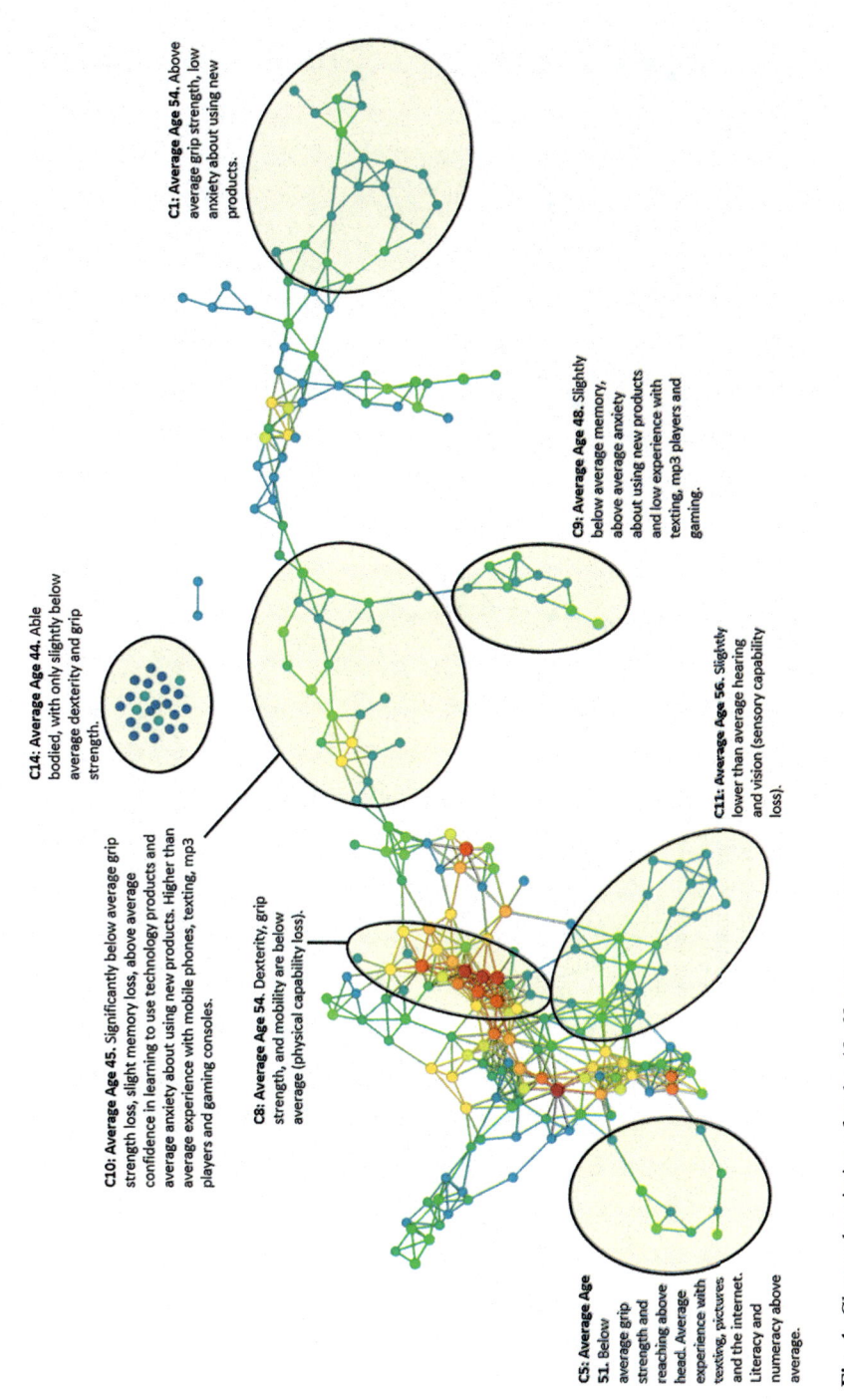

Exploring User Capability Data with Topological Data Analysis 47

C1: Average Age 54. Above average grip strength, low anxiety about using new products.

C14: Average Age 44. Able bodied, with only slightly below average dexterity and grip strength.

C9: Average Age 48. Slightly below average memory, above average anxiety about using new products and low experience with texting, mp3 players and gaming.

C10: Average Age 45. Significantly below average grip strength loss, slight memory loss, above average confidence in learning to use technology products and average anxiety about using new products. Higher than average experience with mobile phones, texting, mp3 players and gaming consoles.

C8: Average Age 54. Dexterity, grip strength, and mobility are below average (physical capability loss).

C11: Average Age 56. Slightly lower than average hearing and vision (sensory capability loss).

C5: Average Age 51. Below average grip strength and reaching above head. Average experience with texting, pictures and the internet. Literacy and numeracy above average.

Fig. 4 Cluster descriptions for the 40–60 year age group

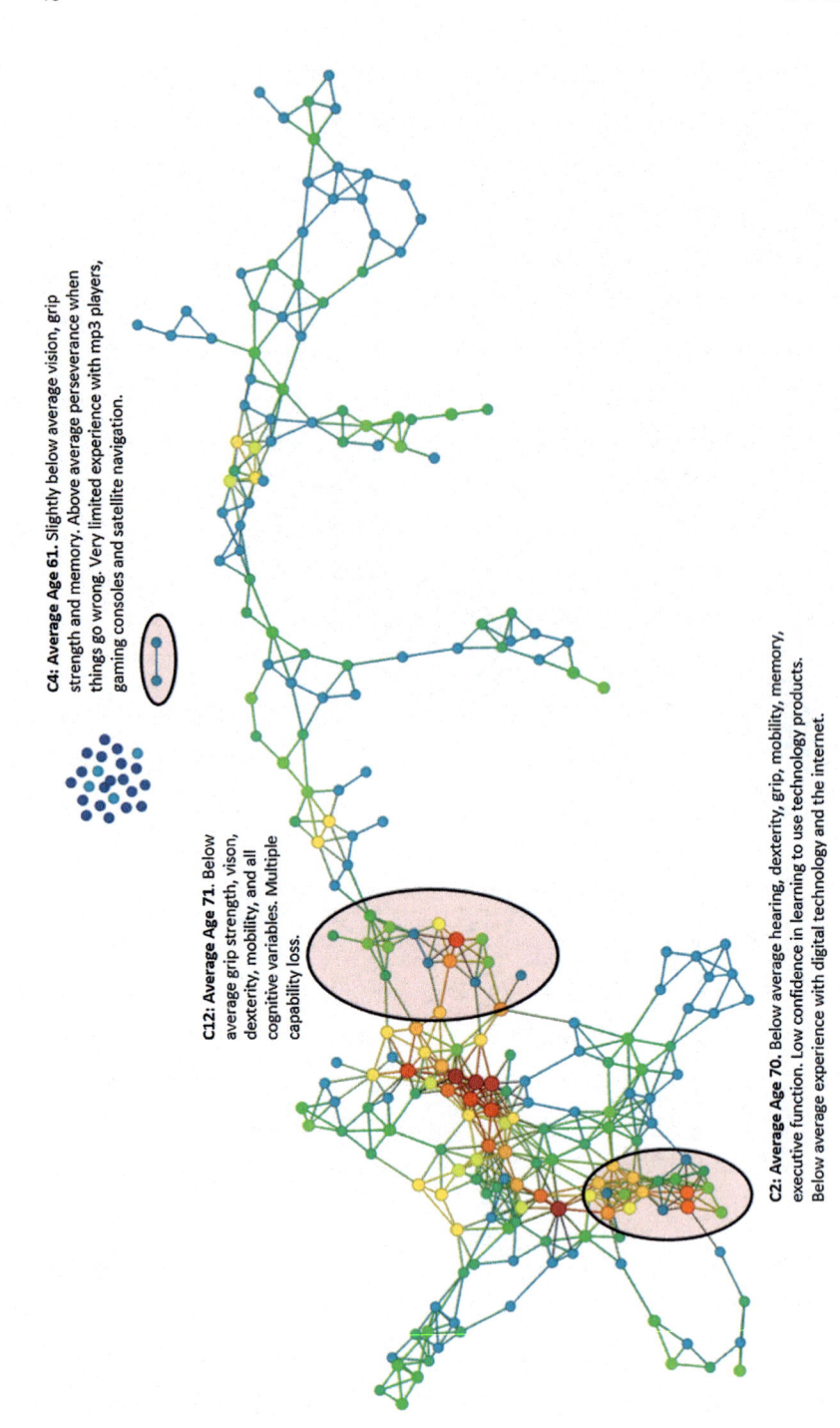

C4: Average Age 61. Slightly below average vision, grip strength and memory. Above average perseverance when things go wrong. Very limited experience with mp3 players, gaming consoles and satellite navigation.

C12: Average Age 71. Below average grip strength, vison, dexterity, mobility, and all cognitive variables. Multiple capability loss.

C2: Average Age 70. Below average hearing, dexterity, grip, mobility, memory, executive function. Low confidence in learning to use technology products. Below average experience with digital technology and the internet.

Fig. 5 Cluster descriptions for the >60 years age group

average sensory, cognitive and motor capability (cluster 1), through the minor capability losses (clusters 9 and 14), to more severe combinations of capability losses (Clusters 10, 8, 11 and 5). Three clusters are shown in Fig. 5 for the greater than 60 years age group. Clusters 2 and 12 highlight moderate to severe multiple capability losses compared to the sample averages, coupled with very limited experience with digital technology and confidence in using new products. Cluster 4, however, shows a tech-savvy subgroup that perseveres with new technology even though they have limited experience and multiple minor capability losses.

5 Discussion and Conclusion

The results presented summarised the Better Design study data in terms of TDA networks and 14 clusters. These clusters provide evidence of the structure of capability distribution in populations. The advantage of the Better Design dataset is that it contained multiple measures across capability domains resulting in rich descriptions of each cluster.

In each age group, there was a spread of capability from single minor capability loss to multiple capability loss. In addition, the attitudes and experience of people in each age group can provide designers with the data that they need to create designs that are usable, accessible and easy to learn. The variation exhibited by the data underscores the importance of Inclusive Design approaches when designing for the wider population. Supporting and capturing the richness of user diversity in design approaches, methods and tools will become more important as populations age and healthcare improvements enable longer life.

The results demonstrate the usefulness of the TDA approach using machine learning and network visualisation to explore and extract insight from user capability data. The data science and machine learning approach show promise for application in future ergonomics/human factors studies that capture large multivariate datasets. The Better Design pilot study points the way to future large-scale data collection efforts with multiple sensory, cognitive and motor variables. Given that analysis and visualisation tools such as TDA will make it easier to see the global structures inherent in data, it will encourage a move to methodologies that allow the data to 'speak for itself' and build new theoretical and practical insights.

So and Joo (2017) demonstrate that creativity in the design process could be improved through the use of personas. Personas capture qualitative details of key users that allow designers to focus on designing for 'real' people rather than a nebulous group (Goodman-Deane et al. 2010, 2014). The cluster information provided in this paper could add a quantitative dimension to the creation of personas by integrating sensory, cognitive and motor capability values in persona descriptions. This data-driven approach could ensure that designers account for the full range of user capabilities while engaging in Inclusive Design. It could also support market segmentation (Goodman-Deane et al. 2010, 2014).

Further work on the Better Design data will focus on relating user capabilities to rated product difficulties with an eye to developing predictive models for analytical product evaluation. In this endeavour, TDA will also play a major role.

References

AYASDI (2017) Ayasdi platform. www.ayasdi.com. Accessed on 15 Sept 2017
Carlsson G (2009) Topology and data. Bull Am Math Soc 46(2):255–308
Goodman-Deane J, Langdon PM, Clarkson PJ (2010) Key influences on the user-centred design process. J Eng Des 21:345–373
Goodman-Deane J, Ward J, Hosking I, Clarkson PJ (2014) A comparison of methods currently used in inclusive design. Appl Ergon 45:886–894
Johnson D, Clarkson PJ, Huppert F (2010) Capability measurement for inclusive design. J Eng Des 21:275–288
Langdon PM, Persad U, Clarkson PJ (2006) Developing a model of capability for inclusive design: the hidden structure of the ONS disability data. In: Disability Studies Association conference 2006: disability studies: research and learning, Lancaster University, Lancaster, UK
Lum PY, Singh G, Lehman A, Ishkanov T, Vejdemo-Johansson M, Alagappan M, Carlsson J, Carlsson G (2013) Extracting insights from the shape of complex data using topology. Sci Rep 3:1236
Persad U, Langdon PM, Clarkson PJ (2011) Investigating the relationships between user capabilities and product demands for older and disabled users. HCI International 2011, Springer, Orlando, FL, US, 9–14 July 2011
So C, Joo J (2017) Does a persona improve creativity? Des J 20(4):459–475
Tenneti R, Goodman-Deane J, Langdon P, Waller S, Ruggeri K, Clarkson PJ, Huppert HA (2013) Design and delivery of a national pilot survey of capabilities. Int J Hum Factors Ergon 2:281–305
Waller SD, Langdon PM, Clarkson PJ (2010) Using disability data to estimate design exclusion. Univ Access Inf Soc 9:195–207

Enhancing the Fashion and Textile Design Process and Wearer Experiences

W. Moody, P. M. Langdon and M. Karam

Abstract Broadly, this research aims to explore technology to create future sustainable and inclusive approaches in the fashion and textiles industry. This paper (1) addresses aspects to enhance the creative digital design process and (2) to facilitate creative and immersive design and emotive sensory wearer experiences, for future-enhanced physical products and virtual experiences. This involves a multimodal experience, and in particular, here the potential of vibrotactile and vibrotactile acoustic devices within this experience. A number of studies have explored wearable vibrotactile interfaces. However, the sense of touch, as a sophisticated and sensitive tool or skill, could be harnessed further. A literature review identifies relevant factors at this early stage of the research that will be used as a basis for developing multimodal design strategies using the sense of touch; and a creative yet functional analysis of this wearable technology.

1 Introduction

This paper explores the potential of the sense of touch within the future of fashion and textile design, and physical and virtual experiences. We question if we can change the way society consumes by developing experiential consumption strategies (Gilovich and Rosenzweig 2012), promoting well-being and reducing hyper-consumption and waste. Broadly, we aim to identify new and more sustainable ways to enhance the physical product and the potential of creating virtual

---

W. Moody (✉)
Cambridge School of Art, Anglia Ruskin University, Cambridge, UK
e-mail: Wendy.Moody@anglia.ac.uk

P. M. Langdon
Cambridge Engineering Design Centre, University of Cambridge, Cambridge, UK
e-mail: pml24@eng.cam.ac.uk

M. Karam
Kings College London, London, UK
e-mail: Maria.karam@kcl.ac.uk

© Springer International Publishing AG, part of Springer Nature 2018
P. Langdon et al. (eds.), *Breaking Down Barriers*,
https://doi.org/10.1007/978-3-319-75028-6_5

wearer experiences of fashion and textiles, much like a service. Retailers and brands are using existing, new and emerging virtual technologies to focus on selling and marketing products, promoting further hyper-consumption and clothing waste. There is the opportunity to simulate and enhance the creative sensory design process and wearer experiences and the imagination, to re-experience clothes and new creative designs in a more sustainable and inclusive way, by creating multiple experiences within any given garment or fabric.

2 Fashion Industry and Sustainability

The UK market value in the fashion industry (British Fashion Council 2017) contributes nearly £21 billion to the UK economy. The global apparel market is valued at 3 trillion dollars and it accounts for 2% of the world's Gross Domestic Product (GDP), with womenswear the highest valued category followed by menswear. However, there are increasing concerns over the amount of waste that is generated at the end of the product lifecycle. WRAP's recent report on the clothing industry in the UK found around 30% of clothing has not been worn in over a year. The cost of this unused clothing is around £30 billion. As a result, collaborative consumption is flourishing (Jiang and Tian 2016). This highlights the need to develop experiential consumption strategies (Gilovich and Rosenzweig 2012). If products had an increase in quality, it would generate higher profits but lower consumer surplus (Jiang and Tian 2016), slow down the life cycle of a garment and encourage people to wear and appreciate clothes for longer (DeLong et al. 2015). Creation of enhanced sensory products and multiple experiences would similarly add product value and extend life cycle.

3 Wearer Behaviour, Emotion and Sensory Factors

Historically, fashion, clothing and textiles have maintained a utilitarian, hedonic and symbolic role in society. Fashion has traditionally been associated with change and sensory stimulation, whereas clothing is defined more with functionality. Jordan (2002) developed a four-pleasure framework for considering product experience. It includes physiological, psychological (cognitive and emotional, e.g. the effective sensation of handling textiles or using products), social and ideological pleasures.

Buyer and wearer behaviour and the multisensory experience of clothing have shown to be used as a social tool for self-development and expression, linking with the self, emotions, moods and memories with the body. Emotions, defined as a set of feelings that affect behaviour, can be evoked, for example, by variable multi-sensory clothing experiences (Arafsha and Alam 2013). In recognising the social significance and role facilitator of clothing, research shows that clothing is used to match, reflect, compensate and manage emotions, moods and personality factors, and the importance of new clothing (Moody et al. 2009, 2010; Kang et al. 2015), highlighting the relationships with well-being, change and desire for enhanced and multiple product experiences.

The vision and touch senses provide the most detailed information about a product experience (Rahman 2012). At variable levels, fashion, clothing and textiles can be traditionally viewed as a more passive tactile experience as they rest and are worn around and on the body for reasons of comfort, fit and function, whereas visual tactile elements are stimulating, along with colour, design shapes, lines and other features. Campbell et al. (1976) found that young consumers rely on sensory and emotional responses, and women are more involved in fashion and exhibit a higher need for tactile input than men. Product aesthetics, aesthetic responses and experiences, both visual and emotional, are important as they may stimulate positive and pleasant sensory responses, arouse emotional feelings and also expressions and create symbolic meanings (Rahman 2012). Schifferstein (2006) found vision the most important sense to identify, recognise and evaluate a product, and the only modality to convey colour. For young consumers, sensory elements are seen as a salient evaluative determinant as they focus on novelty and sensory gratification to satisfy their aspirations (Park and Lee 1999). Sensory or tactile stimulation encourages consumers to imagine how a product will look or feel when in use, whereas visual attributes like colour, style and shape may arouse consumer emotion, communicate value, quality and convey symbolic meanings in users and viewers. Conscious and unconscious tactile feelings, associations and memories therefore play a role in consumer perceptions of clothing and preferences. Tactile inputs strengthen and re-confirm visual perceptions and impressions of a product, and consumers are always searching for multidimensional values in products. Furthermore, designers should pay more attention to multisensory product attributes to connect with their customers, generating more sustainable approaches, i.e. utilising the touch sense (Rahman 2012).

4 Design Thinking

The future designer has an ever-changing role, which draws upon inter- and multidisciplinary approaches to create inspiring, fresh, innovative and creative responses to the current and future world we live in (Gwilt 2014), for different markets or groups of people. In developing enhanced multimodal design strategies, it is important to clarify that traditional approaches used by designers will remain relevant. For example, design elements, such as shape, line, colour, fabric and texture; and principles, such as repetition, rhythm, radiation, contrast, harmony, balance, scale, volume, deconstruction, transparency and bodily sensation (Jones 2005; Volpintesta 2014). In addition, the methods used, for example, drawing, collage, layering, sampling, and the use of digital media and CAD systems, etc. (Eckert and Stacey 2000; Petre et al. 2006). For textiles, this involves knitting, weaving or printing using hand and digital tools. In any case, the fashion and textile designers are stimulated heavily by their senses.

A study by Atkinson et al. (2016) highlighted the importance of tactile properties of fabrics within design thinking. They acknowledged that in this digital age, we need a tool for consumers and designers that can express the needs and ideas of tactile meanings in materials. Based on future-thinking about design tools, manufacture and consumption, Smitheram (2015), amongst others, explored artistic fashion and textile design practices speculatively in the quest to dematerialise fashion and generate more enquiry into future fashion systems. Future design has become more involved with virtual garment simulation and interactive design (Cordier and Magenat-Thalmann 2005). Research into realistic virtual garment simulation, including the mechanical behaviour of cloth, has been highly challenging but achievable (Volino et al. 2005). How the cloth reacts to the body in movement, or other garments and materials, is crucial. Technology has optimised the clothing and fashion industry, benefitting from virtual prototyping and reducing waste. Other innovations in future fashion and textile design, and its relative associations with production and retailing, include

- body scanning technology for sizing;
- digital moving and interactive prints on clothes, accessories or footwear;
- 3D simulated garments reducing over production;
- augmented reality (AR) prints on clothing and in retail to reduce over production;
- virtual reality (VR) and fashion for viewing luxury brand fashion shows; and
- smart wearable clothing, personalisation and consumer interaction, 3D printing and nanotechnology.

None are exploring the potential of touch as part of a multimodal inclusive design system and wearer experience with, for example, VR or AR. The potential future of developing multimodal design strategies, and particularly elements that utilise more tactile approaches could add to the design process, thereby enhancing the wearer experience and their behaviour.

5 Applied Vibrotactile Systems

An analysis of the somatosensory system and vibrotactile technology reveals the potential of the sense of touch further within fashion and textile design thinking, and enhanced sensory wearer experiences.

Touch, as sensations, is aroused through the stimulation of receptors in the skin within two senses: cutaneous (stimulation of the skin) and kinesthetic (signalling from muscles, tendons and joints) (Rahman 2012). The somatosensory system, i.e. perception of touch, pressure, pain, temperature, position, movement and vibration, which arise from the muscles, joints, skin and fascia, is seen as an unexplored area and one where further sensory experience could be investigated and enhanced using products (Harrison et al. 2009; Guler et al. 2016). The skin has many mechanoreceptors to facilitate the sense of touch. The Pacinian Corpuscle, the largest touch receptor, facilitates the vibration sense modality (Toney et al. 2003). The RAII receptors are known to be associated with all the skin afferents. Vibratory discrimination thresholds for touch sensors are dependent on both frequency and amplitude of stimulation. Sensations are dependent on rapidly adapting and slow adapting mechanoreceptors (RA I, SA I, RA II, SA II), embedded in the skin, sensitive to frequencies between 0.5 and 1000 Hz and with receptive field sizes varying from 1 to 1000 mm^2. Sensory perception can be affected by the smallest of changes including tactor area, amplitude or frequency and body location (Toney et al. 2003). Our bodies have variable differences to the sensitivity of touch and are determined by the type of skin. We have glabrous or non-hairy skin that actively interacts with its surroundings (palms, fingers, genitalia, soles of the feet and lips) and non-glabrous or hairy skin that is more passive. Sinclair (1981) found that the glabrous skin is more sensitive to vibrotactile sensations than the hairy; however, this may be determined by the type of display used (Sinclair 1981; Karam et al. 2008).

The existing HMI interaction paradigm relies principally on visual feedback, often supported by sound. This is changing. Although a number of technologies have been tried, including electrode arrays and moving coil transducers, vibrating actuators are more likely to be used routinely as a robust general-purpose interaction device as they are more robust and far less expensive (Wall and Brewster 2006; Chouvardas et al. 2008; Karam et al. 2016). Conventional technology uses sets of tactors. These are configured to operate at around 140 Hz (100–200 Hz) sinusoidal.

There has been a rapid development within accessible technology that utilises the sense of touch and vibrations, e.g. mobile phones, and more recently vibrotactile displays and car interfaces (Karam et al. 2009; Duthoit et al. 2016). Geldard (as cited in Yao et al. 2010) defined four parameters of a simple tactile stimulus to encode information: locus, intensity (amplitude), duration or timing and frequency (Duthoit et al. 2016). Research examining cross-modal displays has shown that they support the presentation of sensory information using a different sensory modality (Karam et al. 2008). These have provided a multisensory experience, augmenting one modality by replacing extraneous information from a second modality or replacing it with another modality, 'sensory substitution' (Karam et al. 2008). Research into sensory substitution has aided the sensory-impaired (Stiles and Shimojo 2015).

Research into vibrotactile displays and wearable vibrotactile devices has been active since the late 1990s. Toney et al. (2003) identified vibration as a good candidate for clothing insert of tactile displays due to the scale and geometry of a vibration device and the fast-adapting, acting and quick response to changing stimuli. Tactile perception parameters include typical size, shape and tactile threshold sensitivities. They recommended that successful integration into clothing must address functional objectives: the culture, tradition and technology but also function, comfort, mobility and levels of social weight (defined as a measure of the social interaction between the user and technology). They also recognised the functional and sensory value of body-worn devices integrated into standard garments that remain hidden.

Vibrotactile displays on different parts of the body have been used as cognitive aids to improve situational awareness, navigation, reckoning, balance and spatial and directional orientation. Those developed for the shoulder were primarily explored for assistive technology for the disabled. The shoulder has been identified as a successful tactile communication channel to mimic social conventions. A shoulder application has been used within video conferencing using, for example, Osamu Morikawa's Hyper Mirror. A remote participant could tap another remote participant on the shoulder (Toney et al. 2003). Toney et al. (2003) integrated a pancake motor-based stimulator in a shoulder pad of a business suit jacket and tested it on 12 people. The outward appearance of the design did not change, the position did not impact on the wearer's mobility or comfort, it could be used to mimic social conventions, e.g. tapping on the shoulder for alerts or guidance, and could be removed for cleaning. This study successfully tested functional factors: comfort levels, levels of detection, quality of vibration, concentration required and ability to distinguish between sensation locations.

In 2002, a Hug Shirt™ was invented to aid remote communication through touch and emotion. The system uses Bluetooth with sensors and actuators and a Bluetooth-enabled smartphone with the Hug Shirt™ App running, then on the other side another smartphone and another shirt. Similarly, the Huggy Pajama is a hugging interface. The doll is the actual hugging interface, and a jacket is the output device. It was designed for parents to communicate with their children while they are away (Teh et al. 2009). In the future, combining emotion and technology could be part of every design process (Cutecircuit 2002).

Touch and music relationships have been examined considerably with our sense of hearing. They are also rather similar, especially their ability to perceive and process vibrations. A majority of the mental images conjured when listening to music are visual and auditory (Gunther and O'Modhrain 2003). Music notes, when visualised using water, have a strong textural quality (Jenny 1967). Based on more creative approaches to using vibrotactile technology, as with visual and tactile texture and the emotional relationships, we know how much music and sound can influence the listeners' emotions. For example, research has shown that vibroacoustic systems on the body can express emotional and characteristic information of an audio signal, indicating the sophisticated levels of sensitivity experienced using a tactile acoustic system, including detection of timbre and other characteristics of music, sounds and emotion (Karam et al. 2009; Russo et al. 2012; Branje et al. 2013). In Karam et al. (2008) research, emotional expression was successfully categorised using vibrations. As in other research exploring application of tactile interfaces, key variables were considered: the detection threshold, vibration frequency range, identification, location on the body, intensity (waveform), duration and how much of it is an integrated fixed system. Further subjective responses, including comfort and thresholds of sensation and pain, were also considered.

Vibroacoustic displays have been used within entertainment chairs (along the back) for tactile stimulation to accompany the sensory experience of a movie or video games (both using primarily music and speech); tactile communication for drivers; and improving somatosensory interactions for automotive applications. The combination of auditory and tactile information has been shown to be very effective for deaf, vision-impaired and sited individuals (Karam et al. 2008).

Other research in the area has explored wearable tactile acoustic vibration interfaces and emotions. However, there is a great deal of scope for further innovation within fashion and textile design, movement of vibrations round the body and wearer experiences. In 2003, Gunther and O'Modhrain explored tactile composition or aesthetic composition for the sense of touch. They were looking for a tool to facilitate tactile composition and the perception of intricate and music patterns of vibration. Much like any source of inspiration for textiles, there are variable patterns—repetitive or abstract. They developed a computer-controlled bodysuit with 13 embedded vibrotactile transducers—three small ones evenly spaced on each limb and a larger one on the lower back. Worn at a concert, users developed a significant 'feel' for the experience with increased exposure to the tactile compositions, appreciating high levels of music complexity and subtlety—calm and soothing compared to jarring music. The concerts provided a novel and enjoyable artistic experience (Gunther and O'Modhrain 2003).

Boudreau et al. (2011, as quoted in Stein 2012) created a garment that uses vibrotactile acoustic stimulation. It allows infants with special needs to detect and interpret sounds through touch enhancing the emotional connection between parents and their children, 'Babyvibe' (yourontarioresearch.ca/game-changer/babyvibe). In 2012, 'VibeAttire' was created to convert audio signals into vibrotactile experiences. A suite of vibration motors was embedded into ordinary clothing that MP3 player or other multimedia device can plug into. Listeners can fully experience music, enhancing the experience. The project was originally created for the deaf and those with hearing difficulties to experience art, relax and to be entertained (Guler 2012).

Hossain et al. (2010) developed interpersonal communication in the game Second Life using a haptic jacket where physical interactions, such as a handshake, hug or a tickle, could stimulate emotions and create emotional reactions. Philips Research Europe developed a jacket that influenced viewers' emotions watching movies using tactile stimulators embedded in a jacket (Jones 2009; Lemmons et al. 2009). Rahman et al. (2010) created a wearable vibrotactile jacket connecting tactile stimulation with YouTube videos. Using a haptic phone or jacket, Alam et al. (2011) used haptic vibrotactile devices to communicate SMS messages using a text-emotion extractor-based server. Boer et al. (2017) recently created a 'Hedonic Haptics Player'—a wearable device to experience vibrotactile compositions. Arafsha and Alam 2013 developed an effective haptic jacket designed for six basic emotions: love, joy, surprise, anger, sadness and fear; using warmth, pressure, vibration and beats from vibrotactile and heat actuators and temperature sensors.

A wearable haptic-based pattern feedback sleeve system was developed using vibro-actuators to encode complex haptic messages (Ranasinghe et al. 2016). Kelling et al. (2016) also explored the impact of haptic patterns within a sleeve design but in this case to test stress levels, 'Good Vibes'. Other research has explored vibrotactile acoustics in gloves to enrich emotional aspects of music in films (Mazzoni and Bryan-Kinns 2016). Neidlinger et al. (2017) developed a creative approach to audio tactile fabric/garments. They used a set of conductive embroidered speakers that play the frequency of goosebumps to tickle the skin and evoke the sensation of excitement (http://sensoree.com/artifacts/awelectric).

A vibrotactile interface was inserted into ballet shoes 'Music-touch Shoes' for hearing impaired dancers responding to a belief that people could learn an invented tactile body language 'vibratese' (Geldard, as cited in Yao et al. 2010). Hertenstein et al. (2009), as quoted in Petreca et al. (2013), developed a coding system to show how people use touch behaviour to communicate emotions to others. Touch behaviour includes patting, squeezing, caressing, etc. However, kinematic qualities also add to this communication of emotion, e.g. speed, duration, pressure, location and direction (Petreca et al. 2013). Furthermore, to emotionally engage with a fabric, touch behaviour kinematic factors are therefore important (Petreca et al. 2013). This indicates that there is a bodily experience or embodied tactile language for experiencing textiles. This could be explored further creatively within fashion and textile design thinking and wearer behaviour.

So far, subjective variables identified as affecting user experiences of wearable vibrotactile devices include body dynamics, body dimensions, body masses, body posture, age, gender, health, experience/training, attitude/motivation, sensitivity and susceptibility (Griffin 1994; Duthoit et al. 2016).

6 Conclusions

An analysis of the wearer experience based on the importance of both vision and touch, the somatosensory system, its relationships with emotions, vibrotactile and vibrotactile acoustic technology, has revealed its potential within design thinking, and its application in fashion and textile design and enhanced emotive and sensory wearer experiences. Key user variables and subjective factors have been identified. What is also interesting here is the proposition of harnessing a rather untouched sensory channel (touch), capable of understanding artistic expressions through fashion and textile design. Acoustic vibrotactile systems show great potential within design and for enhancing wearer experiences, based on the variable emotional tactile sensitivities and tactile patterns expressed within sound and music—sensory aspects that fashion and textiles designers are drawn to. There are opportunities for multimodal analysis within fashion and textile design, and inclusive sustainable design strategies that will extend product lifecycles and enhance emotional well-being. A literature review identified relevant factors at this early stage. This will be used as a basis for future research that will explore with wearers, how vibrotactile experiences can be incorporated into the creative and functional multimodal design process, to generate multiple and immersive designs and experiences within physical and virtual products.

References

Alam KM, El Saddik A, Akther HS (2011) SMS text based affective haptic application. In: Proceedings of VIRC 2011, Laval, France, April 2011

Arafsha F, Alam KM (2013) Design and development of a user centric affective haptic jacket. Multimedia Tools and Application, online 26 November 2013

Atkinson D, Petreca B, Bianchi-Berthouze NL, Baurley S, Watkins P (2016) The tactile triangle: a design research framework demonstrated through tactile comparisons of textile materials. J Des Res 14(2):142–170

Boer L, Cahil B, Vallgarda A (2017) The hedonic haptics player: a wearable device to experience vibrotactile compositions. In: DIS 17 Companion, Edinburgh, 10–14 June 2017

Boudreau JP, Russo FA, Stein R (2011) BabyVibe: A new device for exploring the impact of multimodal stimulation on early development. Poster presented at SRCD Biennial Meeting, Montreal, QC, Canada. In: Stein R (2012) The impact of synchronized tactile stimulation on joint attention in 11 month old infants. Thesis, Ryerson University, Toronto, ON, Canada

Branje C, Nespoil G, Russo F, Fels DI (2013) The effect of vibrotactile stimulation on the emotional response to horror films. Computers in Entertainment (CIE)—Theoretical and Practical Computer Applications in Entertainment 11(1)

Campbell A, Converse PE, Rodgers WL (1976) The quality of American life: perceptions, evaluations and satisfactions. Russell Sage Foundation, New York, NY, US

Chouvardas VD, Miliou AN, Hatalis MK (2008) Tactile displays: overview and recent advances. Displays 29:185–194

Cordier F, Magenat-Thalmann N (2005) A data-driven approach for real-time clothes simulation. Comput Graph Forum 24(2):173–183

Cutecircuit (2002) The HugShirt. The world's first haptic telecommunication wearable. http://cutecircuit.com/the-hug-shirt/. Accessed on 4 Dec 2017

DeLong M, Casto MA, Lee YK, Min S (2015) Sustainable clothing from the user's perspective. In: Proceedings of ITAA 2015 annual conference, Santa Fe, NM, US, 9–11 November 2015, p 118

Duthoit V, Sieffermann J-M, Enrègle E, Blumenthal D (2016) Perceived intensity of vibrotactile stimuli: do your clothes really matter? In: Bello F et al (eds) EuroHaptics 2016, Part I, LNCS 9774. Springer, Berlin, pp 412–418

Eckert C, Stacey M (2000) Adaptation of sources of inspiration in knitwear design. Creativity Res J 15(4):355–384

Gilovich T, Rosenzweig E (2012) Buyer's remorse or missed opportunity? Differential regrets for material and experiential purchases. J Pers Soc Psychol 102(2):215–223

Griffin MJ (1994) Handbook of human vibration. Academic Press, London, UK

Guler SD (2012) http://www.cmu.edu/qolt/AboutQoLTCenter/PressRoom/ces-2012/vibe-attire.html/. Accessed on Sept 2017

Guler SD, Gannon M, Sicchio K (2016) Superhumans and cyborgs. In: Guler SD et al (eds) Crafting wearables: blending technology with fashio. Apress, New York, p 154

Gunther E, O'Modhrain S (2003) Cutaneous grooves: composing for the sense of touch. J New Music Res 32(4):369–381

Gwilt A (2014) Fashion design for living. Routledge, London

Harrison C, Lim BY, Shick A, Hudson SE (2009) Where to locate wearable displays? Reaction time performance of visual alerts from tip to toe. In: Proceedings of CHI' 09, Boston, MA, US, 4–9 April 2009, pp 941–944

Hertenstein MJ, Holmes R, McCullough M, Keltner D (2009) The communication of emotion via touch. Emotion 9(4):566–573

Hossain SKA, Rahman ASMM, El Saddik A (2010) Interpersonal haptic communication in second life. IEEE International Symposium on Haptic Audio-Visual Environments and Games, HAVE 2010, Phoenix, AZ, US, 16–17 October 2010

Jenny H (1967) A study of wave phenomena. MACRO media, San Francisco

Jiang B, Tian L (2016) Collaborative consumption: strategic and economic implications of product sharing. Management Science, Published online on 16 November 2016
Jones SJ (2005) Fashion design, 2nd edn. Laurence King Publishing, London
Jones WD (2009) Jacket lets you feel the movies. IEEE Spectrum. http://spectrum.ieee.org/biomedical/devices/jacket-lets-you-feel-the-movies. Accessed on 20 Nov 2017
Jordan PW (2002) Designing pleasurable products: an introduction to the new human factors. CRC Press, Boca Raton
Kang J-YM, Johnson KKP, Kim J (2015) Clothing functions and use of clothing to alter mood clothing functions and use of clothing to alter mood. Int J Fashion Des Technol Educ 6(1):43–53
Karam M, Nespoli G, Russo F, Fels D (2009) Modelling perceptual elements of music in a vibrotactile display for deaf users: a field study. In: Proceedings of ACHI' 09, Cancun, Mexico, 1–7 February 2009
Karam M, Russo F, Fels DI (2008) Designing the model human cochlea: an ambient crossmodal audio-tactile display. IEEE Trans Haptics 2(3):160–169
Karam M, Wilde R, Langdon P (2016) Somatosensory interactions: exploring complex tactile-audio messages for drivers. In: Nunes I (ed) Advances in human factors and system interactions advances in intelligent systems and computing, vol 497. Springer, Berlin
Kelling C, Pitaro D, Rantala J (2016) Good vibes: the impact of haptic patterns on stress levels. In: Proceedings of the 20th international academic Mintrek Conference, Tampere, Finland, 17–19 October 2016
Lemmons P, Crompvoets F, Brokken D, van den Eerenbeemd J, de Vries G (2009) A body-conforming tactile jacket to enrich movie viewing. In: Proceedings of world haptics 2009, Salt Lake City, UT, US, 18–20 March 2009
Mazzoni A, Bryan-Kinns N (2016) Mood glove: a haptic wearable prototype system to enhance mood music in film. Entertainment Comput 17:9–17
Moody W, Kinderman P, Sinha P (2010) An exploratory study: relationships between trying on clothing, mood, emotion, personality and clothing preference. J Fashion Mark Manage 14(1):161–179
Moody W, Kinderman P, Sinha P, You K-S (2009) Identifying the causal relationships of appearance management through an analysis of one's own clothing and wearing experiences over a 10-day period. J Korean Soc Clothing Text 33(6):841–852
Neidlinger K, Truong KP, Telfair C, Feijs L, Dertien E, Evers V (2017) AW Electric: that gave me goose bumps, did you feel it too? In: Proceedings of TEI 2017, Yokohama, Japan
Park W, Lee S (1999) A market orientated study on the wearing attitude and purchase behavior of jeans. J Costume 43:109–123
Petre M, Sharp H, Johnson J (2006) Complexity through combination: an account of knitwear design. Des Stud 27(2):183–222
Petreca B, Bianchi-Berthouze N, Baurley S, Watkins P, Atkinson D (2013) An embodiment perspective of affective touch behaviour in experiencing digital textiles. In: Proceedings of ACII'13, Geneva, Switzerland, 2–5 September 2013, pp 770–775
Rahman O (2012) The influence of visual and tactile inputs on denim jeans evaluation. Int J Des 6(1):11–25
Rahman MA, Alkhaldi A, Cha J, El Saddik A (2010) Adding haptic feature to Youtube. In: Proceedings of the ACM multimedia 2010, Firenze, Italy, 25–29 October 2010
Ranasinghe A, Althoefer K, Dasgupta P, Nagar A, Nanayakkara T (2016) Wearable haptic based pattern feedback sleeve system. In: Proceedings of the 6th international conference on soft computing for problem solving, Thapar University, Patiala, India, 23–24 December 2016
Russo F, Ammirante P, Fels D (2012) Vibrotactile discrimination of musical timbre. J Exp Psychol Hum Percept Perform 38(4):822–826
Schifferstein HNJ (2006) The perceived importance of sensory modalities in product usage: a study of self-reports. Acta Physiol (Oxf) 121(1):41–64
Sinclair DC (1981) Mechanisms of cutaneous sensation. Oxford University Press, NY, US
Smitheram M (2015) Imagining and imaging future fashion. Craft Res 6(2):241–255

Stiles NRB, Shimojo S (2015) Auditory sensory substitution is intuitive and automatic with texture stimuli. Sci Rep 5:15628

Teh JKS, Cheok AD, Choi Y, Fernando CL, Peiris RL, Fernando ONN (2009) Huggy pajama—a parent and child hugging communication system. In: Proceedings IDC 2009, Como, Italy, 3–5 June 2009, pp 290–291

Toney A, Dunne L, Thomas BH, Ashdown SP (2003) A shoulder pad insert vibrotactile display. In: Proceedings of the 7th IEEE international symposium on wearable computers, White Plains, NY, US, 21–23 October 2003

Volino P, Cordier F, Magenat-Thalmann N (2005) From early virtual garment simulation to interactive fashion design. Comput Aided Des 37:593–608

Volpintesta L (2014) The language of fashion design: 26 principles every fashion designer should know. Rockport Publishers, Beverly

Wall S, Brewster SA (2006) Feeling what you hear: tactile feedback for navigation of audio graphs. In: CHI' 06, Montreal, Quebec, Canada, 22–27 April 2006, pp 1123–1132

Yao L, Ji X, Shi Y (2010) Music-touch shoes: vibrotactile interface for hearing impaired dancers. In: Proceedings of TEI 2010, Cambridge, MA, US, 25–27 January 2010, pp 275–276

Part II
Breaking Down Barriers Between Users, Designers and Developers

Using Inclusive Design to Drive Usability Improvements Through to Implementation

J. Goodman-Deane, S. D. Waller, M. Bradley, P. J. Clarkson and O. Bradley

Abstract There are compelling reasons to improve usability and make designs more inclusive, but it can be a challenge to implement these changes in a corporate environment. This paper presents some ways to address this in practice based on over 15 years experience of inclusive design work with businesses. It suggests that a successful persuasive case can be built with three key components: a proof-of-concept prototype, an experience that enables the stakeholders to engage personally with the issues and quantitative evidence demonstrating the impact of a potential change. These components are illustrated in this paper using a case study that was conducted with Unilever to improve the images used in e-commerce. The ice cream brand, Magnum is one of Unilever's billion-dollar brands that implemented these changes. During an 8-week live trial, comparing the old and new images, the new images experienced a sales increase of 24%.

1 Introduction

Inclusive design has great potential to improve users' experience in an increasingly diverse and ageing population. For example, Waller et al. (2015) argue that 'products that are more inclusive can reach a wider market, improve customer satisfaction and drive business success'.

However, it can be difficult to persuade businesses to engage in inclusive design in practice (Fletcher et al. 2015). Previous researchers have highlighted the key barriers of a lack of resources and guidance, a lack of knowledge and time, the need for a justifiable business case, difficulty in changing business cultures and the perception that inclusive design is expensive (Goodman et al. 2006; Whitney et al.

J. Goodman-Deane (✉) · S. D. Waller · M. Bradley · P. J. Clarkson
Cambridge Engineering Design Centre, University of Cambridge, Cambridge, UK
e-mail: jag76@cam.ac.uk

O. Bradley
Unilever, Leatherhead England, UK

2010; Hussain et al. 2015). They argue that better awareness-raising, training and tools are needed.

We have found that training and tools are valuable, but they need to be integrated within a persuasive case for change. This paper presents such a case to drive inclusive design and usability improvements through to implementation in a real-world business context. This has been developed by the Cambridge Engineering Design Centre (EDC) through over 15 years of inclusive design research and consultancy in a wide range of sectors including consumer goods, digital devices and transport (see, for example, www.cfbi.com/inclusivedesign.htm).

The persuasive case presented in this paper has three key components:

1. develop a proof-of-concept prototype of a better solution that demonstrates in a tangible way that something better is possible;
2. enable business stakeholders to experience the issue, and the difference that the prototype solution makes for them and
3. quantify the number of people that the issue affects, and quantify the extent to which the prototype solution could reduce this number.

Driving change through to adoption involves convincing a wide variety of people in different kinds of roles. Some people are more likely to connect with evidence that is experiential or emotional, while others favour evidence that is analytical. Therefore, the EDC has found that the most successful persuasive cases contain both experiential and analytical elements, comparing a prototype solution against the original design.

The level of detail of each of these components depends on the type and stage of a project. An early-stage consulting project might present rough proof-of-concept prototypes, an artificially created simulated experience and some initial estimates for population numbers. These early-stage outputs can then be used to convince a small project team within a company to allocate further resources to consider the issue in more detail.

At a more advanced stage, a project can produce prototypes that are more refined, with more realistic experiences and more robust quantified evidence. Further down the line, if a project team actually implements the changes, their exemplar solution can become the proof-of-concept prototype that other teams use to inspire them to undertake similar projects. These project teams can experience the actual difference between the exemplar solution and its predecessor, and actual sales results and business cash flows can underpin the quantified evidence.

Ultimately, this can inspire other businesses to rapidly follow the approach, leading to improvements in the accessibility and usability of products or services within an entire category or industry. This has the potential to improve the situation on a wider scale for the population as a whole (Shneiderman and Hochheiser 2001).

This paper describes each of these three components with examples from a detailed case study and other EDC consulting projects. Section 2 describes the use of a prototype solution, Sect. 3 examines the experiential elements and Sect. 4 focuses on the more analytical elements.

1.1 Case Study

The approach in this paper has been used successfully in a variety of projects. However, the details of many of these are confidential. The approach is therefore primarily illustrated in this paper using a project conducted with Unilever, who have kindly agreed to make this case study public.

The project started in August 2013 and focused on the improvement of e-commerce images that are used to represent products on e-commerce websites. At that time, the universally accepted, default form of these images was a photograph of the product (pack shot). However, in many cases, it was difficult or impossible to discern key information from these images, particularly when displayed on a small mobile screen. With more than 50% of e-commerce transactions in the UK being conducted on mobile, this is an increasingly important issue (Criteo 2016). In this use case, some information was completely impossible for all people to read. This was particularly difficult for people with any degree of vision loss including age-related long-sightedness. Thus, this was an issue of inclusive design, but one that impacted large groups in the mainstream population.

The case study involved developing guidelines for new 'hero images'. These are digitally enhanced product images, specially designed for mobile e-commerce. They use digital representations of the product, sometimes enhanced with off-pack communications such as a square containing the product size. More information on hero images can be found at University of Cambridge (2017).

The work was conducted in several phases, each of which involved the three elements of the persuasive case described in this paper. The first part of the work involved assessing early-stage prototypes for a handful of Unilever brands, creating simulated screenshots to show stakeholders directly the difference they made and an expert appraisal technique to quantify this difference. Later stages involved launching the initial prototypes live, professionally producing a video to show the differences with more impact, and conducting a test with 3000 users in a simulated shopping environment. The prototypes were also developed into a set of guidelines for 'Mobile Ready Hero Images' that were made freely available to other companies outside Unilever (University of Cambridge 2017).

By August 2017, several retailers were prepared to publish results from live A/B split tests comparing pack shots and hero images. These are tests conducted with live shoppers, where 50% of the shoppers are shown pack shots and the other 50% hero images. Sales from the two conditions can be compared. Many other global suppliers of consumer products had followed Unilever's approach, including PepsiCo, Nestlé, Kraft and Mondelez. The product identifier global standards body GS1 issued a 'call to action' to form a working group to develop hero images into a new global guideline for best practice e-commerce images.

Throughout the progression from early-stage project to industry-wide adoption, the three components of the persuasive case were critical to promoting the snowball for getting stakeholders engaged in the topic, getting improved solutions developed and getting these solutions launched live with retailers.

The new images greatly increase the numbers of people who can discern key information from them, as shown in Sect. 4. This makes the images more inclusive and works to reduce exclusion from the e-commerce shopping experience. Being able to do your own shopping is one of the Instrumental Activities of Daily Living (IADLs) (Lawton and Brody 1969). Therefore, reducing exclusion in this way may enable more people to live independently, eventually reducing social care costs.

2 Develop a Proof-of-Concept Prototype

Project teams within businesses can often become focused on finding the next cost reduction, or on firefighting things that have gone wrong. In this context, they may assign a low priority to usability and inclusive design issues. Describing such issues and trying to convince stakeholders of their importance may have little impact. We have found that stakeholder engagement is likely to be much higher when starting on a positive note, by showing an example that demonstrates that the usability can be improved and illustrating how this can be done in practice.

An example or prototype provides something tangible that stakeholders can see, feel, interact with or experience (Warfel 2009). It also offers a common talking point for a variety of stakeholders. Prototypes do not have to solve all of the issues, and they do not have to be finished and be ready to implement. They do need to be refined enough to serve their purpose, which typically is to inspire commitment and funding to investigate a problem further and develop a solution that could be implemented.

There are numerous methods for creating prototypes, depending on whether the focus is on the physical shape, the interaction or the look and feel of the solution. For example, one EDC consulting project looked at the packaging for a chocolate box. The client produced a functional and appearance prototype of the chocolate tray, which was used to showcase how changing the tray shape could improve usability. Other EDC projects have used mock-ups of screens drawn in PowerPoint to prototype changes to user interfaces.

2.1 Case Study

In the Unilever case study, the proof-of-concept prototypes were examples of more inclusively designed e-commerce images for a small selection of Unilever brands. The prototypes showed how it is possible to digitally create a hero image that looks like the product, but uses the following principles to increase visual clarity:

- use the full canvas available for a square e-commerce image;
- enhance the size, shape and contrast of key product information in the image (brand, product type, product variant and size) and
- omit everything else to clean up the image.

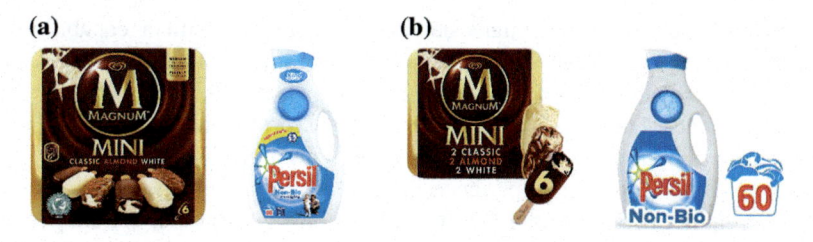

Fig. 1 **a** Original and **b** improved e-commerce images for Magnum and Persil (images © Unilever, used with permission)

Examples of pack shots and hero images are shown in Fig. 1.

To showcase the effectiveness of these images, they were shown within a mock-up of an online retailer store. At different stages in the project, this mock-up was produced at different levels of fidelity, such as:

- taking screenshots of retailer stores and overlaying the new e-commerce images on top of the old ones;
- creating custom desktop and mobile-friendly webpages, copying the look and feel of existing retailer stores and using the new images and
- creating an entire simulated shopping experience for user trials, which replicated the interaction associated with shopping on Amazon.

3 Enable Stakeholders to Experience the Issue

Sometimes stakeholders are initially disinterested in inclusive design issues. We have made presentations to people who are nonplussed, distracted and sometimes even looking for an excuse to escape the presentation to deal with (what they consider to be) other higher priority issues.

It can be very effective to start with something experiential, which gathers interest, attention and enthusiasm from the stakeholders. This first engages the attention and then gives the stakeholders a personal experience of the issues (Kouprie and Visser 2009; Hosking et al. 2015). If they can experience some of the difficulties for themselves, it can move the issue from being 'something that some unknown people experience' to 'something I can imagine experiencing for myself'. In some of our work, this experience has been so successful that previously disinterested stakeholders have been turned around to champion the improvements through to implementation.

There are many different ways to deliver an experience like this. Capability loss simulators are one method that can be very powerful. These are wearable devices or software that give stakeholders a direct experience of what using the original products and the prototypes might be like for someone with a capability loss (Nicolle and Maguire 2003). Stakeholders can wear simulators such as glasses that reduce vision capability and gloves that reduce dexterity, when trying to use physical products. Alternatively, software can be used to manipulate digital images to show what they might look like to someone with a vision impairment.

Other ways to deliver an experience include asking stakeholders to complete a use case scenario, perhaps imagining themselves into the shoes of certain personas (Cooper 1999).

Less direct, but still powerful, are videos of real users struggling with products. These can be used to showcase problems and get stakeholders on board. Combining this with videos of proof-of-concept prototypes can be even more powerful, showing how the prototypes can make a real difference. Where prototypes are not yet functional, acted scenarios can also be used to show how they might work. These are also valuable to engage stakeholders with issues that might be hard to obtain direct video of (Newell et al. 2006).

3.1 Case Study

For the Unilever case study, the EDC created a video that included an embedded shopping challenge (see https://www.youtube.com/watch?v=1223GTQQctE). In the video, the viewer is shown a mock-up of an e-commerce website on a mobile device (see Fig. 2). A set of related products are scrolled vertically in a similar manner to a shopper scrolling through products while shopping online. The viewer is challenged to identify products that meet certain criteria—in this case, packs of Dove bar soap. The challenge is conducted twice—once with the original product images, and once with hero images. On their first try, most people can identify 0 or 1 products (out of 5) with the original images, and 3 to 5 with the hero images. The video is powerful because it enables viewers to experience the difficulty for themselves. If they themselves find it hard to identify images, then they are more likely to admit that something needs to be done.

The video was shown privately to brand teams and retailers across the world, to help to convince them to develop and adopt hero images. In the US, Unilever's vice president of e-commerce announced 'this video is a gift that keeps on giving', in reference to its significance of convincing the US retailers, Walgreens, CVS and Walmart to adopt hero images.

The video was very effective, but it is also possible to deliver a convincing experience with something simpler. In addition to the video, we created PowerPoint slides, one showing an e-commerce pack shot and one showing a hero image of the same product, both with no text (see Fig. 3). Audiences were challenged to discern the brand, the type of product, product variant and product size from these images. Only the brand is really discernible in the first (and then only if the viewer is familiar with the brand), but all four messages are discernible in the second to someone with average eyesight. The authors believe this challenge was the

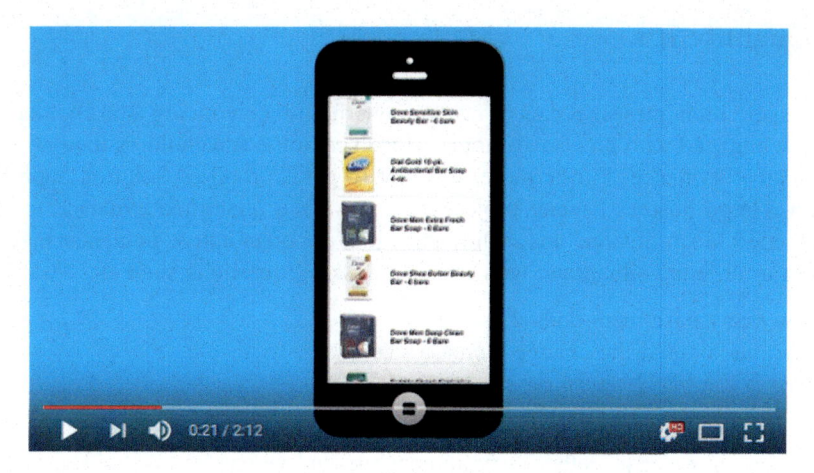

Fig. 2 Still from the Unilever case study video showing the online shopping environment used in the simulated shopping challenge (image © Unilever, used with permission)

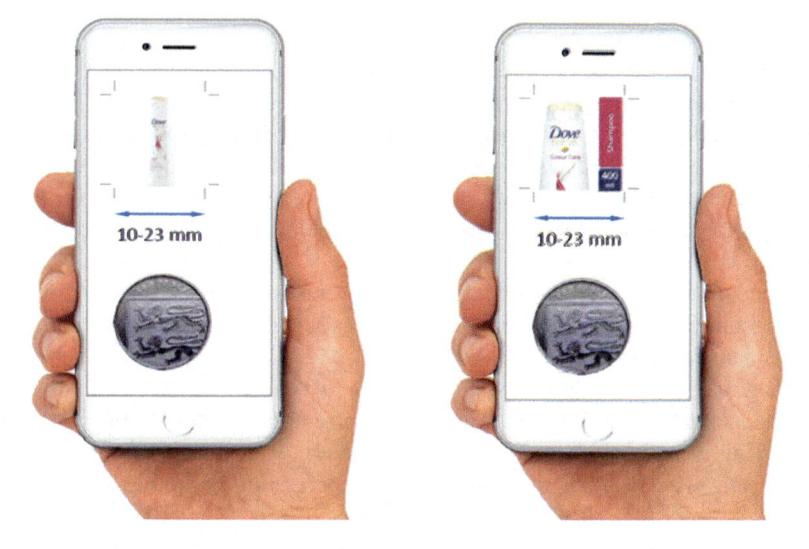

Fig. 3 Images used in presentations to illustrate the difference that hero images make. For the experience to be accurate, the images should be sized so that the 10 pence coin is the correct size

'moment of truth' that convinced many global retailers to support our position. As further evidence of their success and impact, other institutions have replicated and presented these two slides.

4 Quantify It

The experiential message can be very powerful in convincing stakeholders to become engaged with an issue or topic. However, some stakeholders require more quantitative evidence. Furthermore, in order to get a proposed solution approved within a large business, many project managers need quantified evidence for the likely effect on profit and loss. Different kinds of quantitative evidence may be needed in different situations, with managers asking questions such as:

- how many customers does this issue affect?
- how much could the change increase sales?
- what is the likely return on investment?

In many inclusive design projects, some quantitative evidence is required at an early stage, in order to gather some momentum and persuade stakeholders to take proposals further. Full answers to the questions above would require further investment to find out. For example, there is often not enough time or funding at this stage to conduct the large-scale user trials necessary to really determine how many customers would be affected.

Instead, the EDC has developed an exclusion audit process to give early-stage estimations of the number of users unable to access or use the product or service and the proposed prototypes (Waller et al. 2010). In this process, the use of the product is modelled with task analysis, and each task is analysed according to the demands made on the users' vision, hearing, thinking, reach & dexterity and mobility. These levels of demands are then compared with survey data on the UK population to estimate what proportion of the population would be unable to meet the demands.

The exclusion audit helps to relate improvements in usability to the numbers of customers affected. In turn, this can be used to estimate initial answers to questions of sales increase and return on investment.

Having assisted the EDC with a variety of consulting projects involving exclusion audits, Rob Morland from the Centre for Business Innovation says, 'Quantifying user experience in terms of population exclusion provides a common language that designers, managers, usability experts and marketing teams can all relate to'.

Once some more funding is available, more in-depth work can be conducted to gain more detailed quantitative figures. For example, in the Unilever case study, simulated shopping trials were valuable in examining the impact of the hero images. But these could only take place after key stakeholders had been sufficiently convinced by early prototypes.

4.1 Case Study

A key motivator in the Unilever case study was the lack of visual clarity of pack shots. It was much easier to discern key product information from the new hero image proposals than from the pack shots. The experiences in Sect. 3 showed the stakeholders this directly, but some may question whether these experiences apply to the wider population.

To address this, we carried out exclusion audits on the images. There are four critical pieces of product information that consumers typically want to know: brand, product type or format, product variant or flavour and product size. These are conventionally included in the product description. The SEE-IT method (Waller et al. 2016) was applied to the images to estimate the proportion of the UK population who would be unable to determine these critical messages from the images.

SEE-IT is a version of an exclusion audit specifically designed for assessing the visual clarity of flat images that are handheld, such as images shown on a mobile phone screen. It takes account of age-related long-sightedness and the variation in 'normal' vision capabilities, so the exclusion numbers presented are much higher than other methods might predict. In SEE-IT, the assessors determine the furthest distance at which they can discern a particular piece of information or feature in the image. This distance is used together with a measure of the assessors' eyesight and data on vision capability in the wider population to determine what proportion of the population would be unable to discern the information or feature in the image comfortably in normal use.

The results of SEE-IT on an example are shown in Fig. 4. Note that the variant in this example is communicated by the colour blue and the words 'Non-Bio'.

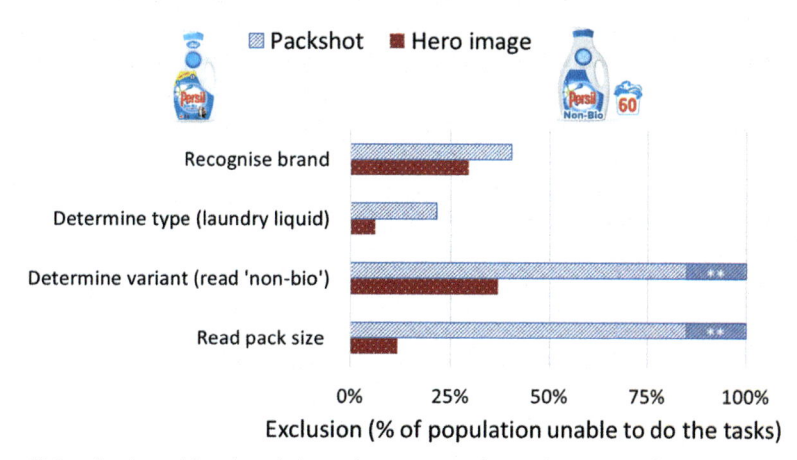

** Note that the model used to calculate exclusion goes out of range above 84.7% exclusion. Exclusion in the starred range lies between 84.7% and 100%

Fig. 4 SEE-IT results for the pack shot and hero image for Persil laundry liquid

The analysis presented here is for reading the text because not all shoppers are familiar enough with the products to distinguish them by colour alone.

Oliver Bradley, e-commerce Director for Unilever, says, 'The exclusion results made a compelling case that the original e-commerce images were not fit for purpose, and the new proposed solution was more effective for a significant proportion of the population. This case was quick to understand, and compelling enough to convince brand teams around the world to develop hero images, and retailers around the world to accept them'.

Following on from our early-stage audits using SEE-IT, some retailers were convinced enough to run live A/B split tests comparing pack shots against hero images. The split test results provided further quantitative evidence which helped to convince other stakeholders on a global basis. For example, Magnum is just one of Unilever's billion-dollar global brands to have benefited from the new images, with a 24% increase in sales measured in an 8-week A/B split test in a French retailer.

5 Conclusion

We propose that a successful persuasive case for usability improvements can be built with three key components: a proof-of-concept prototype, a personal experience and quantitative figures. The experience is important to help stakeholders engage personally with an issue and get them to 'feel' it for themselves. The quantitative part is important to convince business decision-makers to make the change happen. Both experiential and quantitative parts are most successful when they compare a proof-of-concept prototype against the current solution.

These three components have been found to be critically important in over 15 years of experience in working with industry on inclusive design projects. They have been illustrated in this paper using a case study with Unilever, where both experiential and quantitative parts were used to convince brand teams to develop improved e-commerce images and to convince retailers to accept the new images. In August 2017, images that follow these guidelines have been developed by Unilever, P&G, Nestlé, GSK and many other global FMCG suppliers. The images have been accepted by over 68 retailers from 28 countries. In September 2017, GS1 (an independent standards body) issued a call to action to form a working group to develop these image recommendations into a formal set of GS1 guidelines.

Acknowledgements We would like to thank Unilever for allowing us to make this case study public. The work was funded by Unilever, and the standards were developed in collaboration with the Unilever e-commerce team and the design agencies that they worked with.

References

Cooper A (1999) The inmates are running the asylum. SAMS Publishing

Criteo (2016) The state of mobile commerce 2016. http://www.criteo.com/resources/mobile-commerce-report/. Accessed 10 Nov 2017

Fletcher V, Bonome-Sims G, Knecht B, Ostroff E, Otitigbe J, Parente M et al. (2015) The challenge of inclusive design in the US context. Appl Ergonomics 46(B): 267–273

Goodman J, Dong H, Langdon P, Clarkson PJ (2006) Increasing the uptake of inclusive design in industry. Gerontechnology 5(3):140–149

Hosking I, Cornish K, Bradley M, Clarkson PJ (2015) Empathic engineering: Helping deliver dignity through design. J Med Eng Technol 39(7):388–394

Hussain A, Ahmad A, Case K (2015) Inclusive design drivers and barriers - A manufacturing perspective from Pakistan. Prod Manuf Res 3(1):289–309

Kouprie M, Visser FS (2009) A framework for empathy in design: Stepping into and out of the user's life. J Eng Des 20(5):437–448

Lawton MP, Brody EM (1969) Assessment of older people: Self-maintaining and instrumental activities of daily living. The Gerontologist 9(3):179–186

Newell AF, Carmichael A, Morgan M, Dickinson A (2006) The use of theatre in requirements gathering and usability studies. Interact with Comput 18(5):996–1011

Nicolle CA, Maguire M (2003) Empathic modelling in teaching design for all. In: Stephanidis C (ed) International conference on human-computer interaction; Universal access in HCI: inclusive design in the information society 4: 143–147

Shneiderman B, Hochheiser H (2001) Universal usability as a stimulus to advanced interface design. Behav Inf Technol 20(5):367–376

University of Cambridge (2017) Mobile ready hero image guidelines. http://ecommerce.inclusivedesigntoolkit.com. Accessed 10 November 2017

Waller SD, Bradley M, Hosking I, Clarkson PJ (2015) Making the case for inclusive design. Appl Ergonomics 46(B): 297–303

Waller SD, Goodman-Deane JA, Bradley MD, Cornish KL, Clarkson PJ (2016) Walking backwards to quantify visual exclusion. In: Langdon P, Lazar J, Heylighen A, Dong H (eds) Designing around people. Springer

Waller SD, Langdon PM, Clarkson PJ (2010) Using disability data to estimate design exclusion. Univers Access Inf Soc 9(3):195–207

Warfel TZ (2009) Prototyping: A practitioner's guide. Rosenfeld Media

Whitney G, Keith S, Schmidt-Belz B (2010) The challenge of mainstreaming ICT design for all. In: International conference on computers for handicapped persons ICCHP 2010: computers helping people with special needs, Vienna, Austria, pp 583–590, July 2010

Improving Pool Design: Interviewing Physically Impaired Architects

C. M. Pereira, T. V. Heitor and A. Heylighen

Abstract People with a temporary or permanent physical impairment are often excluded from bathing activities due to the difficulties of getting in and out of the water. This paper explores pool design, specifically the design of the access to the tank, which is the key to pools' inclusivity. In trying to break down existing barriers between users, accessibility experts and designers, we interviewed physically impaired architects about their perception of four types of pool access often used by wheelchair users: ramps, transfer walls, transfer systems and lifts. The interviews revealed limitations in all four types of pool access. To compensate for the limitations identified, combining different types of access in one single pool may be of interest. Moreover, the interviews allowed the identification of another type of pool access, designed by one of the interviewees: an upper pool border connected to an underwater bed and seat allows for an easier exit than transfer walls and transfer systems. Another interviewee advanced the idea of a cane holder for physically and visually impaired people, which may contribute to freeing poolside floors from obstacles and reducing the risk of falls. These insights may contribute to making pools more inclusive, by accommodating specific temporary or permanent mobility needs of all of us.

1 Introduction

Aquatic activities are considered a way of promoting health and well-being (Sato et al. 2007; Middlestadt et al. 2015). Pools have the potential of providing freedom to people with impairments, e.g. a wheelchair user or a blind person often do not

---

C. M. Pereira (✉) · T. V. Heitor
University of Lisbon, Lisbon, Portugal
e-mail: carlosmouraopereira@gmail.com

T. V. Heitor
e-mail: teresa.heitor@ist.utl.pt

A. Heylighen
Department of Architecture, Research[X]Design, KU Leuven, Leuven, Belgium
e-mail: ann.heylighen@kuleuven.be

need any assistive device in order to swim. Movements in the water provide freedom and facilitate physical activity, being highly beneficial for some physically impaired people. Paradoxically, non-ambulant people often cannot access pools autonomously due to the design. This study therefore aims to explore inclusive and multisensory design solutions for pool access.

For a pool access to be usable by a non-ambulant person, its design needs to facilitate mobility by centralising the effort in the upper body. As a result, it has the potential to increase haptic comfort for other users allowing less effort to be used in some body parts.

Fletcher (2009) points to the fact that architects have the power to increase or decrease people's disability through their design. Unfortunately, contemporary pools, where entry in and out of the water are facilitated, are rare. We argue that integrating requirements related to usability by physically impaired people may contribute to increasing haptic qualities also for users without physical impairment; e.g. a pool ramp requires less effort than a pool ladder, increasing the sensory comfort in entering and exiting the water.

This study is exploratory and its goal is to understand pool access from the perspective of diverse users, in particular, those with a physical impairment. Moreover, as pools are important spaces for promoting health and well-being, making them more inclusive may increase the quality of life and reduce the need for medical care, thus contributing to a socially sustainable economy. It is important to consider that an inclusive pool is less likely to require future functional adaptations or to be demolished due to obsolescence. This makes it much more durable than a pool without inclusive access and avoids the need for further consumption of building materials, contributing to a more sustainable environment.

Current architectural production is predominantly ocularcentric, paying little attention to the spatial poetics related to integrating other sensory modalities than vision. Moreover, barrier-free spatial components are often designed with neither spatial poetics nor sensory balance in mind. As a result, functionality is perceived by most designers as something with a medical appearance, spoiling the visual poetics of the architecture. According to Guimarães (2011), inclusive sustainability requires a cultural revolution that integrates poetics into the design. Following this premise, we centred our research on the perceptions of physically impaired architects, a group with the potential to break down barriers between the poetics of designers, the inclusivity of accessibility experts and the kinaesthetic experience of physically impaired people.

Pool ramps are usually perceived as an inclusive type of access and mechanical devices as an alternative assistive solution. In order to question this perception, we set out to inventory the advantages and limitations of different types of access, which results in the identification of inclusive pool details unknown in literature.

2 Context

The potential to acquire spatial knowledge through the experience of disabled designers is increasingly recognised (Vermeersch and Heylighen 2011, 2013; Pérez Liebergesell et al. forthcoming). According to Ostroff et al. (2002), the condition of living with an impairment can increase spatial maturity, empathy, determination and social justice. Regarding pool design, Usandizaga (2013) stresses that integrating inclusive premises in the early stages of the design process results in high-quality architecture, as exemplified by the works developed by disabled designers. One of these works is an unusual pool designed by one of the interviewees, which is described in more detail below.

Accessibility standards, including legislation and non-mandatory best practice guidelines, are important documents for achieving inclusivity. Usually, they are based on scientific literature and result from the confrontation with concrete realities that are inherent to the approach adopted in that context. Across the board pool standards in general, and standards on tank access in particular, are poorly developed.

The inclusive principles provided by Story et al. (1998) present a pool ramp as an inclusive spatial component related with equitable use, especially by physically impaired people or children learning to swim.

The accessibility guidelines of SE (2002) recommend a pool ramp, mainly in the shape of a beach, as the best type of pool access. They mention that, for some users, a handrail along the ramp suffices while others require assistance. These requirements reflect an awareness of the loss of autonomy of some users.

The accessibility guidelines of USAB (2004) present a potentially usable tank access, which consists of a pool lift, with the requirement that it must allow users autonomy by being operable both from the deck and from inside the pool, hence users will not have to wait for assistance alone in the water. These guidelines establish a minimum of one access type, specifically a pool lift or ramp, for tanks with walls with a perimeter of less than 91.44 m. Bigger pools require an extra access type, be it a pool lift, pool ramp, pool stairs, transfer wall or transfer system. Using different types of access is recommended in order to permit usability options for impaired users with a diversity of needs.

Transfer walls, also known as low walls, are often found in health and well-being centres, for example, hot tubs. They enable people to transfer from a wheelchair to the top of the wall and rotate to the pool tank. They can be at the pool's edge in the case of pools with a water level over the deck, or partial pool borders accessible by a dry ramp leading to a partially low deck. In these guidelines, transfer walls require a minimum of one grab bar perpendicular to the pool wall and installed on top of the transfer wall.

The transfer system mentioned in these guidelines, also known as transfer steps or transfer tiers, combines pool stairs with a transfer platform with extra steps over the deck. This enables physically impaired people to transfer from a wheelchair to the top of the platform, and to move through the steps in a seated position when entering or exiting the tank.

Howard et al. (2008) present a checklist that facilitates interpretation of the USAB (2004) guidelines. Moreover, they identify the pool lift and transfer system as the means of access that is easier to instal to existing pools.

The American legislation (DJ 2010) is based on the already mentioned USAB guidelines (2004). This legislation does not guarantee pool inclusivity mainly because it allows pools that have only one type of access, a pool ramp, for non-ambulant people, to be acceptable. This ramp access affords less autonomy than a pool lift and excludes people with more severe physical impairments. Still, this legislation was one of the most detailed and inclusive we found.

With regards to the requirements of DJ (2010), Caden (2011) mentions that they allow for the use of portable pool lifts. In our opinion, this condition risks the creation of more operation discontinuities. Pool lifts are less expensive to instal than pool ramps, but the latter are free of the extra maintenance that a mechanical device requires (Caden 2011).

3 Methodology

The exploratory research approach we adopted is based on qualitative inquiry. According to Denzin and Lincoln (2011), current qualitative research explores the hopes and needs of a democratic society. We argue that by exploring inclusivity, the goal of this study can be representative of a democratic approach, focusing on the premise of equitable use by all people.

We interviewed physically impaired architects, combining their user experiences, professional knowledge and expertise on inclusivity. Ostroff (1997) defines a user/expert as anyone who has developed natural experience in dealing with the challenges of our built environment. Confronting the users/experts' perspective is expected to contribute to spatial inclusivity. Therefore, we explore the perspective of a selective group of users with the potential of identifying inclusive design requirements for pool access.

In order to maximise cultural diversity, we recruited participants from ten countries and four continents. We interviewed ten physically impaired architects, namely Christiaan Zandstra (Netherlands), Deepak K.C (Nepal), Francesca Davenport (Australia), Gerasimos Polis (Greece), Karen Braitmayer (USA), Marcelo Guimarães (Brazil), Marta Bordas-Eddy (Spain), Nikola Arsic (Croatia), Silke Schwarz (Germany) and Yoshihiko Kawauchi (Japan).

For reasons of feasibility, we interviewed them via e-mail, an alternative qualitative interview technique applied in similar geographical contexts (Flick 2009). Moreover, given the interviewees' expertise, it is interesting to obtain written reflections, and e-mail interviews have the potential to yield more carefully considered answers. We used a semi-structured format in the questionnaire in order to obtain selective qualitative data without losing the opportunity to extend the interviews, some of which were developed over the course of several e-mails. The starting point was the identification of advantages and limitations of each type of access often used by wheelchair users when entering and exiting pool tanks. We considered both the self-use by the interviewee and the allocentric perception related to inclusive use. A link to the American legislation (USAB 2004; DJ 2010) was sent to most interviewees to help elicit responses. This legislation has been identified in our literature review as a state-of-the-art reference, important for achieving inclusive perceptions that are pertinent for the improvement of pool design. We did not, however, send this link to the American interviewee, as she is familiar with her country's national standards.

None of the participants required anonymisation of the data. Data were analysed using coding to identify similarities and differences of opinion expressed by the interviewees, aiming to achieve generalisable statements related to the usability of pool access.

4 Results

The interviewees identified advantages and limitations in each type of pool access usable by physically impaired people.

Some interviewees preferred the *pool ramp* as means of access for their own use. Advantages they identified include continuous performance, autonomy in use and usability for specific users. 'The ramp may work well for slow walkers who need a support mechanism to enter the pool', an interviewee stated. Other interviewees stressed its usability for people with a temporary physical impairment and for people other than physically impaired. In terms of limitations, an interviewee identified the discomfort of using a bathing wheelchair: 'In order to use the entry ramp, I need to transfer from my wheelchair to the wheelchair for a pool which does not fit my body'. Moreover, regarding its use by other people, he referred to the loss of autonomy in some situations requiring human assistance. Two interviewees mentioned the limitations for some physically impaired people. One of them pointed out: 'The entry ramp works for many but not for complete spinal cord injuries I would say. I understand it requires a waterproof wheelchair, and even if having one, once in the water it might be very difficult to move'.

Pool access through a *transfer system* was considered by some interviewees to be an option for their own use. For one of them, it allowed to avoid the inconvenience of depending on assistance. Moreover, 'the trick is to design a good access point and position it in the right place, so you can use it without having to watch out where your legs are going to end up, or if you are going in some way injure yourself'. Some pointed out, however, that it is usable only for specific users with strong upper limbs. One of them explained: 'The transfer steps require the ability to lift your body up to 6" vertically. Not everyone has that sort of arm strength'. Other identified limitations related to physically impaired people's well-being, as it is not as dignified as other types of pool access. One interviewee mentioned: 'Personally I think accessing a pool by a transfer system is humiliating. It is not a very sexy and elegant way to access a pool'. He also pointed at the difficulty of using the transfer system in the event of an emergency, specifically when exiting the pool.

Some interviewees considered pool access by *transfer wall* to be a means of access that they themselves could use. One explained: 'I prefer to use a quick, simple solution without any further human help'. Another stressed the quality of autonomy in use for a specific impaired condition: 'As a paraplegic, you can manage to do it by yourself without anyone's help (which is always a plus)'. Other interviewees highlighted the transfer wall's usability for a diversity of users, including those with temporary impairments, and appreciated it being continuously operational. However, limitations were identified as well: 'Aging has been a very determining factor for me in abandoning this way of accessing to the water (…) one of the most negative things that a wheelchair user can make that is to lift his body on his arms and specially having all the weight been at the shoulders. Tendonitis and other injuries are guaranteed'. Another interviewee agreed that this form of access is usable only by people with upper limb strength. Some interviewees questioned its usability when exiting the pool and one of them said: 'I'm wondering how and whom people do warn if they need help and want to leave the pool'.

Regarding access by *pool lift*, some interviewees focused on the usability for their own purpose. Its greater usability specifically by physically impaired people with less mobility was also stressed. One of them mentioned: 'It has the advantage of supporting the most significantly limited swimmers'. A limitation was identified in the case of operational discontinuities. One remarked: 'The pool lift has the disadvantage of being the least likely to be operational (any mechanised device is likely to fail)'. Autonomy loss was also identified as a limitation: '[the pool lift] is rarely installed in a manner to be used independently'. Indeed, 'The main disadvantage of it is that we always need someone who is specialised for its operation. Drawing the attention of people while using it is something which I do not like at all'. Another limitation is the 'very slow process to use (to transfer to/from wheelchair, to operate)'. Moreover, pool lifts run the risk of causing accidents: 'I know hoists with chairs (…) for immersion. These chairs can be obstacles to access by other people and can cause accidents' [translated]. One interviewee identified the potential of the platform lift, i.e. a device with a bathing wheelchair for non-ambulant people, which other people can use in a standing position. Another interviewee pointed to a specific type of pool lift, a ceiling-mounted hoist (Fig. 1, left), as being the most adequate pool access for his own use: 'One can enter and exit a pool without assistance. In the case of a severely physically impaired person, we can imagine that person using a life jacket together with the hoist. When it is not in use, the hoist can be put away from the pool, so that the structure does not interfere with the access of other people' [translated].

Another type of pool access was explored by Bordas-Eddy in the design of a home pool in Cabrils (Fig. 1, centre). For the purposes of this study, we name this new type of pool access a *transfer bed*. It combines a transfer wall with an underwater bed on one side of the pool, connected in the corner to a lower underwater seat set in another transverse pool wall. Bordas-Eddy highlighted the usability provided by the underwater bed: 'There's also a bench at different heights:

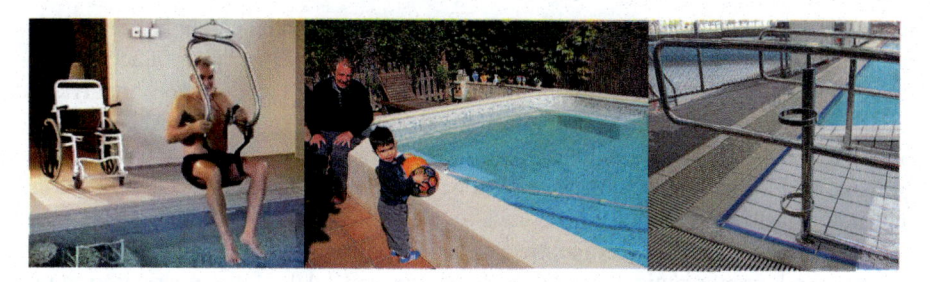

Fig. 1 Ceiling-mounted pool lift (left); Private pool in Spain with transfer bed (centre); Public pool in Australia with cane holder (right) (credits: 1. H.-M.; 2. M. B.-E.; 3. F. D.)

one at 52.5 cm (measured from the inferior limit of the ceramic tile down to the water) to seat down, and one at 22.5 cm to lay down. Specially, the second one is very useful to get out the water'. Moreover, the corner was identified as a spatial component that facilitates entry and exit, and she reflected on her experience of using the transfer bed when pregnant: '(I was heavy and it was difficult to lift my own weight). Instead the pool lift required less effort'.

The importance of a *storage area for assistive objects* for people with reduced mobility was also identified by some interviewees. Davenport sent drawings and pictures of several bathing facilities designed under her consultancy, allowing us to gain information about an unusual detail, a cane holder for pool access (Fig. 1, right). She specified its usability: 'The idea of the cane holder came about when I saw walking sticks, crutches, white canes left on the floor near steps into the pool, creating tripping hazards as well as cluttering the pool perimeter'. She also mentioned the feedback on building performance: 'I originally advised the architect to incorporate the cane holder in one of our earliest projects and since then it has been incorporated in the rest of the projects. In one of the projects, a cylindrical/tubular plastic cane holder was installed instead of the rings. I think the rings are better because the tubular holder has a limited depth and will require cleaning over time'.

In short, some interviewees recommend providing a choice of different pool access types given the diversity of people's needs. One interviewee stated: 'there have to be more than one way of opportunities for the potential users or swimmers to take advantage and make use of it'.

5 Discussion

Regarding the design of pool access, the standards (DJ 2010) are the most detailed legislation found in the literature. They define the criteria for accessible pools under two categories: tanks with a pool wall perimeter of over 91.44 m require two types of access, one of which can be a pool stair; pools with a smaller wall perimeter require only one type of access, often used by wheelchair users, specifically a ramp, a transfer system, a transfer wall or a lift. However, pool stairs can only be used by ambulant people. So, the already mentioned combination of two types of access will leave wheelchair users dependent on one of the four access types analysed. Considering that the interviewees highlighted limitations in all of these, it is pertinent to envisage a minimum of two types of access in order to balance the limitations. Furthermore, this requirement needs to be applied to all accessible pools and not only to large tanks. Small tanks are often used for health and well-being activities, specifically in therapeutic pools for physical rehabilitation or mineral springs, and prophylactic pools at wellness centres. All of these are important facilities for the health and well-being of physically impaired people. Furthermore, equitable use and the possibility of choice for the users are principles of inclusivity (Story et al. 1998). The interviewees also stressed that mechanical devices, such as a pool lift, show fewer limitations than non-mechanical pool accesses, in terms of their usability by people with severe physical impairment. It would be more resilient if pool standards specified the minimum provision of two types of access, mechanical and non-mechanical, considering its usability by non-ambulant people.

We state that the integration of a pool lift has the potential of providing an inclusive pool, if it can be used autonomously by physically impaired people, as required by some standards (USAB 2004; DJ 2010). However, these standards recommend a pool lift with a chair, which in our opinion is a type of assistive device with avoidable medical appearance. Caden (2011) mentions that DJ (2010) standards permit the use of portable pool lifts. Several interviewees warned that pool lifts are not in continuous use. In our opinion, this situation can be improved by insisting on the installation of fixed pool lifts. Portable pool lifts are often used because they can provide access to several pools in the same facility. However, moving the lift to another pool requires assistance and means that physically impaired people have to wait. One interviewee stressed that pool lifts can cause accidents. We argue that, compared to fixed ones, movable pool lifts can increase the risk of collision with other people. It is important to consider that pool decks tend to be slippery when wet. A ceiling-mounted pool lift can be an interesting user-centred option, because it reduces the risk of collision. Aesthetically it has only the presence of a ceiling rail, when not in use, and it can be easily integrated into the pool design. In outdoor pools, it is more difficult to apply this solution. However, it could be interesting to design outdoor pools with partial ceiling areas to provide shade, thus more resilient to avoid ultraviolet radiation injuries.

Regarding non-mechanical pool access, the transfer bed explored by an interviewee has the potential of being more usable than the transfer wall or the transfer system. The underwater bed can be used as a rest platform, facilitating the mobility effort. Another interviewee focused on the risk of a user needing to exit the pool. In this situation, the rest platform can provide more safety than the transfer wall or the transfer system. Moreover, it can also be used by people without impairments, being perceived as more inclusive than the transfer wall or the transfer system. Besides enabling the seating to be used for transfer, the pool border over the deck has the advantage of providing a recognisable spatial component for visually impaired people. Furthermore, they allow for more savings in terms of volume, with fewer built areas below the deck level, and facilitate the cleaning of the pool deck, reducing the risks related with water contamination.

According to the interviewees, a pool ramp shows considerable usability limitations, because it requires a mobility effort that is impossible for some users and it has the discomfort of requiring the use of a bathing wheelchair. Also, in our perception, pool ramps may present difficulties for ambulant people, mainly cane users. This shows why a pool ramp is considered far from being an inclusive spatial component.

The findings of this research show that none of the analysed pool access types as such can be considered inclusive. An inclusive pool design requires different types of access to accommodate as many needs as possible.

Storage provision, in the immediate vicinity of the pool, is required by the accessibility standards SE (2002). We argue that the requirement to provide a cane holder at each pool access, integrated into the proximity of handrails or grab bars, will contribute to people's safety in an inclusive way, as the ones explored by one of the interviewees.

Our findings confirm the potential of the contributions provided by disabled designers, as highlighted by several studies (Ostroff et al. 2002; Vermeersch and Heylighen 2011, 2013; Pérez Liebergesell et al. forthcoming). Specifically, in the case of improving pool design, it confirms Usandizaga's (2013) observation that a physically impaired architect introduces inclusive premises in the early stage of the design process. Physically impaired architects with built works are rare. The already mentioned cases of the swimming pool with a transfer bed and the cane holders, both explored by interviewees, are exceptions and express the premise of inclusivity.

In our opinion, direct commissions and invited competitions to physically impaired architects may result in more inclusive built spaces, with the potential of inspiring other architects to achieve user-centred design solutions.

We argue that a sensory awareness of the potential of spaces usable by physically impaired people can increase comfort, allowing less effort in complex actions, such as entering and exiting the water, for people without impairment, including children and older people.

6 Conclusions

Our findings question the inclusivity of the most advanced legislation standards on pool design in regards to the means of entering and exiting the water. For all the types of pool access analysed, physically impaired architects identified limitations that compromise inclusivity. Therefore, we conclude that for a pool to be inclusive, it will require a minimum of two different types of access, one being non-mechanical and another mechanical, allowing for their continuous autonomous use by non-ambulant people.

Moreover, the findings show the potential for a fixed mechanical access, specifically the ceiling-mounted pool lift. Furthermore, they revealed the transfer bed as a non-mechanical access type, requiring less effort in exiting the water than the transfer wall or the transfer system, and showing two advantages compared to the ramp: it occupies less space and eliminates the discomfort of having to use bathing wheelchairs.

We also highlight the potential of integrating cane holders at all pool access points in order to reduce the risks of falls.

This study adopted an exploratory approach to the improvement of inclusive pool design. The findings presented synthesise observations from individual interviews. In future research, it may be useful to discuss them in a focus group interview. It is also important to study the types of tank access mentioned in this study by conducting walkthrough interviews with a diverse sample of users, including people with cognitive, hearing and visual impairments.

Acknowledgements This research was supported by Fundação para a Ciência e a Tecnologia, reference SFRH/BPD/94371/2013, with joint funding from Portugal and the European Union. We are grateful to Isabella Steffan, Ivor Ambrose, Ljerka Gordić, Sonia Carpinelli and Valerie Fletcher, for their contribution to the interviewees sample, and Daniel C. Gaspar, David M. Correia and Pedro O. Teixeira, for the visual assistance to the first author, a blind person.

References

Caden J (2011) How to apply the Americans with disabilities act. World Aquatic Health conference, Colorado Springs, CO, US, 18–20 October 2017
Denzin NK, Lincoln Y (2011) The SAGE handbook of qualitative research. SAGE
DJ (2010) 2010 ADA standards for accessible design. Department of Justice, Washington, DC, US
Fletcher V (2009) Universal design and multi-sensory environments. Art beyond sight conference, metropolitan museum of art (oral presentation), New York, NY, US
Flick U (2009) An introduction to qualitative research. SAGE
Guimarães MP (2011) Writing poetry rather than structuring grammar: Notes for the development of universal design in Brazil. In: Preiser WFE, Smith KH (eds) Universal design handbook, McGraw-Hill, pp. 14.1–14.9
Howard L, Young LC, Figoni SF (2008) Removing barriers to health clubs and fitness facilities. The Center for Universal Design, Raleigh, NC, US
Middlestadt SE, Anderson A, Ramos WD (2015) Beliefs about using an outdoor pool: Understanding perceptions of place in the context of a recreational environment to improve health. Health Place 34:1–8
Ostroff E (1997) Mining our natural resources: The user as expert. Innov 16(1):33
Ostroff E, Limont M, Hunter DG (2002) Building a world fit for people: Designers with disabilities at work. Adaptive Environments Centre, Boston, MA, US
Pérez Liebergesell N, Vermeersch P, Heylighen A (forthcoming) Designing from a disabled body: the case of architect Marta Bordas Eddy. Multimodal Technologies and Interaction
Sato D, Kaneda K, Wakabayashi H, Nomura T (2007) The water exercise improves health related quality of life of frail elderly people at day service facility. Qual Life Res 16(10 Dec): 1577–1585

SE (2002) Access for disabled people. Sport England, London, UK

Story MF, Mueller JL, Mace R (1998) The universal design file: Designing for people of all ages and abilities. The Center for Universal Design, Raleigh, NC, UK

USAB (2004) Americans with disabilities act and architectural barriers act accessibility guidelines. United States Access Board, Washington, DC, US

Usandizaga M (2013) Learning about universal design: An experience. In: Bordas-Eddy M (ed) Let's open cities for us—LOCUS. Universitat Politècnica de Catalunya, Barcelona, Spain, pp 17–23

Vermeersch PW, Heylighen A (2011) Scaling haptics – Haptic scaling. Studying scale and scaling in the haptic design process of two architects who lost their sight. In: Adler G. et al. (eds) Scale: Imagination, perception and practice in architecture, Routledge, pp. 127–135

Vermeersch PW, Heylighen A (2013) Rendering the tacit observable in the learning process of a changing body. In: Nimkulrat N et al (eds) Knowing inside out. Loughborough University, Loughborough, UK, pp 259–270

Intelligent Support Technologies for Older People: An Analysis of Characteristics and Roles

H. Petrie, J. S. Darzentas and S. Carmien

Abstract For almost two decades, there have been many developments in using intelligent technologies to support older people, with many different terms proposed to describe these technologies including assistive robots, embodied conversational agents and relational agents. Many technologies have been proposed in many different configurations and many assistance roles have been explored. Characteristics of these technologies include tangible or virtual; anthropomorphic, biomorphic, creature or object-like; level of visual realism; paralinguistic abilities; interactivity; adaptability; movement and positioning. The assistive roles proposed include providing information, advice and reminders, helping with physical tasks, monitoring, providing companionship and emotional support. This paper provides an overview of the characteristics and roles of these technologies and attempts to clarify some of the terminology used. It aims to provide a guide for researchers from the wide range of disciplines working on such technologies for supporting older people.

1 Introduction

Intelligent support technologies (ISTs) is the term we have chosen to describe the many forms of technologically based assistance that have been proposed to support older people. The interest in intelligent support for older people has been driven by the growing need for such assistance as a consequence of demographic and societal changes. It is well known that the population throughout the world is ageing.

H. Petrie (✉) · J. S. Darzentas · S. Carmien
Human Computer Interaction Research Group, Department of Computer Science, University of York, York, UK
e-mail: helen.petrie@york.ac.uk

J. S. Darzentas
e-mail: jenny.darzentas@york.ac.uk

S. Carmien
e-mail: stefan.carmien@york.ac.uk

The United Nations (UN) estimates that in 2015, there were 901 million people aged 60 or over (60 years is an inaccurate, but widely accepted threshold for old age; both 60 and 65 years are typically used as the threshold), by 2050 the UN estimates, there will be 2.1 billion older people. As a proportion of the population, that is a rise from 12 to 25%. Currently, Japan, Italy, Finland, France, Germany and Greece and some of the Baltic and East European countries have the highest proportions of older people (over 25% of the population in all cases), but by 2050 it is estimated that the 'oldest' countries will be Japan, Korea, Spain, Greece and Singapore (with over 40% of the population) (UN 2015). So it is not surprising that there is considerable research interest in Europe in this area, but also in Japan, Korea and Singapore. Along with this ageing population, the ratio of people of working age to older people (known as the Potential Support Ratio, PSR), important both in terms of those active in producing wealth and of those available to care for the older generations, is changing. Europe currently has an overall PSR of approximately four younger people for each older one, although many European countries have a PSR of less than 3.0. Japan currently has the lowest PSR in the world at 2.1. As the number of older people increases and the number of younger people decreases, these ratios will decrease and create a major societal issue concerning the availability of people to care for older members of society.

Technological support, in many forms, is widely seen as offering solutions to the growing lack of human power to care for older people. A particular feature of such technological support, beyond performing specific tasks, is that of providing social interaction and emotional support, to overcome the increasing social isolation and loneliness amongst older people. This may explicitly be the purpose of the technology, or it may be epiphenomenal to performing tasks, meaning it is a by-product of the task-based support. One way that much research has addressed the social interaction and emotional support issues, as well as those of the general acceptability of support technology by older people, is by creating technologies which have a tangible or virtual embodiment—whether that is as a humanoid robot, a animal-like robot, a digital pet or an avatar on a screen who converses with the older person. One reason for listing these examples is that there is such a variety of support technologies, and although they share many aims, they have a very wide variety of terminology to describe them. Even a term such as *embodiment* is problematic. There are very many definitions of embodiment (Ziemke 2001; Lee et al. 2006). Fong et al. (2003) use a cybernetics-derived definition: 'that which establishes a basis for structural coupling by creating the potential for mutual perturbation between system and environment' (p. 48). Other researchers, coming from a psychological or communications background, argue that embodiment is not about a relationship between technology and user, but a property of the technology, and whether it has a tangible or visible representation to encourage the user to think of it as a *sentient being* (Reeves and Nass 1996), which is the meaning of embodiment used by researchers in the area of *embodied conversational agents* (e.g. Cassell et al. 2000). This problem of terminology clearly arises from the fact that research on intelligent support technologies for older people is a highly interdisciplinary area of study, bringing together researchers from disciplines as diverse as artificial intelligence, computer science, cognitive science, communications, geriatrics, gerontology, human–computer interaction, psychology and robotics. Thus, there is a great need to explain terms across disciplines.

2 Terminology

Two terms on which there is good agreement are *robot* to refer to tangible technologies, that is objects in the real world, and *agent* to refer to virtual instantiations, often avatars on screens. However, there are many terms within these broad categories (Table 1 illustrates nearly 30 terms we have encountered in relation to technologies for older people), and often the functionality crosses over between terms. For example, Sabelli et al. (2011) evaluated a *conversational robot* which was a human-like physical object, but its functionality was actually identical to an *embodied conversational agent* as defined by Cassell et al. (2000). Even within a particular segment of the research area, there has been considerable fluidity in terminology. Breazeal (2002) coined the term *sociable robots*, but in a subsequent paper noted:

> Traditionally, the term "social robots" was applied to multi-robot systems where the dominant inspiration came from the collective behavior of insects … For this reason, the author coined the term "sociable" to distinguish an anthropomorphic style of human-robot interaction from this earlier insect-inspired work. The author has learned (after recent discussion with Terry Fong) that the term "social" has apparently changed over the years to become more strongly associated with anthropomorphic social behavior. Hence, we shall adopt this more modern use of the term "social" … but still distinguish "sociable" as a distinct subclass of social robots.

(Breazeal 2003, p. 168)

Thus, beyond these broad terms such as *robot* and *agent*, there are many terms used for ISTs and it may not be clear to new researchers what characteristics or roles they are attempting to distinguish. In the next section, we set out a classification of some of the key characteristics and roles that should be considered and discuss how these terms map onto those characteristics and roles.

But first, let us consider some of the commonly used terms listed in Table 1. *Service robots* are defined by ISO 8373:2012 as robots that 'perform useful tasks for humans' (ISO 2012). Fong et al. (2003) divided *service robots* into *assistive robots* which assist with physical tasks and *socially interactive robots* which interact with humans (but not necessarily assist them with tasks). Feil-Seifer and Matarić (2006) defined *socially assistive robots* (SARs) as the intersection of these two types of robots. The purpose of SARs is to assist humans, but to do this in a socially interactive way. The assistance might be by doing physical tasks but it might also be by providing information.

However, in another often cited definition, Broekens et al. (2009) use the terms *social robot* and *assistive social robot*. They distinguish these types of robots from

Table 1 Terms for intelligent support technologies (ISTs) for older people

Term	Used by
Affective communication robot	Khosla and Chu (2013)
Affective embodied agent	Tsiourti et al. (2014)
Assistive robot	Fong et al. (2003)
Assistive social robot	Broekens et al. (2009)
Assistive social agent	Heerink et al. (2010)
Conversational robot	Sabelli et al. (2011)
Companion robot	Broekens et al. (2009), Dautenhahn et al. (2007)
Conversational agent-based system	Ring et al. (2013)
Embodied conversational agent (ECA)	Cereghetti et al. (2015), Tsiourti et al. (2014, 2016)
Healthcare robot	Sabelli et al. (2011)
Listener agent	Sakai et al. (2012)
Relational agent	Bickmore et al. (2005)
Relational artefact	Turkle et al. (2006)
Robotic companion	Sidner et al. (2014)
Screen agent	Heerink et al. (2010)
Service (type) robot	Broekens et al. (2009), Pearce et al. (2012)
Sociable robot	Breazeal (2002)
Social agent	Lee et al. (2006), Heerink (2010)
Socially assistive robot (SAR)	Feil-Seifer and Matarić (2006), Johnson et al. (2014), Tapus et al. (2007)
Social embodied agent	Spiekeman et al. (2011)
Socially intelligent robot	Fong et al. (2003), Dautenhahn (2007)
Socially intelligent virtual agent	Tsiourti et al. (2016)
Socially interactive robot	Fong et al. (2003)
Social robot	Breazeal (2003), Fong et al. (2003), Bartneck and Forlizzi (2004), Lee et al. (2006), Broekens et al. (2009)
Virtual assistive companion	Tsiourti et al. (2014, 2016)
Virtual carer	Garner et al. (2016)
Virtual companion	Sidner et al. (2014)
Virtual (support) partner	Cereghetti et al. (2015)

service robots, which aid in physical tasks such as helping people to move around, and *companion robots*, such as PARO the robotic seal which was developed purely to imitate a real pet (Wada and Shibata 2007).

Researchers interested in *sociableness* of robots can search using the term SARs (Feil-Seifer and Matarić 2006; Tapus et al. 2007; Johnson et al. 2014), recognising that one of the main application areas for these has been for older people.

In addition, the search term *social robot* (Breazeal 2003; Lee et al. 2006; Broekens et al. 2009; Heerink et al. 2010) is still very current.

Turning to virtual ISTs, *embodied conversational agent* (ECA) is a term that has been inherited from earlier research for wider audiences (Cassell et al. 2000). These refer to screen-based computer-animated characters, usually human-like, which simulate a conversation with the user. ECAs were originally conceived to be easier to interact with than a graphical user interface, but as they have been developed in ISTs for older people, the social and emotional roles that these may play have come to the fore. Thus, Bickmore et al. (2005a, b) proposed the term *relational agent* to indicate ECAs that are designed to 'build and maintain long-term social-emotional relationships with users' (Bickmore et al. 2005b, p. 712). Other researchers have used terms such as *virtual partners* (Cereghetti et al. 2015) and *virtual assistive companions* (Tsiourti et al. 2014, 2016) for ECAs with very similar goals. Further terms are used to indicate different goals, such as *virtual carer* (Garner et al. 2016) to indicate caring and communicative goals and *listener agent* (Sakai et al. 2012) to indicate an ECA which can detect the cognitive status of older people with dementia.

This wide variety of terminology may be confusing for researchers when trying to understand the literature and does not clarify the important similarities and distinctions between different ISTs. Therefore, we have created a classification of both robot and virtual ISTs to try to highlight some of the important properties of these technologies.

3 A Classification of Intelligent Support Technologies (ISTs) for Older People

Although robots and agents seem very different as ISTs for older people, they share many characteristics and roles. A classification of these characteristics and roles is useful for research as the question being investigated is often what is the most acceptable, useful and usable form of IST for older people. Both when discussing particular studies and when comparing different studies, it is useful to have a clear picture of what characteristics and roles the technology has and what properties and roles have been manipulated.

We have found the following characteristics useful when considering ISTs. In each case, any IST will have a value on each of these characteristics, as illustrated in Fig. 1 (which does not show all possible combinations, it illustrates some combinations):

Tangible versus Virtual: As mentioned above, many ISTs are instantiated as tangible objects in the world (*Tangible*, terms in brackets refer to nodes in Fig. 1), usually termed *robots*, while others are *virtual agents* on a computer screen or *smart speakers* which are simply a voice (e.g. Siri or Alexa) (*Virtual*).

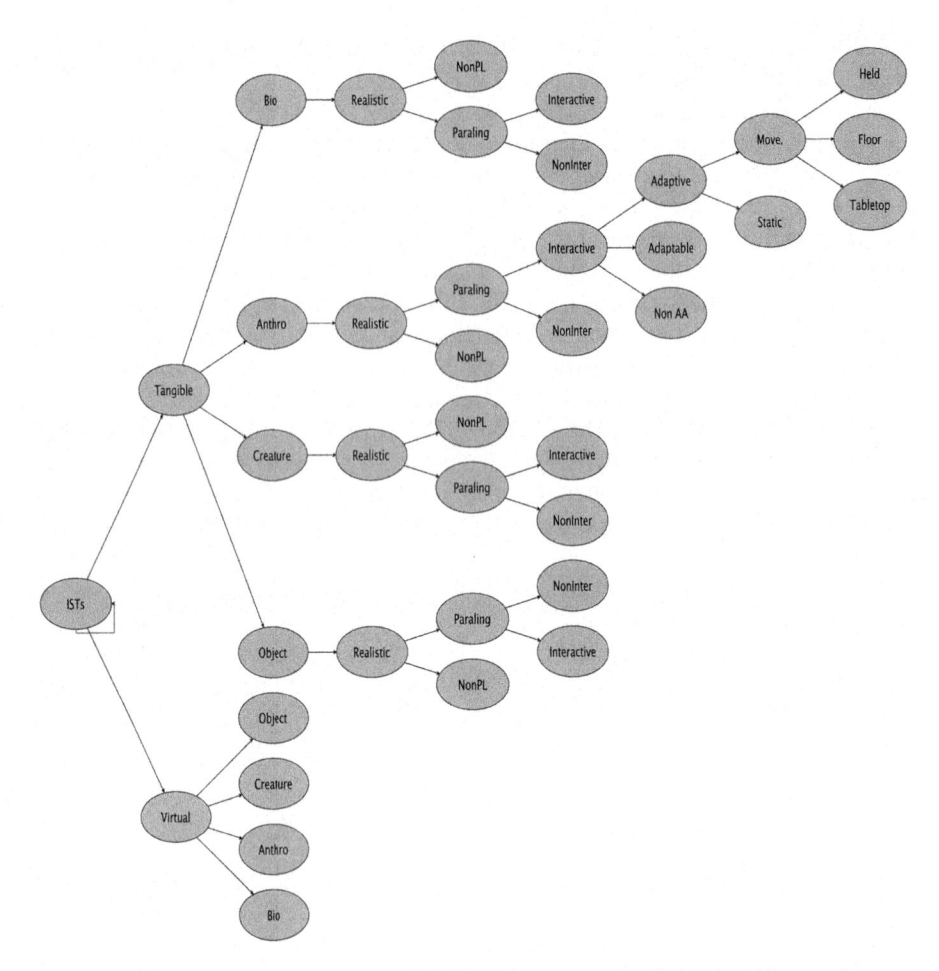

Fig. 1 Classification of characteristics of intelligent support technologies for older people

Type of Representation: Some ISTs attempt to be human-like (anthropomorphic, *Anthro*), some attempt to be animal-like (biomorphic, *Bio*), some represent new creatures which are not like any known animal (*Creature*) and some represent other non-biological real-world objects (*Object*). Many robots and agents are designed to look human and many robots look like animals (e.g. the seal-like PARO robot, Wada and Shibata 2007). Examples of 'new creatures' include the Reeti robot (www.reeti.fr), (Sidner et al. 2014) and ElliQ which is a featureless, moving 'head' (https://www.intuitionrobotics.com/elliq/). An example of a non-biological object is the IST investigated by Iwamura et al. (2011) who compared an anthropomorphic robot which carried a shopping basket to assist older shoppers in the supermarket with a robot which consisted simply of the shopping basket on a column. So the latter makes no attempt to look like any kind of human, animal or other creature.

Level of visual realism: For the anthropomorphic and biomorphic ISTs, the level of visual realism varies greatly. This is a deliberate strategy, presumably to deal with the problem of the 'uncanny valley' (Mori 2012). Some ISTs strive to create a very realistic representation, for example, the *virtual assistive companion* developed by Tsiourti et al (2014, 2016). Other ISTs use more cartoon-like or schematic representations, whether it is of a human (e.g. Bickmore et al. 2013 exercise coach for older people or Yasuda et al. 2013 cartoon-like grandchild for older people with dementia) or an animal. Clearly, this characteristic is a continuum from totally realistic to a cartoon, but for purposes of simplicity, in Fig. 1, we indicated a dichotomy (*Realistic* and *Cartoon*).

Paralinguistic behaviour including gestures: A further property related to realism is the extent to which ISTs use human or animal-like paralinguistic behaviour. This can include a number of visual and verbal behaviours such as making appropriate gestures when speaking, moving the eyes (if relevant) or other features appropriately and using realistic pitch changes (e.g. for questions) and tone of voice. Clearly, this characteristic could be broken down into a number of more specific categories, depending on the interest of researchers. Often it is hard to understand from research papers how much paralinguistic behaviour an IST is capable of. Tsiourti et al. (2016) mentioned that a set of facial expressions have been integrated into their *virtual assistive companion* and the Nao robot in the KSERA Project (Johnson et al. 2014) used a range of paralinguistic phenomena to attract the user's attention and make its recommendations more persuasive (in Fig. 1, we indicate simply *Paraling* or *NonPL*).

Interactivity: Most ISTs now aim to be interactive, that is accept input from the user and react to it appropriately. Some ISTs do this only in a limited way, and often it is not clear from research papers what the level of sophistication of the interaction is. For example, the evaluation of a robot by Sabelli et al. (2011), involved a Wizard-of-Oz-like implementation of interactivity, with a human operator using both pre-scripted and improvised interactions, but these appear to have been only single responses to questions and comments from older people (again in Fig. 1, we indicate simply *Interactive* or *NonInter*).

Adaptive and adaptable behaviour: The behaviour of the IST may be adaptive or adaptable. Adaptable technologies can be tailored by the user (or in the case of older users, a family member or carer) to suit the needs and personal preferences of the user. Adaptive technologies alter their behaviour by learning from the user's behaviour (van Velsen et al. 2007). For example, Bickmore et al. (2005b) virtual exercise coach used a simple process of adaptive behaviour in that the coach became more friendly the more times the user undertook exercises.

The final two properties are only applicable to the robot ISTs:

Movement: The IST may move around the environment. The classic idea of a robot is that it does move, but numerous studies have recently investigated robots which are static. For example, Brian (McColl et al. 2013) is a robot with just a head, torso and arms which sits in front of the user. Some IST robots also move in a manner to entertain, rather than to perform tasks. For example, Matilda can dance for users to entertain them (Khosla and Chu 2013).

Position: The robot ISTs can be floor-standing objects, which typically move around the environment, but not always; Sabelli et al. 's (2011) floor-standing robot was moved from place to place by human operators. Other robot ISTs sit on a table or other surface such as Matilda (Khosla and Chu 2013) or the iCAT (Herrink et al. 2010) standing 38 cm tall. Other robots, such the Nao, are not too tall to stand on a table at 58 cm, but can also be floor-standing. Finally, there are robots that are designed to be held, particularly robot pets, such as PARO (Wada and Shibata 2007).

Turning to roles, we make a distinction between social roles as used by Dautenhahn et al. (2005) such as that of a butler, and described using the sociological model of social roles (Huber et al. 2014) and task-based roles. The main task-based roles are as follows:

Providing information, advice and reminders: The iCat was programmed to initiate conversation, to set reminders, get directions to the supermarket and provide next day weather forecasts (Heerink et al. 2008); Karen (a virtual agent) and Reeti (a robot) were programmed to offer nutrition and health tips (both from Sidner et al. 2014).

Motivational support or coaching: For example, encouraging people to take physical exercise by a virtual agent (Bickmore et al. 2013) or robot (Fasola and Matarić 2012).

Monitoring: Working in cooperation with sensors in the environment, or worn on clothing, potentially risky behaviours can be detected, such as wandering or not drinking, and the agent, for instance the CareOBot (Sorrell and Draper 2014), can warn the older person.

Providing companionship and entertainment: Playing card games with Brian (McColl et al. 2013), and Bingo with Matilda (Khosla and Chu 2013), while Karen and Reeti offered short humorous anecdotes to the user (Sidner et al. 2014).

Providing emotional support: Interaction with PARO improved people's moods, making them more active and more communicative, both with each other and their caregivers (Moyle et al. 2017; Wada and Shibata 2007).

4 Conclusions

In studying robotic and virtual ISTs developed for older people, we were aware of the many questions regarding the nature of robots and virtual agents, and whether the latter can in fact be considered as robots. Other questions concern the tasks that these technologies are designed to carry out the style of interaction, and what are the technologies, or aspects of technologies, that make the interaction successful. The field has long been aware that it is difficult to draw meaningful distinctions between their characteristics and roles. In our paper, we expose some of problems that raise barriers to understanding, such as the proliferation of terminology and confusing distinctions. Our current contribution is to offer a conceptualisation with which to categorise and understand these technologies, that isolates characteristics and roles that are generic to both robotic and virtual agents. We believe that this contributes a working tool for thinking about these questions.

References

Bartneck C, Forlizzi J (2004) A design-centred framework for social human-robot interaction. In: Proceedings of the IEEE international workshop on robot and human interactive communication, Kurashiki, Okayama, Japan, 20–22 September 2004, pp 591–594

Bickmore TW, Caruso L, Clough-Gorr K (2005a) Acceptance and usability of a relational agent interface by urban older adults. In: Proceedings of CHI'05, Portland, OR, US, 2–7 April 2005, pp 1212–1215

Bickmore TW, Caruso L, Clough-Gorr K, Heeren T (2005b) It's just like you talk to a friend: Relational agents for older adults. Interact Comput 17(6):711–735

Bickmore TW, Simmiman RA, Nelson K, Cheng DM, Winter M, Henault L et al (2013) A randomized controlled trial of an automated exercise coach for older adults. J Am Geriatr Soc 61(10):1676–1683

Breazeal CL (2002) Designing sociable robots. MIT Press, Cambridge, MA, US

Breazeal CL (2003) Toward sociable robots. Rob Autono Syst 42:167–175

Broekens J, Heerink M, Rosendal H (2009) Assistive social robots in elderly care: a review. Gerontechnol 8(2):94–103

Cassell J, Sullivan J, Prevost S, Churchill E (eds) (2000) Embodied conversational agents. MIT Press, Cambridge, MA, USA

Cereghetti D, Kleanthous S, Christophorou C, Tsiourti C, Wings C, Christodoulou E (2015) Virtual partners for seniors: Analysis of the users' preferences and expectations on personality and appearance. In: Proceedings of european conference on ambient intelligence 2015 (AmI-15), Athens, Greece, 11–13 November 2015

Dautenhahn K (2007) Socially intelligent robots: Dimensions of human-robot interaction. Philosophical transactions of the royal society B: Biological sciences 362(1480):679–704

Dautenhahn K, Woods S, Kaouri C, Walters ML, Koay KL, Werry I (2005) What is a robot companion-friend, assistant or butler? In: Proceedings of the IEEE/RSJ International conference on intelligent robots and systems (IROS'05), Alberta, Canada, pp 1192–1197

Fasola J, Matarić MJ (2012) Using socially assistive human-robot interaction to motivate physical exercise for older adults. In: Proceedings of the IEEE, special issue on quality of life Technology, pp. 2512–2526

Feil-Seifer D, Matarić MJ (2006) Defining socially assistive robotics rehab robotics, pp 465–468

Fong T, Nourbakhsh I, Dautenhahn K (2003) A survey of socially interactive robots. Rob Auton Syst 42(3–4):143–166

Garner TA, Powell W, Carr V (2016) Virtual carers for the elderly: A case study review of ethical responsibilities. Digital Health 2:1–14

Heerink M, Krose B, Wielinga B, Evers V (2008) Enjoyment intention to use and actual use of a conversational robot by elderly people. In: Proceedings of HRI '08, Amsterdam, The Netherlands, 12–15 March 2008, pp 113–12

Heerink M, Kröse B, Evers V, Wielinga B (2010) Assessing acceptance of assistive social agent technology by older adults: The almere model. Int J Soc Robot 2:361

Huber A, Lammer L, Weiss A, Vincze M (2014) Designing adaptive roles for socially assistive robots: A new method to reduce technological determinism and role stereotypes. J Hum-Rob Interact 3(2):100–111

ISO (2012) ISO 8373:2012—Robots and robotic devices—Vocabulary. International Organization for Standardization, Geneva, Switzerland

Iwamura Y, Shiomi M, Kanda T, Ishiguro H, Hagita N (2011) Do elderly people prefer a conversational humanoid as a shopping assistant partner in supermarkets? In: Proceedings of Human Robot Interaction (HRI'11), pp 449–456

Johnson DO, Cuijpers RH, Juola JF, Torta E, Simonov M, Frisiello A et al (2014) Socially assistive robots: A comprehensive approach to extending independent living. Int J Soc Rob 6:195

Khosla R, Chu M T (2013) Embodying care in Matilda: An affective communication robot for emotional wellbeing in older people in Australian residential care facilities. ACM Trans Manag Inf Syst 4(4): Article 18

Lee KM, Jung Y, Kim J, Kim SR (2006) Are physically embodied social agents better than disembodied social agents? The effects of physical embodiment, tactile interaction, and people's loneliness in human–robot interaction. Int J Hum Comput Stud 64(10):962–973

McColl D, Louie WG, Nejat G (2013) Brian 2.1: A socially assistive robot for the elderly and cognitively impaired. IEEE Robot Autom Mag 20(1):74–83

Mori M (2012) The uncanny valley (translated by MacDorman KF, Kageki N). IEEE Robot Autom 19(2):98–100

Moyle W, Beattie ER, Draper B, Shum D, Thalib L, Jones C (2017) A social robot called Paro and its effect on people living with dementia. Innov Aging 1:344

Pearce AJ, Adair B, Miller K, Ozanne E, Said C, Santamaria N et al. (2012) Robotics to enable older adults to remain living at home. J Aging Res 2012: Article 538169

Reeves B, Nass C (1996) The media equation: How people treat computers, television, and new media like real people and places. Cambridge University Press

Ring L, Barry B, Totzke K, Bickmore T (2013) Addressing loneliness and isolation in older adults. In: Proceedings of ACII'13, Geneva, Switzerland, 2–5 September 2013, pp 61–66

Sabelli AM, Kanda T, Hagita N (2011) A conversational robot in an elderly care center: an ethnographic study. In: Proceedings of Human-Robot Interaction (HRI'11), pp 37–44

Sakai Y, Nonaka Y, Yasuda K, Nakano YI (2012) Listener agent for elderly people with dementia. In: Proceedings of HRI'12, Boston, MA, US, 5–8 March 2012

Sidner C, Rich C, Shayganfar M, Behrooz M, Bickmore T, Ring L et al. (2014) Robotic and virtual companions for isolated older adults. AAAI Fall symposium: Artificial intelligence for human-robot interaction, Arlington, VA, US, 15–17 November 2014

Sorrell T, Draper H (2014) Robot carers, ethics and older people. Ethics Inf Technol 16(3): 183–195

Spiekeman ME, Haazebroek P, Neerincx, M (2011) Requirements and platforms for social agents that alarm and support elderly living alone. In Mutlu et al. (eds): ICSR 2011, LNAI 7072: pp 226–235

Tapus A, Matarić MJ, Scassellati B (2007) Socially assistive robotics [Grand challenges of robotics]. IEEE Robot Autom Mag 14(1):35–42

Tsiourti C, Joly E, Wings C, Moussa MB, Wac K (2014) Virtual assistive companions for older adults: qualitative field study and design implications. In: Proceedings Pervasive Computing Technologies for Healthcare (PervasiveHealth'14), pp 57–64

Tsiourti C, Moussa MB, Quintas J, Loke B, Jochem I (2016) A virtual assistive companion for older adults: design implications for a real-world application. In: Proceedings SAI Intelligent Systems Conference, pp 1014–1033

Turkle S, Taggart W, Kidd CD, Daste O (2006) Relational artifacts with children and elders: the complexities of cybercompanionship. Connection Sci 18(4):347–361

UN (2015) World population prospects: Key findings and advance tables (2015 revision). United Nations, New York, NY, US

van Velsen L, van der Geest T, Klaassen R, Steehouder M (2007) User-centered evaluation of adaptive and adaptable systems: A literature review. The Knowl Eng Rev 23(3):261–281

Yasuda K, Aoe J-I, Fuketa M (2013) Development of an agent system for conversing with individuals with dementia. In: Proceedings of JSAI 2013, Toyama, Japan, 4–7 June 2013

Wada K, Shibata T (2007) Living with seal robots—Its sociopsychological and physiological influences on the elderly at a care house. Trans Robot 23(5):972–980

Ziemke T (2001) Are robots embodied? In: Balkenius C et al. (eds) Proceedings of the first international workshop on epigenetic robotics: Modeling cognitive development in robotic systems, Lund university cognitive studies, vol 85. Lund, Sweden

Participatory Design Resulting in a 'Do-It-Yourself Home Modification' Smartphone App

C. Bridge

Abstract While the numbers of Do-It-Yourself (DIY) home modifications have increased, there is little available information that assists people to do their own home modifications. This is in the context that the traditional Australian home has generally been built with little consideration for anyone who may be less agile or who may have any other ability issues. For instance, someone may find themselves no longer able to step into a bath or have difficulty standing up from the toilet and need to make changes to their home to remain independent and safe. Home modifications describe these types of changes in the home typically made in response to loss of ability and are designed to help people to remain independent and safe whilst reducing any risk of injury to their carers and care workers. This paper outlines the participatory design process used to create the smartphone App and reports on its beta testing and final launch.

1 Introduction and Background

Modifications to the home include changes to the structure of the dwelling, e.g. widening doors, adding ramps, providing better accessibility, etc., and the installation of assistive devices inside or outside the dwelling e.g. grabrails, handrails, lifts, etc. Home modifications is a key to being able to '*aging in place*', in other words, living independently at home. To '*age in place*' means that you can remain in your own home rather than being forced to relocate or enter assisted living, or a retirement community, etc. Home modifications assist people with disability and older people to be more independent and may reduce the need for ongoing assistance (https://www.homemods.info/about). Population wise, there are more people living alone and most older people and people with impairments of ability have a strong desire to choose where they live.

C. Bridge (✉)
UNSW, Sydney, Australia
e-mail: C.Bridge@unsw.edu.au

This research project aimed to support and enhance life for people with impairments of ability and those who are ageing by production of a Do-It-Yourself (DIY) resource App known as '*DIYmodify*'.

The *DIYmodify* project builds from previous research undertaken in 2015–2016 (Bleasdale et al. 2014; Bridge et al. 2016) that explored the phenomena of DIY modifications from a literature, consumer, industry and economic perspective. This scoping research found that there were significant DIY installations of grab rails, handrails, handheld showers, shower infills and small ramp installations undertaken annually by older or disabled people in New South Wales (NSW). The cost offset to health and aged care services of these activities amounted to more than $15 million dollars based on our analysis of consumer direct sales data from Australia's largest national hardware chain. The annual savings cited in this initial report were based on product selection, purchase, installation or construction being undertaken by privately funded individuals or their families. The data analysis revealed that the number of people doing their own home modifications comprised a significant and growing market segment within the existing home hardware enterprise.

Where home modifications are made of necessity, for example before being able to return home from hospital, the home modifications are likely to be instigated by a health professional, with often little thought for aesthetics or the emotional impact on the household, family and friends. Additionally government services offering home modification assessment and/or intervention funding often have long waiting lists. Unsurprisingly, given that nearly all wealthy countries have an ageing population doing home modifications without professional input in such circumstances, is a growing trend. However, it is also because there are greater numbers of people deciding that they would like more choice over the quality, appearance, cost and timing of these support types. Additionally, those that undertook DIY home modifications stated that they took pride in the results they achieved and this sense of self-efficacy enhanced their sense of wellbeing and capacity. This is unsurprising as previous research has shown that home modifications can improve quality of life and reduce care (Carnemolla and Bridge 2011, 2016).

Our previous research revealed that while most participants reported a positive experience of the DIY process, most negative aspects of the DIY experience were attributed to a serious lack of information on the process and products available for undertaking DIY home modifications. It was also noted that there were also often issues in communicating the needs of the person to tradespeople who might be undertaking the project on their behalf (Bridge and Barlow 2016). Further, there was rarely any information available either online or at the Point of Sale (POS) in the hardware shop to help them. The process of home modifications empowers people and helps to maintain independence over their lives (McNamarra et al. 2014) and the DIYmodify App and its associated factsheets needed to ensure the experience of modifying a home DIY was a safe and positive one.

It was found that DIY participants were likely to have a broad range of skills and information needed from the very basic to the highly technical and thus the resources developed had to be able to cover this knowledge range. The information needed to be tailored so that different groups could access it and it needed to be available in a variety of formats (Bridge and Barlow 2016). It was considered especially important that appropriate resources be available at Point of Sale (POS).

The five home modification types for including in the initial POS resources were

- grabrails;
- handheld showers;
- level access shower alcoves;
- handrails and
- ramps.

Factsheets were the overall preferred resources for obtaining information by seniors, with websites coming second. Although Apps may still not be the preferred means of resources for seniors, there is a significant number of people who do use their smartphones and who access Apps on a daily basis (Berenguer et al. 2017). The decision to develop a hybrid App gives a wider access across a greater range of resources as smartphones can link to factsheets and additional information. Factsheets then can be printed. Also, information is accessible via a website.

2 Aims and Methods

The primary aim of the participatory design research funded by the NSW government was development of Point of Sales (POS) resources for DIY home modifications. This project set out to develop and curate the resource(s) needed to assist people with impairments of ability of all ages and their carers. It also aimed to facilitate people to be able to make more informed decisions in relation to their needs, skills, home situation and resources, so as to undertake home modifications with confidence and greater autonomy.

This participatory part of the research project reported in this chapter was directed by the following research questions:

1. What are the design requirements for accessible POS resources for undertaking DIY modifications?
2. What type of online formats are required to cover the product decision-making, installation and maintenance processes?
3. What are the required design elements and information content to ensure that the App is effective in assisting consumers to access DIY home modification information?

The overall project used a mixed method research approach where the research tasks were divided into several interlocking tasks:

1. review of existing resources;
2. review of App and smartphone resources;
3. resource review update—home modifications;

4. new resources development and
5. resource design—design of the App and factsheets; and the Participatory Action Research (PAR) was used as a vehicle throughout all of the tasks to review research findings and to inform decision-making.

3 Participatory Action Research Sessions

Participatory Action Research (PAR) seeks to understand and improve the world by changing it. It includes collective, self-reflective inquiry, which researchers and participants undertake iteratively usually in a number of cycles so that together they can understand and improve the practices in which they are involved. The same process is often used for research that seeks to create new computational outputs or objects (Bridge and Carnemolla 2014). Some of the values of PAR are empowerment, support and relationships, learning and social change. PAR affirms that experience can be a basis of knowing and that experiential learning can lead to a legitimate form of knowledge that influences practice (Bostock and Freeman 2003).

Three workshops were undertaken as a part of the POS material development in order to formulate, and provide feedback on development of the *DIYmodify* App. To undertake the project, a team involving researchers, an App developer, and participants with ability impairment and some experience in home modifications, was established.

The participants shared their knowledge, skills, expectations and experiences regarding home modifications and their aspirations for a DIYmodify App. The team included three critical key stakeholder groups: home modification policymakers; home hardware and construction industry and people with impairments of ability. The final PAR team included some of the participants from the previous 'World Café', a creative group interaction method focused on conversations for leading collaborative dialogue, sharing knowledge and creating possibilities for action that was organised as a part of an initial DIY home modification scoping research (Bridge et al. 2016) as well as new invitees from the three key stakeholder groups with an emphasis on end users with impairments.

Involvement in the PAR team was completely voluntary, unpaid and all members committed to the three, two and half hour workshops. All workshops were fully compliant with our Human Ethics Clearance (HC 16578) and involved informed consent for photos, video and audio recording. The workshops comprised 8–11 people: two researchers, an App developer and 6–8 participants. Workshops were audio recorded, and all discussion transcribed. The transcriptions were searched for keywords or synonyms using standard content analysis techniques to clarify and inform all key decisions. A brief overview of the three PAR workshops is detailed so some of the decision-making and tasks undertaken in the DIYmodify App development can be better understood.

3.1 Workshop 1—Formulation of the Design Brief for the App

The findings from previous scoping research were presented, although some of the PAR team were already familiar with them having agreed to participate in the most recent work or having already participated in the earlier research. As a preliminary activity, some of PAR participants spoke of the value of DIY projects to themselves and why someone might launch into such a project. They spoke of people doing their own home modification projects due to time, cost and for doing it 'properly'. For example, *'Realistically, that's why they are doing it themselves—to save money'* (Participant 02) and *'A lot of it is to save time'* and *'They don't do post-occupancy checks and if they're wrong, you're in a very dangerous position—and you have to get it done again privately.'* (Participant 01)

A DIY matrix adapted from the original Enabler Model (Steinfeld et al. 1979) was presented as a way of illustrating how peoples' abilities might inform both project selection and an understanding of matching resources and abilities to make undertaking a home modification project in a DIY manner more successful. The matrix in this model focused on DIY tasks and used a self-assessment of ability. It was decided that the App would address 'abilities' and through their own self-assessment, a person would be advised if they would be able to complete the required task for example, installing a grabrail or whether they should be advised to seek assistance from a family member or friend or perhaps employ a tradesperson to do this installation for them. While some members of the PAR team were concerned about physical installation risks, it was decided that the physical installation was merely one part of the total project. Final group consensus was that a Task Analysis that 'advised' you would be unable to complete the installation task of 'installing' a grabrail failed to appropriately acknowledge other options, i.e. included having a relative, friend or neighbour assist with a project. For example, someone might easily accomplish all the pre-installation steps, i.e. choosing which sort of grabrail they needed, deciding which direction it should be installed, and how high it should be installed, etc., for the grabrail home modification type or any of the other of the four home modification types, yet may be unable to physically instal it themselves.

As a team, they felt the App should lead users through the decision-making process using a set of self-reflective questions. For instance, one PAR member said it should commence with *'What do I need? A grabrail. What do I need it for? What type of grabrail do I need? Then, how do I install it?'* (Participant 03). Another PAR members stated *'You just need to remember that a grabrail in the bathroom isn't going to help you get into bed'*. (Participant 02). Following the discussion on the Enabler Model and Task Analysis Matrix (Steinfeld et al. 1979), a brief overview of smartphone App's, their current vogue and importance was given. After that there was an opportunity to work on an App prototype, using the information gained from the workshop.

It was also identified that there needed to be somewhere in the process the possibility of accessing assistance, perhaps the advice of an occupational therapist,

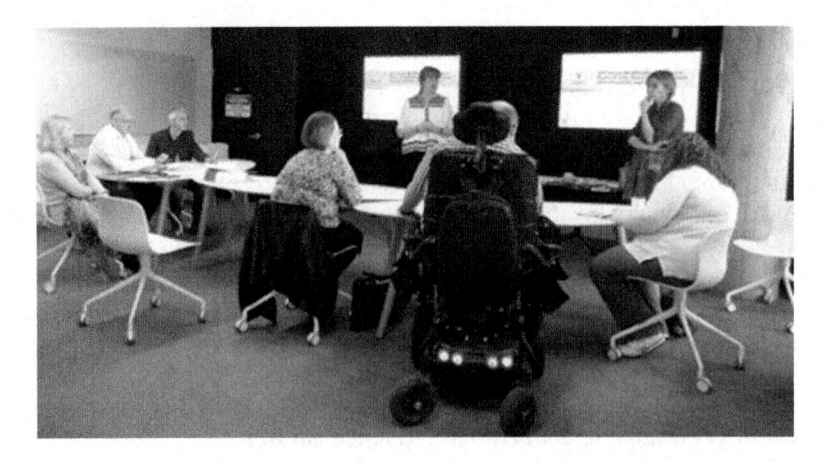

Fig. 1 Participatory Action team at workshop one, problem-solving the decision framework

a building advisory service or additional help from a tradesperson, as it may not always be the case that the instigator of the home modification project would be completing all of the installation themselves. Figure 1 illustrates the participants of first workshop reflecting on current information summaries.

Key learnings from the first workshop used to inform the next stages of resource development were that:

- resources need to be straightforward, explaining why a particular home modification might be needed and by whom.
- language needed to be direct and clear.
- screens/pages should be uncluttered and should be accessible for people with visual impairment, colour blindness and other types of disability.
- While there was a lot of information that people might need to know, if it is stepped through clearly, it need not be overwhelming.
- there should be links to other sources of information if this will assist people to understand what is needed and would help them throughout the DIY process.

3.2 Workshop 2—Feedback on Initial Framework for the DIYmodify App

By the second workshop, the App programmer had been engaged and progress on the thinking for the App had substantially developed. The PAR team was invited to be involved in the decisions around the icons and language to be used in the App, as well as the logic sequencing for the screens.

A significant chunk of time within the workshop time was spent on brainstorming the name of the App. The names suggested by the PAR members were developed into a list—and each suggestion was checked for availability. Once checked the short list of available names was forwarded to each PAR team member for them to vote on. '*DIYmodify*' was by far the preferred name. This included all the necessary aspects including 'Do-It-Yourself', as well as 'modification' and was short enough to be suitable to use as a title under the logo.

The longest discussion however surrounded organising framework or modified Task Analysis that drew on the idea of a matrix integrating environmental variables impacting DIY performance and an ability framework known as the Enabler model (Steinfeld et al. 1979) which was designed to assist decision-making around potential barriers/enablers impacting an individual's capacity for undertaking the chosen home modification task. Figure 2 illustrates the participants in workshop two wrestling with the best way to lead users through the information so that there was no wrong door and that the information could be kept up to date effectively.

By the end of workshop two, there was still no clear agreement on how to proceed on this issue, yet it was considered an important aspect of the content that would be on the App and it would form the basis of leading a consumer through the App to the relevant solution. A standard technique in PAR is critical reflection of a method often associated with undertaking design activities to improve practice. Its use has been shown to lead to a deeper and more complex understanding of experience and 'reflection on experience and past actions' which the process enables draws out understandings that would be otherwise difficult to obtain (Fook 2011). As part of this reflection on the Task Analysis, a paper outlining the possible alternatives to the Task Analysis was forwarded to each PAR member for them to reflect on and provide input on prior to attending workshop three.

Meanwhile the App Developer and the researchers continued on the Information Architecture for the App and the content of the App itself. In this stage of the App

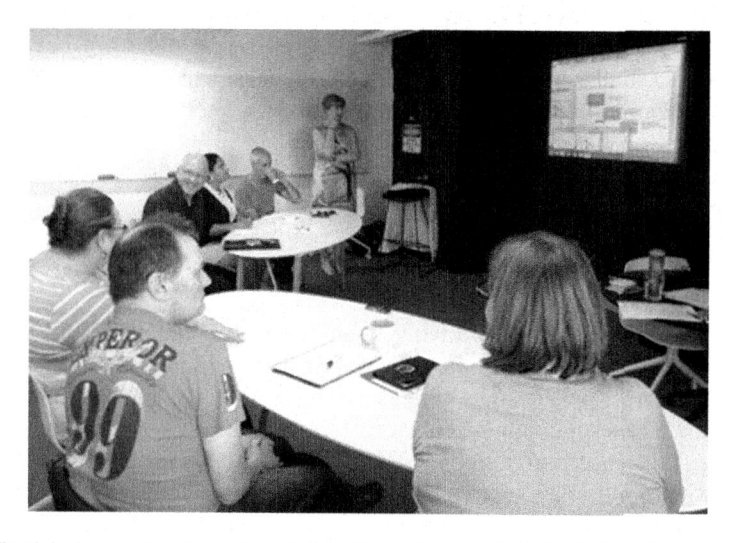

Fig. 2 Participatory action team at workshop discussing the Task Analysis options

development, it was realised that by shifting the thinking away from the task analysis as a 'deciding factor' and having it instead as a checklist on the factsheets, many of the issues would be solved.

3.3 Workshop 3—Feedback on the User Interface for the App

By workshop three, as the App was further advanced the PAR team was able to make very explicit decisions on content, including colour and words and information order. Including how the App was operating, e.g. swiping or clicking screens to move forward or back, etc. An issue that continued to be extremely important to the PAR team was that of language, i.e. how it was used, who the App was targeting and therefore, whether the language was appropriate for that specific group. Other issues addressed included:

- The appearance of the App.
- The use of colour.
- A desire for the App to go back one page at a time rather than returning as it did at that time back to opening page and main menu.
- More images were also requested.

The PAR team stated that they found the prototype App to be uncluttered and generally easy to read, despite some content requiring further development. For example, the video segments were considered too long and further editing was requested. The launch and marketing were also discussed. Other issues raised at the PAR workshops included the words and language used throughout, the colours, the name of the App and how the App pages were moved from one page to the next instead of using scrolling or a 'next' button). Each decision in the App development was treated in a similar manner with reasoned and considered analysis, a systematic process, time for reflection and development and amendment or further planning for the next cycle, when necessary.

4 Beta Testing

App development typically also involves: alpha testing and beta testing. Initially, alpha testing usually by the people involved in its development such as our PAR team, leads to larger beta testing. In this case, our PAR team were included in both the alpha and beta testing of the App. However, Beta testing involved a much larger and broader audience and tested whether the *DIYmodify* App was working as expected without mistakes on end users smartphones, as well as making sure it is suitable for its intended audience, people with impairments. Beta testing is standard and is carried out to ensure any glitches in the operating of the App are resolved before forwarding the App to the respective App stores for download.

Originally, the Apple and Android versions of the App were to be developed alongside each other but the App Development team advised that as it can take substantial lead time for an App to be approved for release by the Apple Store that the Apple version of the App be developed first and then the Android version be developed in order to achieve the completion target dates.

Once the Apple version was at a suitable stage for beta testing, a range of people from peak bodies and organisations whose clientele might find an App on home modifications useful, and who had agreed to be 'beta testers' and who had Apple operating system phones or iPads were sent a link to the app to test. After the beta testing feedback was received for the Apple version, the Android version of the updated App was sent to those who had an Android device and expressed an interest in the Android beta testing. It was, however, more difficult for people with Androids to access the test App from their Android phones.

Each person contacted was sent a package explaining the process of beta testing. Of those contacted, 42 agreed to be 'beta testers' with only four negative responses received and these mostly concerned wanting more items, difficulty with the download or feeling that the DIY option was not for them. For example, one beta user commented that '*it would have been good to have other types of ramp addressed, not only the doorway ramp*' (Beta tester).

Additionally, the last 500 users of the 'Home Modification Information Clearinghouse' website were sent invites to test the App in either its Apple or Android form prior to its official launch, with no significant negative responses being received, both the Android and Apple Apps were officially launched on the 16 July 2017. *DIYmodify* has been downloaded 2639 times, with 2373 downloads from the Apple store and 266 from Google play. This appears to indicate that despite both smartphone types having accessibility features, Apple devices appear to be more generally used by people with disability.

5 Conclusions

As originally intended, and with the assistance of our PAR team it appears that the *DIYmodify* App 'supports consumer decision-making and in-store purchasing'. It addresses issues involved for those who are renting their home, as well as for those whose home is purchased under Strata Title, i.e. a home where permission to modify is required from a body corporate or similar. It explains what to look out for when undertaking the home modification, how to choose, and then maintain and clean the home modification. It does not, however, go into detail on how to physically instal the home modification as existing material is already readily available online to explain how to do this.

The *DIYmodify* App is the world's first in that, it curates existing resources and knowledge in a novel decision-making frame to provide guided decision-making for selected home modification products. It was designed with no animation to accommodate those who may have photosensitive epilepsy. It targets a marginalised group—people with impairments of ability, as well as those who are ageing, with the intent of empowering them and recognising that while they may be requiring assistance in some areas of their life, they are essential members of society and that they can be responsible for their decisions in what they want in their home to help with daily life.

The 21 associated evidence-based factsheets developed for and curated by the *DIYmodify* Apps extend the knowledge that was previously available. They include checklists to assist the DIY-er in organising how they will undertake the project and provide letter templates to send to the owner of the property if the user is not the property title owner. For those requiring installation assistance, there is a factsheet on how to ask for a quote on a project, what to tell the tradesperson and what to look for when comparing quotes. These factsheets extend the knowledge base for each of the five home modifications and provide valuable additional information. A more extensive evaluation of the *DIYmodify* Apps was outside the scope of the original POS development reported here but is planned as a part of future extension work yet to be undertaken.

References

Berenguer A, Goncalves J, Hosio S, Ferreira D, Anagnostopoulis T, Kostakos V (2017) Are smartphones ubiquitous? IEEE Consum Electron Mag 6(1):104–110

Bleasdale M, McNamara N, Zmudzki F, Bridge C (2014) Positioning paper: DIY home modifications: point-of-sale support for people with disability and their carers. Home Modification Information Clearinghouse, UNSW, Sydney, Australia, published 6th August 2014. www.homemods.info. Accessed on 14 Nov 2017

Bostock J, Freeman J (2003) 'No limits': doing participatory action research with young people in Northumberland. J Community Appl Soc Psychol 13:464–474

Bridge C, Barlow G (2016) Co-design of point-of-sale resources for do-it-yourself (DIY) home modification. Presented at the 6th international conference for Universal Design, Nagoya, Japan, 9–11 December 2016

Bridge C, Carnemolla P (2014) An enabling BIM block library: an online repository to facilitate social inclusion in Australia. Constr Innov 14(4):477–492

Bridge C, Maalsen S, Zmudzki F, O'Neil S, Carnemolla P (2016) DIY home modifications: what information is required at point of sale? Home modification information clearinghouse, UNSW, Sydney, Australia, published 4th April 2016. www.homemods.info. Accessed on 14 Nov 2017

Carnemolla P, Bridge C (2011) Home modifications and their impact on waged care substitution. Home modification information clearinghouse. UNSW, Sydney, Australia, published. www.homemods.info. Reprinted version accessed on 14 Nov 2017

Carnemolla PK, Bridge C (2016) Accessible housing and health-related quality of life. Int J Architectural Res 10(2):38–50

Fook J (2011) Developing critical reflection as a research method. In: Higgs J, Titchen A, Horsfall D, Bridges D (eds) Creative spaces for qualitative researching. Practice, education, work and society, vol 5. Sense Publishers, Rotterdam

McNamarra N, Bridge C, Zmudzki F (2014) Consumer choice and DIY home modifications: exploring universally designed housing. Presented at the 5th international conference for Universal Design, Fukushima and Tokyo, Japan, 11–13 November 2014

Steinfeld E, Schroeder S, Duncan J, Faste R, Chollet D, Bhisop M et al (1979) Access to the built environment: a review of literature. US Dept of Housing and Urban Development, Washington, DC, US

Identifying Barriers to Usability: Smart Speaker Testing by Military Veterans with Mild Brain Injury and PTSD

T. Wallace and J. Morris

Abstract Emerging technologies need to be tested for usability and usefulness by target users in the context in which they would likely use these technologies. This is especially true for people with disabilities who may have specific use cases and access needs. This paper describes the research protocol and results from usability testing of smart speakers with home hub capability—Amazon Echo and Google Home—by military combat veterans with mild traumatic brain injury (mTBI) and post-traumatic stress disorder (PTSD). Research was conducted with eight clients in a rehabilitation program for military service members at Shepherd Center in Atlanta, Georgia, USA. Smart speakers and two smart plugs were installed in residences owned by Shepherd Center and occupied by clients undergoing rehabilitation. Participants tested each device for 2 weeks, including set-up and daily use, and completed electronic diary entries about their experience. Additionally, they completed a summative questionnaire interview about their experience at the end of each phase. The goal of the research is to identify usability opportunities and challenges of each device in order to inform development of in-home therapeutic solutions using emerging smart home technologies for this population.

1 Introduction

Smart home technology (smart speakers, smart plugs, smart thermostats, etc.) has emerged as a new category of consumer electronics that offers potential as assistive technology (AT) for people with disabilities. These Internet of Things (IoT) technologies connect to Wi-Fi networks, or smartphones via Wi-Fi or

---

T. Wallace · J. Morris (✉)
Shepherd Center, Atlanta, GA, USA
e-mail: john.morris@shepherd.org

T. Wallace
e-mail: tracey.wallace@shepherd.org

© Springer International Publishing AG, part of Springer Nature 2018
P. Langdon et al. (eds.), *Breaking Down Barriers*,
https://doi.org/10.1007/978-3-319-75028-6_10

Bluetooth. IoT technologies offer substantial assistive and accessibility benefits to users, including multiple ways to collect and retrieve data and control the environment using voice, touch and gesture.

Amazon Echo and Google Home are Internet-connected smart speakers equipped with far-field microphones to support voice recognition and hands-free interaction with voice-enabled smart assistants (e.g. Amazon Alexa and Google Assistant). They provide information or assistance, play music or control smart home devices in response to voice commands. Both can add 'skills', much like adding smartphone applications, and connect to third-party smartphone apps to add functionality.

2 Smart Speakers: PTSD and Mild TBI

Smart speakers sit at the intersection of in-home intelligent personal assistants (IPAs, including Alexa, Siri, Cortana and Google Assistant) and home automation. They are particularly useful for their combination of access to information (news, weather, sports scores, trivia, etc.) and entertainment (music, games, etc.), and access to environmental controls (lights, thermostat, door locks and other devices).

PTSD and mTBI frequently co-occur in combat veterans returning from Iraq and Afghanistan, often impacting independent living and quality of life (Tschiffely et al. 2015). Common features of PTSD include anxiety, perceived threat, avoidance behaviours and hyper-vigilance (American Psychiatric Association 2013). Combat veterans with persistent mTBI symptoms often experience challenges with memory, attention and executive functioning. Those experiencing both PTSD and mTBI also commonly report depression, sleep problems and emotional disturbances (Tanielian and Jaycox 2008; Chen and Huang 2011).

The considerable AT potential and rapid pace of development of smart speakers points to the need for systematic assessment of usability by people with specific functional difficulties, including difficulties confronting combat veterans with PTSD and mTBI. Such assessment will help designers and developers ensure equitable access to these increasingly important technologies and will help inform and guide AT consumers.

Amazon has promoted the assistive and accessibility capabilities of the Echo at disability conferences and has won favourable coverage for its potential as assistive technology (St. John 2017). Both Echo and Home show potential to support independent living of people with disabilities (Capan 2016; Woyke 2017). However, only limited investigation of the usability, user preferences and potential to meet the unique needs of users with disabilities has been conducted, particularly for users with cognitive and psychological disability. A literature search of research on the usability of Echo and Home yielded limited results, and none addressed usability by military service members with TBI and PTSD.

3 Consumer Technology: Accessibility as a Fundamental Need

Usability of mainstream consumer electronics (information and communications technology or ICT) has been a central concern of rehabilitation researchers and engineers. Each new generation of technology—personal computers (Kessler Foundation/National Organization on Disability 2010), cellphones, smartphones and tablets (Fox 2011; Morris and Mueller 2014), wearable technology (Wallace et al. 2017)—has prompted new lines of investigation and rehabilitation engineering.

The literature on access and use of consumer technology by people with disabilities comprises a number of themes, often focused on so-called 'divides', including most centrally the disability divide. This line of inquiry was energised in the United States by the publication of two seminal reports published in the early years of the smartphone era: the Kessler Foundation/National Council on Disabilities survey research report on technology access (2010) and the U.S. Federal Communications Commission working paper on broadband adoption (Horrigan 2010). There has also been research into age, education and income divides for both the general population (Blumberg and Luke 2017); and people with disabilities (Morris et al. 2014). Morris and Mueller (2014) have also documented differences in the use of consumer technologies across disability types, specifically blind and deaf individuals.

At the core of research into these divides—including the 'disability divide'—is concern for equitable access to technology. Increasingly, access to information and communication technology is essential to community participation, education and employment. For people with disabilities, these concerns are enshrined in public policy on the national level in the United States (Americans with Disabilities Act of 1991, 21st Century Communications and Video Accessibility Act of 2010, for example), and on the international level (UN Convention on the Rights of Persons with Disabilities, CRPD). CRPD's Article 9 (UN 2006) on "Accessibility" stresses that signatory partners should take appropriate measures:

> To promote access for persons with disabilities to new information and communications technologies and systems, including the Internet.

> To promote the design, development, production and distribution of accessible information and communications technologies and systems *at an early stage* (emphasis added), so that these technologies and systems become accessible at minimum cost.

4 Smart Speakers and Usability

Their versatility and the centrality of voice control in their operation endow smart speakers with considerable potential as assistive technology. But usability challenges remain for smart speakers/smart assistants. Controlling multiple smart speakers/smarthome hubs (e.g. Echo's and Echo Dots) can be confusing on a single mobile app. The use of multiple connected devices in your smart home can make learning their 'dialogue path' (e.g. 'Alexa, etc.') and device names complicated and confusing for users, family members and guests (Stinson 2017).

Other usability challenges identified for specific devices have been documented. Google Home cannot set reminders (Murnane 2017)—a potentially key assistive function for people with difficulty remembering. One product reviewer noted that a requested list of ingredients for cooking recipes was spoken too fast (even at the optional slower rate) to be useful (McGregor 2017). For the recently released updated version of the primary Echo device, Amazon has replaced the twist-top volume ring found on the original Echo device with harder-to-find unlighted buttons, just like those on the cheaper and smaller Echo Dot.

More fundamental questions about ease of set-up and use by people who may have uneven or limited speech, dexterity, hearing or vision also need to be answered. Can Alexa and OK Google understand slurred, slow or halting speech? Can users hear and distinguish the various tones and other audio output? What are the physical interactions like with these devices and do they provide sufficient flexibility of use as recommended by principles of Universal Design (Center for Universal Design 1997)? The present focuses on user experiences and preferences from real-world use. More in-depth laboratory testing will follow.

5 Methodology

An in-home usability diary study of Amazon Echo and Google Home smart speakers was conducted with eight military service members with PTSD and mTBI. Information about the accuracy, reliability and usability, user acceptance, user preference and potential for future development of skills for the smart home speakers was gathered.

Participants were recruited from the SHARE Military Initiative program at Shepherd Center, a rehabilitation hospital for people with spinal cord injury, brain injury and other neurological disorders. The SHARE program is a comprehensive outpatient day rehabilitation program for military service members with mTBI and PTSD. Participants live in an apartment complex owned by Shepherd Center while receiving intensive physical, cognitive and behavioural outpatient therapy for up to 12 weeks. The structure of the SHARE program provided a unique opportunity for this in-residence usability testing of smart speakers.

Purposive sampling was undertaken to identify participants with mTBI and PTSD with functional language, speech, hearing and vision. The research team consulted with the SHARE psychologists and speech-language pathologists to identify appropriate candidates for in-residence technology testing. Fourteen potential participants were identified. Two declined to participate in the study; one reported discomfort with having a speaker in his apartment that was 'listening to everything' while the other stated he was 'not big on technology' because he found learning to use new technology was often frustrating.

In all, eight individuals, seven males and one female, completed testing of both devices. Participant age ranged from 30 to 57 years with time since initial onset of injury ranging from 1 to 24 years. Most reported experiencing multiple mTBIs resulting from direct fire or explosive blasts, falling and/or motor vehicle accidents. All reported one or more trauma events resulting in PTSD. Difficulties with anger, anxiety, depression, aggression, isolation, memory, attention, back pain and headache were reported by more than half of the participants.

Information on experience with computers and smart technology was collected for each user prior to initiation of technology testing (Table 1). All owned a smartphone, an inclusion criterion for participation in the study, which are needed to set up and use these two smart speakers.

Participants tested each smart speaker, either Amazon Echo or Google Home, in their apartment for 2 weeks using a crossover design for a total of 4 weeks testing of the two devices per participant. Half of the participants tested Echo first and half tested Home first to minimise bias related to which smart speaker was experienced first. Each participant was also given two TP-Link mini-smart plugs. Participants were asked to set up the technology in their apartments and were provided with assistance if they were unsuccessful. Participants completed one-on-one interviews on their experience setting up each device.

They were also asked to complete electronic diary entries about their experience twice weekly. And they completed a summative questionnaire interview about their experience at the end of each phase. Guiding questions in each interview and electronic diary entry were aimed at identifying usability opportunities and challenges of each device to illustrate usability for this population and to inform future development of in-home therapeutic solutions using emerging smart home technologies.

For usability questions, a 5-point Likert scale was used that ranged from 'very hard' to 'very easy'. Questions related to preferences for either device or the voice input/output used other formats. Additionally, the questionnaires for study intake,

Table 1 Participants experience with and use of technology ($n = 8$)

Do you use any of the following on a regular basis?	
Smartphone	100%
Laptop of desktop computer	50%
Fitness tracker	50%
Tablet	38%
Regular cell phone	13%
Smartwatch	13%
Amazon Echo, Dot or Tap	13%
Google Home	0%
Mp3 player (separate from another device)	0%
Google Glass	0%

set-up, use diary and exit interview relied on numerous open-ended question formats to encourage unstructured user feedback. These were more suited to the exploratory nature of the research. The small sample size also supported including many qualitative questions. The questionnaires were brief in order to ensure that cognitive load was minimised and to avoid causing emotional frustration.

6 Results

Most users found Amazon Echo easier to set up than Google Home, mainly because of difficulties connecting the latter to the Wi-Fi network maintained by Shepherd Center for apartment complex provided to SHARE program clients. Google Home required considerably more assistance, apparently the result of difficulties using the required two-step authentication process of the devices with the shared secure network. Also, three of participants required assistance setting up the smart plugs.

Some users reported frustration with the lack of written instructions provided by Amazon, Google and TP-Link for setting up these smart devices. Their makers state set-up of the devices is intuitive and guided by the apps installed during the set-up. However, this user testing indicates set-up may be less intuitive for users with cognitive and/or psychological dysfunction. Some users may benefit from access to supplementary written instructions. A written description of possible error messages (and associated changes in light colour or blinking patterns) for each device may also be helpful.

During and after use of the smart speakers, 75% of participants reported Amazon Echo was easy or very easy to use compared to 71% (one observation missing) for Google Home (Table 2). One participant reported difficulty manually controlling the volume on Google Home, which requires fine motor use of a finger to swipe clockwise or counterclockwise on the top of the device. Participants reported Home correctly understood their voice commands more often than Echo, rating Home as understanding what the users were saying an average of 93% of the time, versus 81% for Echo.

Table 2 User assessment of the set-up process and use of Amazon Echo and Google Home

	Amazon Echo	Google Home
How easy/hard was it to set up each device?	Easy or very easy—75%	Easy or very easy—25%
How easy/hard has it been to use each device in last 3–4 days? (Final diary entry)	Easy or very easy—75%	Easy or very easy—71% (1 missing observation)
How useful has each device been in your life over the past 3–4 days? (Final diary entry)	Somewhat or very useful—88%	Somewhat or very useful—71%

Participants also reported a preference for the sound of the Alexa smart assistant's voice on Echo, compared to Google Assistant's voice on Home, rating the former at average of 8.1 out of 10, versus 7.5 for the latter (Table 3). Several participants reported they preferred the Echo's wake word (Alexa) to Google Home's (OK Google or Hey Google), noting that it felt more personal. Participants also preferred Echo's look and aesthetic design, rating it at an average 7.4/10 versus a 6.8/10 for Home. Overall, at study conclusion, seven of the eight participants said they preferred Amazon Echo to Google Home.

Participants made numerous suggestions about things or activities they wish the devices could do or things they would change about the devices (Table 4). Some referred to improving set-up process and minimising connectivity issues. Many mentioned that they wish they could access other media and devices with the smart speakers, including their iTunes library and other, the television and voice calling.

Many of the participants used the devices for alarms and reminders, for which they made several suggestions on how they want those reminders to function, with

Table 3 User assessment of the design of Amazon Echo and Google Home

	Amazon Echo	Google Home
How do you feel about the sound of smart assistant's voice on each device?	8.1/10 average rating	7.5/10 average rating
How do you like the look of each device?	7.4/10 average rating	6.8/10 average rating

Table 4 What would you change about each device? /What else do you wish each device could do?

Amazon Echo	Google Home
I would like for the Echo to be more active in being used as a reminder for people with memory problems, more uses such as alarms and or appointments, and to be more sensitive to commands. Sometimes the device could not process commands	When an alarm goes off I want the details. I don't just want an alarm sound. I want it to be like hey—you gotta do … now. Or hey, it's time for you to do …
Have a repeating alarm. I had to set one every day for medications	I wish it could automatically call a contact. If a timer was set and I wish it could tell me my daily schedule
Connect to and control a firestick. Ask permission of owner/operator before allowing drop ins. Better voice recognition and learning	Turn on the TV for me, hook it up with more things in my house
Choices for different voices	A different voice
A few times I got the red ring and it had trouble connecting. I wish that didn't happen because I didn't know what was going on	Make the set up easier
Improve the lag time between having to say "Hey Alexa" or "Alexa" and the statement of what it is I am needing	Its appearance, configuration, and smartphone app

specific requests for more details on what the alarm is for or for reminders of items on their daily calendars. Additionally, several wanted improved voice interaction. Some wished that the smart speakers understood what they were saying better. Others complained of the need to speak slowly or of the need to use specific vocabulary for commands. Additionally, one participant complained of the perceived required lag between saying the 'wake-up' word ('Alexa', or 'OK Google') and being able to voice the desired command.

Participants reported similar uses for both devices. Nearly all participants used them to stream music regularly and most commented on how useful that feature was for helping them relax. Other functions commonly performed by most participants included turning lamps off or on (with connected smart plugs), asking for information (e.g. the time, date, weather or sports scores) and using timers, alerts or calendar integration to recall and complete planned tasks. All participants reported that the smart speakers were useful in their daily life and all reported they would like to continue to use the smart speakers at study conclusion (Table 5).

When asked if they thought smart speakers could help them or if they had helped them, participants were unanimously positive. Specific areas identified were support for relaxation, memory and communication or sharing of important information with family and caregivers (Table 6).

Table 5 What do you think overall about the smart home devices you tested?	The Google Home was good at reminders, music, and a great sleep therapy device. I used it with my grounding technique from therapy to relax and wind down for sleep. I was able to increase my sleep by an hour and a half. I also liked the idea of the reminders for appointments, medication, and wake-ups
	Something I would continue to use in my own home. The Alexa was much easier to connect and use than the Home device. It aided me on scheduling, alarms, timers, music, tasks, reminders, information
	I thought it was really cool. It made me feel not so alone
	It was interesting. I think I'm going to get one

Table 6 Do you see this type of technology as something that could help you? Did it help you? How?	Yes, it was very helpful for assisting me with my memory problems about dates and events. It also helped with relaxation from the different music options
	It aided me on scheduling, alarms, timers, music, tasks, reminders, information
	Yes. To distract me with music or games. And to set alarms
	Yes, it can help. With things around the house it could help me control things. Now that I'm more into schedules, when I have time I can apply that to the device and it can keep me on track. I could track when finances are due and have it notify me

7 Conclusions

This study identified insights into the usability, needs and user preferences for smart speakers by military veterans with PTSD and mTBI. It also indicates further exploration of the usability challenges of smart speakers for this population is needed.

Overall, it showed that most participants found both devices easy to use, which is critical for this population, which can have difficulty handling added stress and frustrations. Both devices were also reported to have high reliability in recognising spoken commands by these users. On the other hand, it showed that set-up is not as seamless as it needs to be, particularly for Google Home.

From a research design perspective, the study proved challenging. Testing technology over an extended period in the user's place of residence adds considerable logistical requirements. Set-up and troubleshooting required considerable time on the part of the research team, an investment that would have been greatly reduced with a sit-by testing design in the lab with its ideal conditions.

Additionally, in-residence testing required more careful screening of participants to make sure that they would be in the rehabilitation program long enough to complete the study. Enrolling new participants early in the program became a key strategy, but was not fail-safe, as the personal lives of a number of participants interrupted our carefully planned testing schedule. Vacations, holidays, family emergencies and other unanticipated events required regular readjusting of testing schedules.

Our experience conducting this pilot study has encouraged us to explore developing a more detailed study for this population, and has inspired us to consider testing with other disability populations. The rapid pace of consumer technology innovation—including smart speakers—requires ongoing testing to ensure accessibility and usefulness by consumers with disabilities.

Acknowledgments This research was supported by The Rehabilitation Engineering Research Center for Information and Communications Technology Access (LiveWell RERC), which is funded by a 5-year grant from the National Institute on Disability, Independent Living and Rehabilitation Research (NIDILRR) in the U.S. Department of Health and Human Services (grant number 90RE5023). The opinions contained herein are those of the authors and do not necessarily reflect those of the U.S. Department of Health and Human Services or NIDILRR.

References

American Psychiatric Association (2013) Diagnostic and statistical manual of mental disorder, 5th edn. American Psychiatric Publishing, Washington, pp 271–280

Blumberg SJ, Luke JV (2017) Wireless substitution: early release of estimates from the National Health Interview Survey, July–December 2016. National Center for Health Statistics. http://www.cdc.gov/nchs/nhis.htm. Accessed on 10 Nov 2017

Capan F (2016) Why Amazon device is a gift for healthcare. Med Mark Media 51(1):20

Center for Universal Design (1997) Principles of universal design. Center for Universal Design, North Carolina State University, NC, US. https://projects.ncsu.edu/ncsu/design/cud/about_ud/udprinciplestext.htm. Accessed on 10 Nov 2017

Chen Y, Huang W (2011) Non-impact, blast-induced, mild TBI and PTSD: concepts and caveats. Brain Inj 25(7–8):641–650

Horrigan JB (2010) Broadband adoption and use in America. https://apps.fcc.gov/edocs_public/attachmatch/DOC-296442A1.pdf. Accessed on 29 Oct 2017

Kessler Foundation and National Organization on Disability (2010) The ADA, 20 years later. http://www.nasuad.org/sites/nasuad/files/hcbs/files/195/9739/surveyresults.pdf. Accessed on 29 Oct 2017

McGregor J (2017) An honest review of Google Home and Amazon's Alexa. Forbes, 11 April 2017. https://www.forbes.com/sites/jaymcgregor/2017/04/11/an-honest-review-of-google-home-and-amazons-alexa/#21177a5d5fd4. Accessed on 12 Sept 2017

Morris J, Mueller J (2014) Blind and deaf consumer preferences for Android and iOS smartphones. In: Langdon PM, Lazar J, Heylighen A, Dong H (eds) Inclusive designing: joining usability, accessibility and inclusion. Springer, Berlin, pp 69–79

Morris J, Mueller J, Jones M (2014) Wireless technology uses and activities by people with disabilities. J Technol Persons Disabil 2:29–45

Murnane K (2017) Alexa, remind Google that home needs reminders. Forbes. https://www.forbes.com/sites/kevinmurnane/2017/06/08/alexa-remind-google-that-home-needs-reminders/#5eb7c92c1675. Accessed on 12 Sept 2017

St. John A (2017) Amazon echo voice commands offer big benefits to users with disabilities. Consumer Reports, 20 January 2017. https://www.consumerreports.org/amazon/amazon-echo-voice-commands-offer-big-benefits-to-users-with-disabilities/. Accessed on 15 Nov 2017

Stinson L (2017) Alexa is conquering the world. Now Amazon's real challenge begins. Wired. https://www.wired.com/2017/01/alexa-conquering-world-now-amazons-real-challenge-begins. Accessed on 12 Nov 2017

Tanielian T, Jaycox LH (eds) (2008) Invisible wounds of war: psychological and cognitive injuries, their consequences, and services to assist recovery. RAND Corporation Center for Military Health Policy Research, pp 35–82. https://www.rand.org/content/dam/rand/pubs/monographs/2008/RAND_MG720.pdf. Accessed on 15 Nov 2017

Tschiffely AE, Ahlers ST, Norris JN (2015) Examining the relationship between blast-induced mild traumatic brain injury and posttraumatic stress-related traits. J Neurosci Res 93(12):1769–1777

United Nations (2006) Convention on rights of persons with disabilities. https://www.un.org/development/desa/disabilities/convention-on-the-rights-of-persons-with-disabilities.html. Accessed on 11 Nov 2017

Wallace T, Morris J, Bradshaw S, Bayer C (2017) Breathe Well: developing a stress management app on wearables for TBI & PTSD. J Technol Persons Disabil 5:67–82

Woyke E (2017) The octogenarians who love Amazon's Alexa. MIT Technol Rev 120:17

Part III
Removing Barriers to Usability, Accessibility and Inclusive Design

Breaking Down Barriers: Promoting a New Look at Dementia-Friendly Design

J. Kirch, G. Marquardt and K. Bueter

Abstract The ageing of the population is proceeding rapidly and the prevalence of people living with dementia is rising. Dementia is a syndrome caused by a variety of diseases and injuries that primarily or secondarily affect the brain. It is characterised by deterioration in cognitive function and therefore influences people's memory, thinking, behaviour and their ability to perform activities of daily living independently. A great number of studies have established a relationship between the built environment and outcomes of people with dementia. However, the importance and potential of this topic are still not fully recognised. In Germany, building regulations rarely depict dementia-friendly design. It is underrepresented in the education of architectural students and existing guidelines often do not cover the full range of design interventions. Further, a one-sided interpretation of design principles resulted in a preconceived image of dementia-friendly design, which often does not meet aesthetical standards or is at risk of stigmatising users. In this literature-based introductory chapter, the authors argue that dementia-friendly design does not need an obviously different look but a sensitive and user-centred design approach instead. To promote the realisation of inspiring and innovative concepts, it will be important to break down current prejudices among architects and to take a step towards an integrated, inclusive understanding of dementia-friendly design.

J. Kirch
Network Aging Research, Heidelberg University, Heidelberg, Germany
e-mail: kirch@nar.uni-heidelberg.de

G. Marquardt · K. Bueter (✉)
Faculty of Architecture, Technische Universitaet Dresden, Dresden, Germany
e-mail: kathrin.bueter@tu-dresden.de

G. Marquardt
e-mail: gesine.marquardt@tu-dresden.de

© Springer International Publishing AG, part of Springer Nature 2018
P. Langdon et al. (eds.), *Breaking Down Barriers*,
https://doi.org/10.1007/978-3-319-75028-6_11

1 Introduction

Dementia is *'one of the biggest global public health challenges'* our generation is facing (ADI 2013, p. 5). Old age is considered the main risk factor for getting dementia (Wallesch and Förstl 2005). Due to the phenomenon of an ageing population (United Nations 2017), the number of people with dementia is increasing worldwide (ADI 2013). In 2017, around 47 million people worldwide were known to have dementia (WHO 2017). It is estimated that by 2030 this number will be 66 million increasing to 115 million people with dementia by 2050.

Dementia is a syndrome caused by a variety of diseases and injuries that primarily or secondarily affect the brain. It leads to deterioration in cognitive function and therefore influences people's memory, thinking, behaviour and their ability to perform activities of daily living independently (WHO 2017). Dementia is one of the major causes of disability and dependency in old age.

To promote people's independence as well as to relieve caregivers' burden, different measures are considered to be supportive. As stated below, the design of the built environment is one important influencing factor. By taking into account the specific needs of people with dementia, the built environment can contribute to the compensation of cognitive decline and physical constraints while disease progresses. However, there are different barriers to the conception and implementation of dementia-friendly design. The aim of this chapter is to identify these barriers and elucidate which aspects make design dementia-friendly and which do not.

2 Why Do We Need Dementia-Friendly Design?

Theories from the field of environmental psychology demonstrate the relationship between the built environment and the user. An individual's ability to function is affected by the fit between their level of abilities and the demands of their environment (environmental press). Due to cognitive decline, the ability of people with dementia to deal with environmental press decreases. Too much press from the outside could make them unable to cope and negative effects, such as maladaptive or challenging behaviour, could evolve (Lawton and Nahemow 1973; Kolanowski 1999). Therefore, people with dementia are more sensitive to their surroundings and their dependency on the environment rises (Hall and Buckwalter 1987; Gutzmann 2003):

> The basic premise of environmental-based strategies is that achieving a proper environmental fit can optimize the abilities, health, and morale of the person with dementia.
>
> (Calkins et al. 2011, p. 22.6)

Numerous studies prove the success of environmental strategies showing that a built environment, which is adapted to the needs of people with dementia, positively influences behaviour, cognition, functionality, well-being, orientation and social abilities (Marquardt et al. 2014).

3 What Is Dementia-Friendly Design?

So far, no precise definition of the term *dementia-friendly design* exists. Design recommendations usually consider age- and dementia-related impairments. Further efforts have been made to move aged care away from the medical model to a more person-centred approach (Van Steenwinkel et al. 2017a). Instead of deficit-oriented approaches, now, person-centred goals serve as directives for dementia-friendly environmental strategies (Calkins et al. 2011): *Awareness and Orientation* refers to the necessity to support orientation in terms of space, time and situation among people with dementia, whereas *Safety and Security* considers possible hazards within the built environment due to cognitive and physical impairments. People's need for *Privacy, Personal Control* as well as for *Social Contact* demonstrates the demand for a supportive and manifold spatial performance, which offers options to make meaningful choices. A competence-inducing environment will support people's *Functional Abilities* and a familiar atmosphere can even contribute to affirm *Continuity of Self*.

To meet these goals a set of design principles has been defined and each goal may be realised through various spatial measures (Fleming et al. 2012; ACI 2014; Van Hoof and O'Brien 2014; Waller et al. 2017):

- ensure safety and security;
- provide appropriate stimulation (avoid unhelpful and highlight useful stimulation);
- promote independent functioning (assure people's mobility and activity);
- facilitate spatial orientation (e.g. by enabling visual access);
- built in human scale;
- create a homelike and familiar atmosphere;
- strike a balance between private and social spaces.

Familiarity is one key principle in dementia-friendly design. It is based on the theory that since long-term memory remains intact for a longer period of time, it may be easier to remember and recognise environments and elements from the past. Therefore, utilising environments and features familiar to people with dementia may enhance their autonomy and memory.

Much research on dementia-friendly design was conducted in long-term care facilities. Here, the systematic review of Marquardt et al. (2014) shows that effective dementia-friendly design interventions are manifold and reach from architectural features, such as building typologies and spatial layouts, to interior design elements. A straight circulation system, visual access to relevant places and the integration of meaningful reference points are examples of supportive spatial features. Environmental attributes, on the other hand, refer to sufficient lighting, appropriate acoustic measures to avoid high noise levels and comfortable room climate (see Table 1).

Table 1 Dementia-friendly design recommendations for long-term care facilities based on the systematic review of Marquardt et al. (2014)

Design category	Recommendations regarding the built environment
Basic design decisions	Small-scale environments
	Low social density: efforts should be made to enable people with dementia to regulate the degree to which they wish to interact with other residents and staff
	Building layout: supportive spatial features include a straight circulation system, visual access to relevant places and the integration of meaningful reference points
Environmental attributes	Sufficient lighting: higher luminance level during the day Good acoustics: highlight pleasant sounds, avoid high noise levels by appropriate acoustic measures
	Comfortable room climate
	Informed application of colours, including a strong colour contrast, avoid using patterns and dark lines on flooring
Ambience	Environment that does not have an institutional design but a homelike appearance, personalised character and allows for individual transformations
	Provide sensory stimulation through visual, auditory, tactile and olfactory stimuli
	However, the degree of sensory stimulation has to be controlled in order not to trigger any adverse outcomes through overstimulation
Environmental information	Apply signposting, room numbers and colours: Signs, for instance should contain icons and text
	Personalised cues such as nameplates, portrait-type photographs or personal memorabilia can be placed outside of rooms
	Visual barriers on intended objects, such as camouflaged doors or doorknobs, reduce the attempts of people with dementia to leave the facility

4 Barriers to the Creation and Implementation of Dementia-Friendly Design

There are several barriers in the conception and realisation of dementia-friendly design concepts: First, the importance and potential of this topic are still not fully recognised. In Germany, building regulation rarely depicts dementia-friendly design. A few DIN-standards (Deutsches Institut für Normung = German Institute for Standardisation) mention the need for this type of design, however, without defining precise suggestions (DIN 18040-1:2010-10, DIN 13080:2016-06). For healthcare facilities, such as nursing homes and hospitals, it is not obligatory to implement relevant measures. In addition, dementia friendly, as well as accessible designs, are underrepresented in the education of architectural students (Marquardt 2015) resulting in knowledge gaps and architects not being sensitised to this important challenge (Van Steenwinkel 2015). Further, available planning guidelines often do not cover the full range of design interventions. They usually focus on interior decorations rather than architectural features, such as building typologies or the spatial layout (ACI 2014; Alzheimer's WA 2015; Waller et al. 2017). Therefore, *'architects' core business of form and spatial organisation'* is hardly addressed (Van Steenwinkel et al. 2017b, p. 1). Dementia-friendly design appears to be only about choosing the right colours or pictures on the wall, which can be done without including an architect in the planning process. As a result, realised concepts often do not follow a holistic approach.

Second, dementia-friendly design seems to be an unattractive topic with a negative connotation for architects. The number of realised examples, which could serve as inspirational sources, is limited. Many realised examples work with similar elements and in an antiquated style pretending to be mandatory in dementia-friendly design. However, this type of style might be due to a one-sided interpretation of the design principle *Familiarity*. The creation of a familiar environment is important for people living with dementia who experience short-term memory loss while their long-term memory remains intact longer. Design features familiar to the person from an earlier part of his/her life may be more recognisable, more easily understood and more usable. People with dementia, however, are a very heterogenic group based on different ages, cultural and social backgrounds, as well as their degree of physical and cognitive impairments, and the type of dementia they have. Dementia-friendly design needs to consider this diversity. Otherwise commonly applied stereotypical elements, such as, for example, floral wallpaper or plush sofas, lead to a stigmatising design. A nonreflective interpretation of other design principles can also be recognised. For example, for *Safety and Security*, illusory elements, such as hidden exit doors or artificial bus stops in nursing homes' hallways, prevent residents from eloping. This leads to the risk of disrespecting residents' dignity. Ethical as well as architects' aesthetical standards are often unmet and creative leeway seems to be limited. This might result in prejudices against dementia-friendly design tasks.

5 Breaking Down Barriers: Does Dementia-Friendly Design Have to Look Different?

Physical environments for people with dementia do not necessarily need a fundamentally different appearance. It is not about applying a specific style of furnishing or making use of a certain set of colours on walls. It should be the small inconspicuous details, which make the difference in dementia-friendly design rather than an obviously different look, which may lead to stigmatisation and which works against social inclusion. Designing for dementia means to create a sophisticated design, which focuses on users' needs. Environments need to be clear and legible, easy to understand and interpret (Marquardt 2011). *"People with dementia need beautiful buildings, as we all do. They need space and light and art."* (Marshall and Delaney 2012, p. 26). Fundamental human demands such as the need for safety, privacy and self-control have to be considered (Lawton and Nahemow 1973; Radzey 2014), characteristics which are beneficial for many users.

To promote dementia-friendly design, psychological barriers need to be broken down. First, the establishment of an individual and modern image of ageing, which reflects the actual diversity of our ageing population, should be pushed forward. Second, the picture of an old-fashioned, stereotypical architecture, as the primary way to design for dementia needs to be removed. We have to show that dementia-friendly design is a creative challenge, which implies a high aesthetical quality and designer's sensibility. *Familiarity* as a key principle in dementia-friendly design has substantially influenced the appearance of care home environments so far. The often one-sided interpretation resulted in a preconceived image of dementia-friendly design. Care homes seemed to follow rather stereotypical design guidance, where quite often anything old was considered to evoke a feeling of familiarity among the residents. To counteract this image we need to encourage an individual and flexible interpretation of the design principle *Familiarity*. Both the individual with dementia to whom we are designing for, as well as, the setting the design is applied to, need to be considered. We also need to acknowledge that *Familiarity* represents a human value which cannot be described in a solely objective way through certain design elements (Van Steenwinkel et al. 2017a). Instead, it needs a holistic approach.

In an increasingly diverse and multi-cultural society, creating familiar environments represents a challenge. Features considered typical or familiar for a 90-year-old person in one culture may be unusual and disorientating for a 70-year-old person from another background. Still, due to their dementia, they may be using the same environment, e.g. when living together in a nursing home. Through a user-centred design approach, we can overcome the use of stereotypes and, hence, prevent a stigmatising design. Especially getting to know the people we are designing for, and integrating them into the design process, is important. People with dementia are sensitive about aesthetics in their surroundings (Halpern and O'Connor 2013) and they are able to express their opinions on potential design (Godwin 2014; Hung et al. 2017). Further, research shows that people with dementia do not necessarily want to live in the past but show the wish to create new things (Van Steenwinkel et al. 2014). Communication with them might be difficult especially when words fail. In addition, participatory research often requires higher efforts due to ethical issues (Sherratt et al. 2007; Novek and Wilkinson 2017). However, giving voice to them directly is highly relevant for a user-centred design approach, not only because studies show that opinions and preferences of people with dementia can differ systematically from those of staff and family members (Harmer and Orrell 2008; Godwin 2014). A user-centred approach becomes particularly challenging when architects do not know the individual user, e.g. when designing collective housing. Here a range of case studies with an open and rich character may help architects to gain a better understanding of the diverse experiences of living with dementia (Van Steenwinkel et al. 2017b). The diverse range of needs should be incorporated in the building while room is left for personalisation and adjustment to suit the specific *individual needs* as required (Pierce et al. 2015).

A highly sensitive interpretation of the design principle *Familiarity* is needed in regard to the type of *setting* we are designing. On the one hand, we have to differentiate in terms of setting's function. For example, in hospitals, creating a familiar environment may need a different approach than in living environments. Common rooms designed as homelike living rooms are rather unusual in hospitals and therefore may be disorientating for people with dementia. On the other hand, a balance needs to be struck between design that caters for the specific, complex needs of people with dementia, such as specialised dementia care units, and design, which will be used by a variety of people. In environments not exclusively designed for dementia, an appropriate course of action could be to apply a universal design approach (Calkins et al. 2011). Universal Design (UD) is about creating an environment that can be used by all people, regardless of their age, size, disability or ability (Preiser and Ostroff 2011). Many of the UD principles are closely connected to those of dementia-friendly design (Pierce et al. 2015). In case of Familiarity, Calkins et al. (2011) argue that the UD principle *Simple and Intuitive* promotes design that meets users' expectations and thus in some ways supports the principle of *Familiarity*. Mäki and Topo (2009) propose that the principle *Simple and Intuitive* eliminates unnecessary complexity. Therefore, the use of design is easily understood regardless of users' knowledge, experience, language skill or current concentration levels.

6 Conclusions

Even when an environment is created in a modern way, it can refer to the needs of people with dementia. The actual task is to keep in mind users' sensitiveness and vulnerability. It is important to break down current prejudices among architects and to take a step towards an integrated, inclusive understanding of dementia-friendly design. Environments need to be tailored to users' needs as well as to setting requirements and follow a holistic concept, so that a unique and coherent ambience may evolve. Further, dementia-friendly design represents an opportunity to study the built environments' usability (Zeisel 2011). It considers a diverse range of needs: Age-related and dementia-specific as well as fundamental psychological needs, such as the need for safety, privacy, self-control and aesthetics. Therefore, dementia-friendly design can be beneficial for many other users. However, it is important to promote a high aesthetical quality and to prevent the use of stereotypical and stigmatising design elements. Only then dementia-friendly design will be commonly accepted and can represent the principles of Universal Design.

References

ACI (2014) Key principles for improving healthcare environments for people with dementia. ACI Aged Health Network, Chatswood, NSW, Australia. https://www.aci.health.nsw.gov.au/__data/assets/pdf_file/0019/280270/ACI_Key_Principles_for_Improving_Healthcare_Environments_for_People_with_Dementia.PDF. Accessed 15 Nov 2017

ADI (2013) Policy brief for heads of government: The global impact of dementia 2013–2050. Alzheimer's Disease International. https://www.alz.co.uk/research/GlobalImpactDementia2013.pdf. Accessed 15 Nov 2017

Alzheimer's WA (2015) Dementia care environment audit tools. https://www.enablingenvironments.com.au/audit-tools–services.html. Accessed 2 Aug 2017

Calkins M, Sanford J, Proffitt M (2011) Design for dementia: challenges and lessons for universal design. In: Preiser W, Ostroff E (eds) Universal design handbook, 2nd edn. McGraw-Hill, New York, NY, US, pp 22.1–22.24

Fleming R, Crookes P, Sum S (2012) Dementia design audit tool. Part 3: literature review. A review of the empirical literature on the design of physical environments for people with dementia, 3rd edn. Dementia Services Development Centre, University of Stirling, Scotland, UK

Godwin B (2014) Colour consultation with dementia home residents and staff. Qual Ageing Older Adults 15(2):102–119

Gutzmann H (2003) Therapeutische Ansätze bei Demenzen. In: Wächtler C (ed) Demenzen. Thieme, Stuttgart, Germany, pp 51–71

Hall GR, Buckwalter KC (1987) Progressively lowered stress threshold: a conceptual model for care of adults with alzheimer's disease. Arch Psychiatr Nurs 1(6):399–406

Halpern AR, O'Connor MG (2013) Stability of art preference in frontotemporal dementia. Psychol Aesthetics Creativity Arts 7(1):95–99

Harmer BJ, Orrell M (2008) What is meaningful activity for people with dementia living in care homes? A comparison of the views of older people with dementia, staff and family carers. Aging Mental Heal 12(5):548–558

Hung L, Phinney A, Chaudhury H, Rodney P, Tabamo J, Bohl D (2017) Little things matter! Exploring the perspectives of patients with dementia about the hospital environment. Int J Older People Nurs 12:3

Kolanowski AM (1999) An overview of the need-driven dementia-compromised behavior model. J Gerontol Nur 25(9):7–9

Lawton MP, Nahemow L (1973) Ecology and the aging process. In: Eisdorfer C, Lawton MP (eds) The psychology of adult development and aging. American Psychological Association Washington, DC, US, pp 619–674

Marquardt G (2011) Wayfinding for people with dementia: A review of the role of architectural design. HERD 4(2):55–90

Marquardt G (ed) (2015) MATI Mensch—Architektur—Technik—Interaktion für demografische Nachhaltigkeit. Fraunhofer IRB Verlag, Stuttgart, Germany

Marquardt G, Bueter K, Motzek T (2014) Impact of the design of the built environment on people with dementia: an evidence-based review. HERD 8(1):127–157

Marshall M, Delaney J (2012) Dementia-friendly design guidance for hospital wards. J Dementia Care 20(4):26–28

Mäki O, Topo P (2009) User needs and user requirements of people with dementia: Multimedia application for entertainment. In: Topo P, Östlund B (eds) Dementia, design and technology: time to get involved. IOS Press, pp 61–75

Novek S, Wilkinson H (2017) Safe and inclusive research practices for qualitative research involving people with dementia: a review of key issues and strategies. Dementia (London), Jan 2017

Pierce M, Cahill S, Grey T, Dyer M (2015) Research for dementia and home design in Ireland looking at new build and retro-fit homes from a universal design approach: key findings and recommendations report 2015. Dublin, Ireland

Preiser W, Ostroff E (2011) Universal design handbook, 2nd edn. McGraw-Hill, New York, NY, US

Radzey B (2014) Lebenswelt Pflegeheim. Eine nutzerorientierte Bewertung von Pflegeheimbauten für Menschen mit Demenz, Mabuse, Frankfurt am Main, Germany

Sherratt C, Soteriou T, Evans S (2007) Ethical issues in social research involving people with dementia. Dementia 6(4):463–479

United Nations (2017) World population prospects: the 2017 revision. Key findings and advance tables. Working Paper No. ESA/P/WP/248. Department of Economic and Social Affairs, Population Division. United Nations, New York, NY, US. https://esa.un.org/unpd/wpp/Publications/Files/WPP2017_KeyFindings.pdf. Accessed 15 Nov 2017

Van Hoof J, O'Brien D (2014) Designing for dementia. Evid Based Des J 1(1):1–38

Van Steenwinkel I (2015) Offering architects insights into living with dementia: three case studies on orientation in space-time-identity. PhD thesis, University of Leuven, Leuven, Belgium

Van Steenwinkel I, Van Audenhove C, Heylighen A (2014) Mary's little worlds: Changing person–space relationships when living with dementia. Qual Health Res 24(8):1023–1032

Van Steenwinkel I, Dierckx de Casterlé B, Heylighen A (2017a) How architectural design affords experiences of freedom in residential care for older people. J Aging Stud 41:84–92

Van Steenwinkel I, Van Audenhove C, Heylighen A (2017b) Insights into living with dementia: Five implications for architectural design. In: Proceedings of Arch17—3rd international conference on architecture, Research, Care, Health, Aalborg University Copenhagen, Denmark, 26–27 April 2017

Waller S, Masterson A, Evans SC (2017) The development of environmental assessment tools to support the creation of dementia friendly care environments: innovative practice. Dementia 16 (2):226–232

Wallesch C-W, Förstl H (eds) (2005) Demenzen. Thieme, Stuttgart, Germany

WHO (2017, May) Dementia. Fact sheet. World Health Organization, Switzerland. http://www.who.int/mediacentre/factsheets/fs362/en/. Accessed 15 Nov 2017

Zeisel J (2011) Universal design to support the brain and its development. In: Preiser W, Ostroff E (eds), Universal design handbook, 2nd edn. McGraw-Hill, New York, NY, US, pp 8.1–8.14

Usability of Indoor Network Navigation Solutions for Persons with Visual Impairments

G. A. Giannoumis, M. Ferati, U. Pandya, D. Krivonos and T. Pey

Abstract The United Nations (UN) Convention on the Rights of Persons with Disabilities (CRPD) obligates States Parties to ensure personal mobility and independence for persons with disabilities by promoting access to and the development of assistive technology (AT)—i.e. products and services that enhance daily living and quality of life for persons with disabilities. Research has examined the experiences of persons with different disabilities using ICT and AT for indoor navigation and wayfinding. However, in the last year, ICT developers have made substantial strides in deploying Internet of Things (IoT) devices as part of indoor network navigation solutions (INNS) for persons with visual impairments. This article asks, 'To what extent do persons with visual impairments perceive INNS as usable?' Quantitative and qualitative data from an experimental trial conducted with 36 persons with visual impairments shows that persons with visual impairments largely consider INNS as usable for wayfinding in transportation stations. However, the results also suggest that persons with visual impairments experienced barriers using INNS due to the timing of the instructions. Future research should continue to investigate the usability of INNS for persons with visual impairments and focus specifically on reliability and responsivity of the instruction timing.

G. A. Giannoumis (✉) · M. Ferati · D. Krivonos
Oslo and Akershus University College of Applied Sciences, Oslo, Norway
e-mail: gagian@hioa.no

M. Ferati
e-mail: Mexhid.Ferati@hioa.no

D. Krivonos
e-mail: krivonosdaria@gmail.com

U. Pandya
Wayfindr, London, UK
e-mail: ume@ustwo.com

T. Pey
Royal Society for Blind Children, London, UK
e-mail: tom.pey@rsbc.org.uk

© Springer International Publishing AG, part of Springer Nature 2018
P. Langdon et al. (eds.), *Breaking Down Barriers*,
https://doi.org/10.1007/978-3-319-75028-6_12

1 Introduction

The United Nations (UN) Convention on the Rights of Persons with Disabilities (CRPD) obligates States Parties to ensure personal mobility and independence for persons with disabilities by promoting access to and the development of assistive technology (AT), which typically refers to products and services that enhance daily living and quality of life for persons with disabilities (ATIA 2015). AT for navigation enables persons with disabilities to plan and travel to a destination using a variety of technologies for wayfinding, such as electronic white canes, computerised vision and semi-autonomous robots (Yanco 1998; Levine et al. 1999; Hameed et al. 2006; Faria et al. 2010; Fernandes et al. 2010; Cowan et al. 2012).

Research shows that wayfinding involves decision-making—i.e. planning an action; decision execution—i.e. putting plans into action; and information processing—i.e. sensing and understanding new information for decision-making and execution (Passini 1996; Golledge 1999). Since the 1990s, research on wayfinding has adopted a user-centred design (UCD) perspective, and has argued that wayfinding design involves creating environments where people can interact with complex environments and perceive, select and understand information and environmental characteristics to make decisions and reach destinations (Passini 1996; Carpman and Grant 2003; Gibson 2009; Calori and Vanden-Eynden 2015).

Research has examined the experiences of persons with different disabilities using ICT and AT for indoor navigation and wayfinding (Yanco 1998; Kulyukin et al. 2006; Chang et al. 2008). However, in the last year, ICT developers have made substantial strides in deploying Internet of Things (IoT) devices as part of indoor network navigation solutions (INNS) for persons with visual impairments (Ready 2015; Munkås 2016; Transport for London 2016). IoT refer to interconnected devices embedded in ordinary objects, and INNS use IoT devices to augment the physical environment using audio wayfinding information. These solutions use low energy Bluetooth (BLE) beacons and mobile applications to enable persons with visual impairments to navigate complex indoor environments independently (ITU 2017).

BLE beacons, used in conjunction with mobile applications, broadcast wayfinding information about various elements in the built environment—e.g. entrances and exits, toilets, stairs and other points of interest. Thus, INNS provide a more accurate, precise, efficient and low-cost investment for service providers compared with traditional forms of indoor wayfinding for persons with visual impairments—e.g. personal assistance, braille signs, tactile maps or GPS-enabled mobile phones. Industry analysts have also argued that BLE beacons are in the process of disrupting several major industries (Industry Arc 2015).

As research has yet to examine fully the experiences of persons with visual impairments using INNS, this article aims to fill this gap by investigating the usability of a BLE beacon network that uses audio wayfinding instructions for persons with visual impairments to navigate complex environments. This article asks, 'To what extent do persons with visual impairments perceive INNS as usable?' This article uses qualitative and quantitative data from an experimental trial conducted at the Pedestrian Accessibility Movement Environment Laboratory (PAMELA) at University College London. The results show that persons with visual impairments largely consider INNS as usable for wayfinding in transportation stations.

This article proceeds in three sections. First, it details the methods used for data collection and analysis. Second, this article analyses the results in terms of overall usability, effectiveness, efficiency and satisfaction. Third, it discusses the results in relation to further development of INNS, and concludes by summarising the results and suggesting new opportunities for future research and development.

2 Methods

2.1 Sample

This article uses quantitative data gathered from a convenience sample of 36 participants ($n = 36$). Forty-six persons with visual impairments were initially recruited, but ten participants withdrew from the trial for reasons not stated. Participants identified as blind ($n = 32$) or partially sighted ($n = 4$) used different mobility aids including white cane ($n = 16$), a guide dog ($n = 8$), both ($n = 6$), and neither ($n = 6$). Participants' ages ranged from 21 to 77. The majority ($n = 15$) of participants' ages were between 21 and 29, and seven participants' were over 65. The majority of participants were identified as male ($n = 21$) as opposed to female ($n = 15$) and no participants were identified as non-binary. The majority of the participants ($n = 15$) had a congenital visual impairment. Other participants acquired a visual impairment from age 2 to 10 ($n = 6$), age 11 to 19 ($n = 11$) and over 20 ($n = 4$). Participants lived with a visual impairment from 1 to 77 years with the majority having lived with a visual impairment from 20 to 29 years ($n = 12$). Some participants ($n = 5$) were identified as having multiple disabilities including autism, diabetes, depression, anxiety, epilepsy, hearing loss, emphysema and chronic obstructive pulmonary disease.

Participants also reported their activity, use of assistive technology on mobile devices and their general confidence. While the majority of participants reported that they left the house daily ($n = 28$), some participants ($n = 3$) reported only leaving the house four times a week. Participants were also asked about their familiarity with screen reading software on mobile phones. Screen readers use text-to-speech synthesisers to convert text information to sound. Two of the most popular screen reader applications for mobile devices are TalkBack and VoiceOver. The former is available on Google's Android and the latter is available on Apple's iOS operating systems. The majority of participants were familiar with VoiceOver ($n = 30$) and some participants ($n = 4$) were not familiar with either TalkBack or VoiceOver. Finally, participants were asked about their confidence in completing the trial. The participants reported that they were very confident ($n = 16$), somewhat confident ($n = 14$) or neither confident nor unconfident ($n = 6$).

2.2 Protocol

The trials ran for 2 weeks in the Spring of 2017. Each participant was briefed on the trial's aims and procedures and informed consent was obtained orally. The trials were conducted at PAMELA where four routes were created to simulate different features of a transportation station. Each route was embedded with a series of BLE beacons and adhered to the international standard for audio navigation (ITU 2017). The BLE beacons were programmed to work with a mobile application to provide audio instructions for wayfinding. When a Bluetooth-enabled mobile device passes near a BLE beacon, the mobile device receives an identity (ID) number. The ID number is sent over the Internet to a database where the instruction is selected that corresponds with the ID number. The instruction is sent back to the device and the screen reader converts the instruction to audio.

Participants were first asked a series of demographic questions and then were taken to the beginning of first of four routes (Fig. 1). Participants were then given a bone-conducting headset and a mobile phone with a demonstration application pre-installed. The demonstration application was developed by Wayfindr for Apple's iOS operating system, and the source code is available online (Wayfindr 2017). Bone conduction headphones were used because they are more accessible

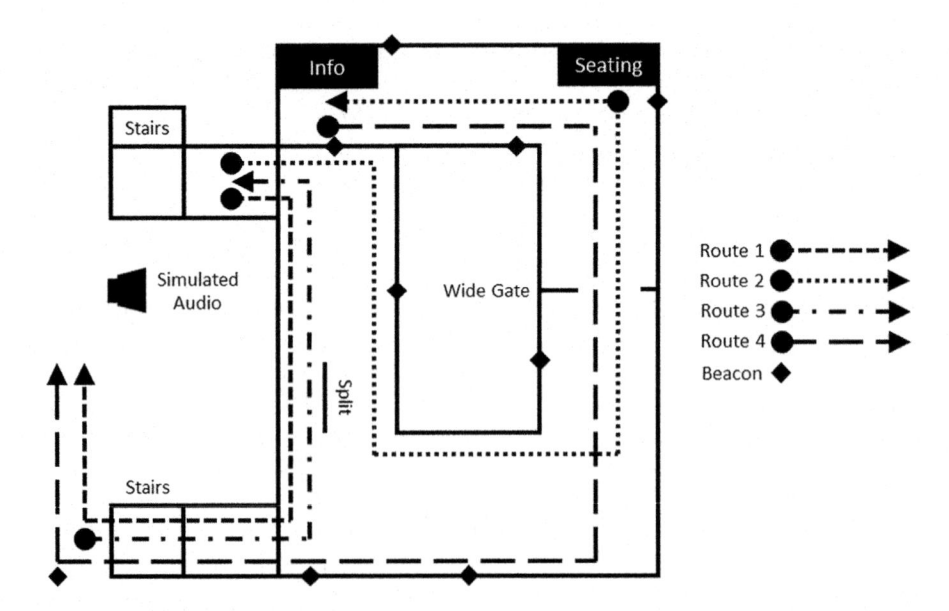

Fig. 1 Route map

for persons with hearing impairments and they allow the participants to hear both the audio instructions and the ambient simulated sound (Fig. 1, audio simulation).

Figure 1 details the four routes and the environmental features. Route 1 (Fig. 1) begins on a platform and the first beacon instructs the participant to turn right and keep to the right of the pedestrian barrier (Fig. 1, Split). The second beacon instructs the participant to turn right and proceed down the stairs. The third beacon instructs the participant to turn right and that their destination is ahead. Route 2 begins on the same platform as Route 1. The first beacon instructs the participant to turn right and keep to the left of the pedestrian barrier. The second beacon instructs the participant to turn left and the third to turn left and proceed through the wide gate. The wide gate is intended to simulate a wheelchair accessible ticket gate used in transportation stations. The fourth beacon informs the participant that they have reached the seating area on the train. The participant is then instructed to proceed to the information booth by turning left and the fifth beacon informs the participant that they have reached the information booth. Route 3 begins on another platform and the first beacon instructs the participant to proceed up the stairs. The second beacon instructs the participant to turn left and keep to the left of the pedestrian barrier. The third beacon instructs the participant to turn left to reach their destination. The fourth route begins near the information booth. The first beacon instructs the participant to turn right and proceed through the wide gate. The second beacon instructs the participant to turn right and continue down the stairs. The third beacon instructs the participant to turn right to reach their destination.

Approximately six participants completed the trial per day and participants were scheduled to arrive in two groups that met in either the morning or afternoon. Participants used their preferred mobility aid during the trial. Participants were allowed 1 hour to complete the routes with a 1-hour break between routes two and three. All routes were completed in order and the ordering of the routes aimed to minimise the potential for the participants to mentally map their environment and reduce learnability. Eight fixed cameras installed in the lab captured video recordings. A technician who noted their overall performance followed participants. After completing the trial, participants were compensated for their participation.

2.3 Measuring Usability

The International Organization for Standardization (ISO) defines usability in relation to three criteria including effectiveness, efficiency and satisfaction (ISO 2002, 2010). While this article adopts the ISO definition of usability, we recognise that scholars have posed other definitions of usability that include criteria such as learnability (Nielsen 1994). In order to measure usability, this article uses three measures including observation of users, performance-related measures and questionnaires. Observations were conducted on the video recordings to validate the performance measures. The performance measures were conducted by a technician who noted the time it took each participant to complete each route, the number of errors made during wayfinding and the number of times wayfinding was abandoned.

The questionnaires included a series of demographic questions completed before the trial, and after completing each route, the system usability scale (SUS) was administered orally. The SUS is a validated survey instrument for measuring perceived usability of ICT products and services for sample sizes as low as 20 (Sauro 2011). The SUS consists of ten questions scored using a Likert scale from one to five. The results are converted to a score ranging from zero to 100. Scores are typically interpreted based on additional qualitative data. The SUS was supplemented with two additional questions. The first question asked about the participant's confidence in using INNS for wayfinding in the future and was scored using a Likert scale from one to five. The second question was qualitative and asked about the participant's overall experience.

3 Analysis

3.1 Effectiveness

Qualitative performance measures were used to assess effectiveness. A technician observed and upon completion of each route documented whether and to what extent the participant navigated the route accurately and completely (ISO 2010). The qualitative data was coded according to themes that emerged from the observers' comments (Miles and Huberman 1994). Of the 132 records on effectiveness, 67 results showed that the participants experienced a barrier to effectiveness.

The results showed that the barriers to effectively navigating the routes led to a variety of outcomes. Participants sometimes failed to complete the route (i.e. the participant gave up). They sometimes failed to follow (e.g. went to right instead of the left side of pedestrian barrier or turned left instead of right) or complete the instruction (e.g. they did not arrive at the destination or did not follow the instruction). Participants also repeated steps to complete instruction (e.g. participant retraced their steps). They also frequently hesitated during the route—according to one technician 'the participant hesitated because [they] did not hear any instruction' and at times experienced confusion or disorientation—according to one technician '[the participant] was confused after going [down]stairs'.

The results showed that the timing of the instructions posed the principle barrier to participants' effectively navigating the route. This article argues that the timing of the instructions refers to when and where, in relation to the desired action, a user receives the instruction. According to ITU (2017), users should receive an instruction 8 ± 1 m before a decision point such as making a turn. Technicians observed that the participants received the instructions sometimes too early and sometimes too late. For example, during one route, technicians observed, '[the participant's] walking was slow and the instructions came early'. Another technician observed 'the instruction to turn left [...] came late and [the participant] had to wait'. Technicians also observed that the participants' walking speed affected the timing of the instructions. For example, one technician noted, '[the participant's] movement was relatively slow, so the instruction [...] was not synchronised'. Another technician noted, 'instructions were not well synced with [the participant's] movement'. Technicians also noted that a delay occurred between the participant receiving an instruction and taking an action (e.g. 'there was time delay between instruction and response').

3.2 Efficiency

Quantitative performance measures were used to assess efficiency. A technician timed how long each participant completed each route. Figure 2 shows the frequency distribution for the time participants took to complete all routes (Fig. 2a) and each route individually (Fig. 2b).

Table 1 shows that on average, the participants took 54 s to complete a route. While participants took on average much less time to complete route one (50 s) and route three (47 s), route four took on average the longest (61 s), potentially owing to the distance the participant had to travel. The spread of the scores around the mean of route three (17 s) was concentrated, in comparison to routes two (25 s), one (26 s) and four (32 s). The results do not appear to relate to the number of beacons or instructions given along a route. However, the data, only to a limited extent, provide a useful basis for examining the relationship between the number of

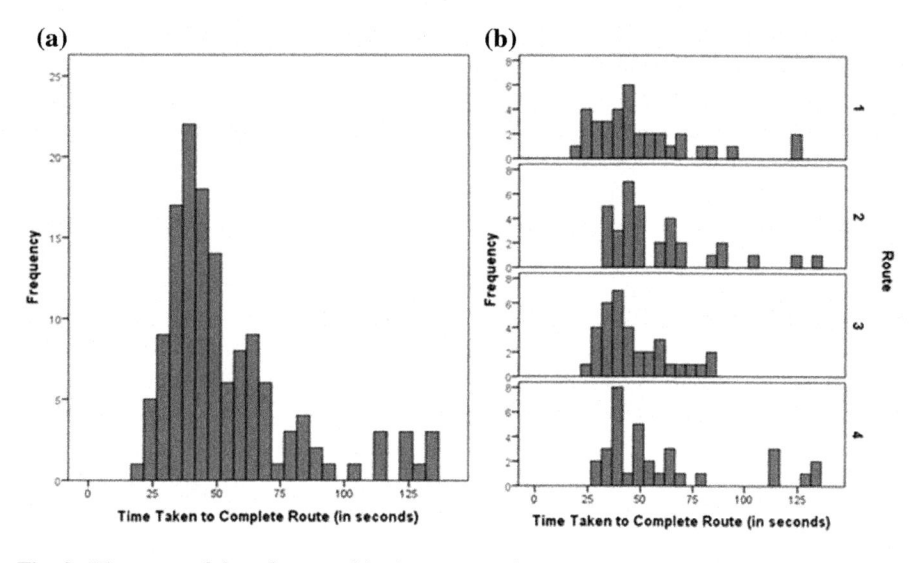

Fig. 2 Histogram of time (in seconds) taken to complete routes

Table 1 Descriptive statistics for time taken to complete routes (in seconds)

Route	N	Min	Max	Mean	Standard deviation
All	137	19	134	54	26
1	35	19	123	50	26
2	34	32	134	58	25
3	35	24	86	47	17
4	33	30	132	61	32

instructions and time taken to complete the route. Hypothetically, a higher number of instructions may result in an increased amount of time for decision-making and longer routes. The distance that the participants travel may also explain some of the variation in time taken to complete the route. Nonetheless, the results provide a useful basis for conducting further research on the efficiency of INNS using BLE beacons.

3.3 Satisfaction

The SUS questionnaire was used to assess satisfaction and it was analysed using boxplots to represent the overall and broken out scores by route (Fig. 3). The quartiles in the boxplot were interpreted using qualitative data drawn from questions about the participants experience using the system. The boxplot shows that the median of all SUS scores for all routes ($n = 132$) was 85. Research suggests that SUS scores above an average of 68 are considered usable (Sauro 2011). The median SUS scores remained stable across all routes and ranged from 83 to 92.

Overall SUS scores in the first interquartile (Q1–MIN) ranged from 75 to 45 (Fig. 3a). Comments for scores in this range typically focused on instruction timing. According to one participant, 'the instruction should come just before actions are needed'. Another participant noted 'the instructions weren't delivered at right place … it's difficult to know if it's working or not as no instruction came … feedback of the distance to the next point is needed'. A third participant suggested that 'the device should be customised [for] faster walking … I didn't get correct information to the destination'.

SUS scores in the second interquartile (Q3–Q1) ranged from 95 to 75 (Fig. 3a). Comments for scores in this range also noted that the instruction timing posed a barrier to usability. However, participants also commented on their satisfaction with the system. According to one participant 'apart from the fact [that] I got stuck and the instruction came late, the whole function was good … the instruction that did not arrive confused me'. A second participant commented, 'it is nice after understanding how to use it'. Another participant also noted their satisfaction stating the system was 'easy to use and I enjoyed it' and followed up by noting, 'it's better to repeat instructions automatically'. Finally, a fourth participant commented on their

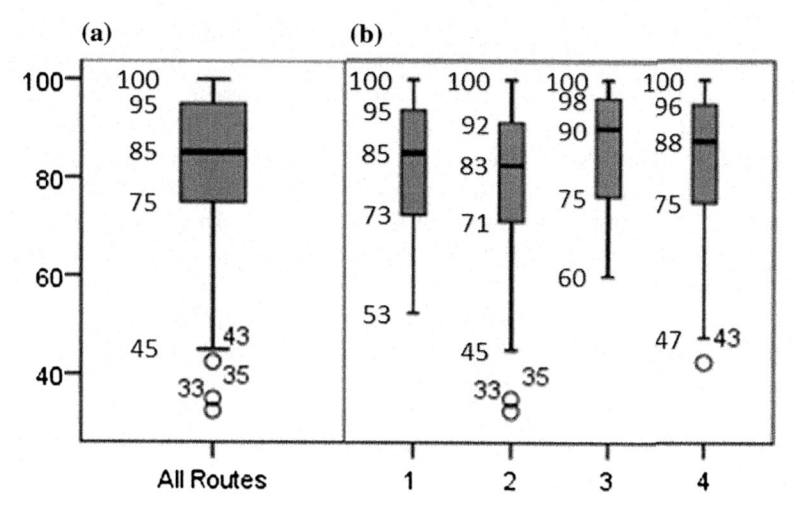

Fig. 3 Boxplot of SUS scores

satisfaction stating it was a 'good experience overall' and stated that the testing area was small and that 'a larger setting … could be better'.

SUS scores in the third interquartile (MAX–Q3) ranged from 100 to 95 (Fig. 3a). Comments for scores in this quartile were generally very positive—e.g. participants commented 'good experience', 'easy to understand and follow' and 'exciting to experience this kind of technology'. One participant commented 'the instruction[s were] really useful and valuable' and went on to state that with the system they were able 'to safely negotiate the stairs'. Another participant noted, 'the instructions were clear and made me able to get from "A" to "B"'. However, participants also had suggestions for improving the system—e.g. one participant commented, 'it would be good if [the] instructions sent more detailed information like which side the hand rail is [on]'.

The boxplot also provides evidence of three outlier scores in routes two and four (Fig. 3b). According to one of the participants, 'The system did not provide information to make a decision; [it] failed three times to tell me where I was'. Another participant stated, 'It tells me at wrong time and … I couldn't find [the] stairs as [the] instruction didn't come properly'.

4 Discussion and Conclusion

The results show that persons with visual impairments broadly perceive INNS as usable. However, in terms of effectiveness, persons with visual impairments experience barriers using INNS. In terms of efficiency, the skewed distribution of the time taken to complete the routes suggests that while most participants took approximately 50 s to complete the routes, several participants took 2–2.5 times as long to complete the routes. The time taken to complete the routes may be related to a person's specific impairment or other demographic characteristics. However, the data did not show a conclusive relationship. Although the SUS scores revealed a high level of usability, participants' satisfaction with the INNS was mixed.

Overall, the results suggest that persons with visual impairments experienced barriers using INNS due to the timing of the instructions. This article suggests that future research should continue to investigate the usability of INNS for persons with visual impairments and focus specifically on the timing of the instructions. While this article uses data from a convenience sample of persons with visual impairments, future research could extend the results of this article by investigating the relationship between perceived usability and other variables such as impairment type, age, confidence and experience using ICT. This article also recommends that future developers of BLE beacon hardware and INNS software focus on promoting the reliability and responsivity of instruction timing.

References

ATIA (2015) What is assistive technology? How is it funded? https://goo.gl/aMvuRz. Accessed 8 Nov 2017

Calori C, Vanden-Eynden D (2015) Signage and wayfinding design: a complete guide to creating environmental graphic design systems. Wiley, Berlin

Carpman JR, Grant MA (2003) Wayfinding: a broad view. In: Bechtel RB, Churchman A (eds) Handbook of environmental psychology. Wiley, USA

Chang Y-J, Tsai S-K, Wang T-Y (2008) A context aware handheld wayfinding system for individuals with cognitive impairments. In: Proceedings of the 10th international ACM SIGACCESS conference on computers and accessibility, Halifax, Nova Scotia, Canada, 13–15 October 2008

Cowan RE, Fregly BJ, Boninger ML, Chan L, Rodgers MM, Reinkensmeyer DJ (2012) Recent trends in assistive technology for mobility. J Neuroeng Rehabil 9(1):20

Faria J, Lopes S, Fernandes H, Martins P, Barroso J (2010) Electronic white cane for blind people navigation assistance. In: World Automation Congress (WAC), Kobe, Japan, 19–23 September 2010

Fernandes H, Costa P, Filipe V, Hadjileontiadis L, Barroso J (2010) Stereo vision in blind navigation assistance. In: World Automation Congress (WAC), Kobe, Japan, 19–23 September 2010

Gibson D (2009) The wayfinding handbook: information design for public places. Princeton Architectural Press, USA

Golledge RG (1999) Human wayfinding and cognitive maps. In: Golledge RG (ed) Wayfinding behavior: cognitive mapping and other spatial processes. Johns Hopkins University Press, USA

Hameed O, Iqbal J, Naseem B, Anwar O, Afzal S (2006) Assistive technology-based navigation aid for the visually impaired. In: Proceedings of the 2006 international symposium on practical cognitive agents and robots, Perth, Australia, 27–28 November 2006

Industry Arc (2015) Indoor positioning and navigation market: by system type (satellite based, hybrid, network based, sensors), by application (navigation, positioning, others), by vertical (aviation, advertisement, others), by geography-forecast (2016–2021)

ISO (2002) ISO/TR 16982 Ergonomics of human-system interaction—usability methods supporting human-centred design, ISO

ISO (2010) 9241-210:2010 Ergonomics of human-system interaction, ISO
ITU (2017) F.921 Audio-based network navigation system for persons with vision impairment, ITU
Kulyukin V, Gharpure C, Nicholson J, Osborne G (2006) Robot-assisted wayfinding for the visually impaired in structured indoor environments. Auton Robots 21(1):29–41
Levine SP, Bell DA, Jaros LA, Simpson RC, Koren Y, Borenstein J (1999) The NavChair assistive wheelchair navigation system. IEEE Trans Rehabil Eng 7(4):443–451
Miles MB, Huberman AM (1994) Qualitative data analysis: an expanded sourcebook. Sage Publications, U S A
Munkås Ø (2016) Med ny appteknologi vil de hjelpe deg å finne veien. https://goo.gl/MQPjiR. Accessed 8 Nov 2017
Nielsen J (1994) Usability engineering. Elsevier Science, Amsterdam
Passini R (1996) Wayfinding design: logic, application and some thoughts on universality. Des Stud 17(3):319–331
Ready F (2015) IBeacon helps visually impaired students find their way around Penn State campus. https://goo.gl/ugCTGG. Accessed 8 Nov 2017
Sauro J (2011) Measuring usability with the system usability scale (SUS). https://measuringu.com/sus/
Transport for London (2016) Wayfindr. https://goo.gl/HCuUrM. Accessed 8 Nov 2017
Wayfindr (2017) Wayfindr demo app. https://goo.gl/KnjDBw. Accessed 8 Nov 2017
Yanco HA (1998) Wheelesley: a robotic wheelchair system: indoor navigation and user interface assistive technology and artificial intelligence. In: Mittal V, Yanco H, Aronis J, Simpson R (eds) Lecture notes in artificial intelligence: assistive technology and artificial intelligence—application in robotics, user interfaces and natural language processing. Springer, Berlin, pp 256–268

Physical Barriers to Mobility of Stroke Patients in Rehabilitation Clinics

M. Kevdzija and G. Marquardt

Abstract Regaining independent mobility and general independence is the main goal of physical rehabilitation in stroke patients. The patients requiring rehabilitation stay as inpatients in rehabilitation clinics for a period of several weeks to several months. During this time, mobile patients are required to go to therapies and other scheduled appointments on their own. The aim of this study is to provide evidence that specific architectural design features of rehabilitation clinics hinder the independent mobility of stroke patients and to identify the main issues caused by the building design. Patients ($n = 50$) and staff members ($n = 46$) from five large German rehabilitation clinics participated in the study. Three methods were used to collect the data: patient questionnaire, staff questionnaire and patient shadowing (observation). Both staff and patients identified the major issues that stroke patients encounter in the built environment of rehabilitation clinics: wayfinding problems, insufficient dimensions of spaces (corridors), physical obstacles, uneven floor surfaces and large distances between patient rooms and therapy rooms. Shadowing data showed that the patients in the earlier stages of rehabilitation, mainly using a wheelchair, encounter the most barriers related to the built environment. Design recommendations for more mobility supportive rehabilitation clinics are made based on the study findings.

1 Introduction

Stroke is a disease predominantly occurring in the population above the age of 65. It is also one of the leading causes of death in the developed world and a major cause of disability in adults (Adamson et al. 2004). Stroke survivors are a diverse group with various consequences: from one-sided paralysis to speech and cognitive

---

M. Kevdzija (✉) · G. Marquardt
Technische Universität Dresden, Dresden, Germany
e-mail: maja.kevdzija@tu-dresden.de

G. Marquardt
e-mail: gesine.marquardt@tu-dresden.de

© Springer International Publishing AG, part of Springer Nature 2018
P. Langdon et al. (eds.), *Breaking Down Barriers*,
https://doi.org/10.1007/978-3-319-75028-6_13

impairments. In many cases, rehabilitation is necessary for the patients to re-train their muscles and regain as much as possible of the abilities they had before stroke (Dobkin 2005). The most common impairment caused by stroke is motor impairment, which restricts function in muscle movement or mobility. Recovery of mobility is one of the most important rehabilitation goals after a stroke (Langhorne et al. 2009).

Physical activity, not only in therapies, but also during free time in the rehabilitation clinic is important for patients' faster recovery and for regaining independence (Luker et al. 2015). The outcome of research studies on the time use of patients in rehabilitation (De Wit et al. 2005; Skarin et al. 2013; Anåker et al. 2017) is that patients are inactive in their rooms for more than 50% of the day on average. A large amount of inactivity reported in all research studies is in contrast with the main goal of rehabilitation: recovering mobility.

There is a significant amount of studies providing evidence that the design of healthcare environments has an influence on the well-being of patients. Stroke patients, with their physical and cognitive impairments, are a group whose spatial needs are not investigated enough. The recent study on the patient activity in a Swedish stroke unit before and after the reconstruction demonstrates that the activity levels of stroke patients changed significantly after modifications in the stroke unit's floor plan configuration and interior design (Anåker et al. 2017).

This research study investigates the variety of mobility barriers that stroke patients encounter in the built environment of rehabilitation clinics. The goal is to identify the most common issues that patients encounter in the existing clinics and to provide knowledge for their redesign and for the design of future clinics.

2 Context

Neurological rehabilitation in Germany is divided into five rehabilitation phases: A, B, C, D and E phase. Patients are sorted into these phases based on their Barthel Index (BI), a scale used to measure performance in activities of daily living (ADL). Phase A is an acute phase and starts in a hospital, immediately after the onset of stroke. The patients who require rehabilitation continue their recovery through phases B, C and D as inpatients in rehabilitation clinics, for several weeks to several months. Afterwards, they become outpatients in the E phase.

There are significant differences between the mobility levels of patients in different phases. Patients in B phase are often bed confined and have functional impairments in the vital domain. In the C phase, the main issue is the missing ADL competence and the patients in the D/E phase have limitations in the social and vocational competencies (Schönle 2000).

Stroke patients in Germany stay in neurological rehabilitation clinics as inpatients for 4 to 6 weeks on average. During this time, the goal is to restore as much of the independence as possible. As the independent mobility is especially important during the stroke recovery, the policy of the rehabilitation clinics is to encourage patients to be more mobile. Most of the patients who are not bed confined are expected to go to therapies/meals alone. Therapy rooms are usually placed outside of the patient wards, the common dining area is on the ground floor, etc. When going there on their own, patients encounter different environments and cover large distances each day. According to the medical staff, this is beneficial for their well-being and mobility training.

At the same time, patients have various internal barriers to mobility such as hemiplegia, hemiparesis, cognitive impairments, etc. These internal barriers cause difficulties for patients when moving independently in the clinic. A large number of patients require additional equipment to be able to walk/move, such as a wheelchair or a walker. In addition to the internal barriers caused by the disease, stroke patients encounter the barriers in the physical environment of the rehabilitation clinics.

3 Methods and Participants

The goal of this study is to determine which features of the built environment of rehabilitation clinics act as barriers to stroke patients' mobility. Three complementary research methods were used: staff questionnaire, patient questionnaire and patient shadowing.

Staff and patient questionnaires accessed two different perspectives on the role of the clinics' physical environment in the independent mobility: expert perspective and participant perspective. For this reason, they were treated as two separate methods in this study. Staff questionnaire was focused on the professional opinion of the medical staff in the participating clinics. Staff members treat and observe a large number of patients and have the experience of the most common mobility issues that patients encounter every day. Patient questionnaires were focused on the personal daily experience of the rehabilitation participants. The answers from both patient and staff questionnaires were coded and analysed using NVivo 11 Pro.

The information on the daily routine of patients in rehabilitation clinics and the physical obstacles they encounter was obtained by the shadowing method. Every issue with the physical environment that the patient experienced during the observation day was noted down. The issues were then sorted into categories and counted. A Pearson correlation coefficient was computed to assess the relationship between the number of physical environment categories, in which the patient encountered issues and their mobility level.

The research study was carried out in five German neurological rehabilitation clinics. The average surface area of the participating clinics was $16,586.20 \pm 2350.05$ m^2 and the average number of patient beds in each clinic was 214 ± 19.6. In total, 50 patients were included in the study.

The researcher spent 2 weeks in each clinic (ten working days) observing the patients and collecting the questionnaires. Ten patients were chosen for the study by each clinic. The inclusion criteria were: the patient had suffered a stroke, is over 60 years old and is able to move independently in the clinic (with or without the use

Table 1 Characteristics of the participating patients

Category	Number of patients ($n = 50$)		
Gender	Male: 26	Female: 24	
Rehabilitation phase	B: 3	C: 30	D: 17
Mobility level	Wheelchair: 13	Walker: 20	Ind. walking: 17
Barthel index for mobility	5 points: 10	10 points: 13	15 points: 27

of wheelchair, walker or other equipment). The exclusion criteria were any of the following: dementia, severe communication and cognitive impairments, severe multi-morbidity and significant mobility impairment prior to stroke.

Table 1 shows the characteristics of the participating patients, focusing on their level of mobility on the day of observation.

Barthel Index for mobility is a part of the BI scale that describes the patient's mobility on level surfaces. The categories are: immobile (0 points), wheelchair independent (5 points), walks with help of one person (10 points) and independent (15 points). BI for mobility was not used as a measure of mobility level in this study since the points did not indicate the patient's current way of moving in the building. For instance, the patient was able to walk (15 points), but was still using a walker. The mobility aid used was taken as a measure of the mobility level.

This research study was approved by the Ethical Committee at the Technische Universität Dresden (no. EK 452102016). All participants gave their written consent for the study.

4 Findings from Patient and Staff Questionnaires

Patients and staff members (nurses: $n = 42$ and therapists: $n = 4$) from five rehabilitation clinics responded to questions concerning the obstacles and barriers in their rehabilitation clinic. The patients who completed the questionnaires were the same patients who were shadowed in each clinic. Four patients were not able to fill in the questionnaire, which resulted in 46 respondents. For each observed patient, one member of the medical staff in charge of that patient completed a different questionnaire. The response rate was 92%, which resulted in 46 completed staff questionnaires in total. Both questionnaires consisted of yes/no and open-ended questions. The answers to open-ended questions were later divided into categories by the researcher.

4.1 Staff Perspective

The questionnaire for the medical staff was divided into two parts. The first part addressed the importance of the independent mobility for the patients' well-being.

The second part addressed the most frequent barriers to mobility that patients encounter in the clinic, observed by the staff members.

4.1.1 Importance of Patients' Independent Mobility

The official policy of the participating rehabilitation clinics is that the majority of patients are encouraged to go to therapies on their own. The staff members were asked the following question: 'Do you think that it is beneficial for the patients to move independently in the clinic? Why do you think that?' The question was answered positively by 87% of the respondents and 13% were neutral. The second part of the question provided a report on different reasons why independent mobility is beneficial for the patients. Table 2 summarises the answers to this question. The respondents reported the most common reasons why independent mobility is important: it is an additional exercise for patients and it promotes and maintains independence. The staff members who answered with 'not beneficial' were mostly concerned about the patients, who are not able to move independently in the building. The policy of the clinics is that only the patients who are physically and cognitively capable of being independent are allowed to go to the therapies alone.

Table 2 Reasons why patients' independent mobility is important

Category	Prevalence % (n)	Comments made by questionnaire respondents
Independence	57.4 (31)	'Rehabilitation means that the patient learns to become self-sufficient again' 'To strengthen the capabilities and prepare for home, independence is important' 'Especially in neurology and in elderly patients, it is important to maintain and promote independence and to train orientation'
Exercise	29.6 (16)	'The patient can exercise movements (primarily the ones learnt in therapy), work on increasing the mobility and walking safety, patient feels more independent and more comfortable' 'I see it as a further therapeutic activity for orientation, movement and mobility'
Not beneficial	5.5 (3)	'Different depending on the disease. In the case of dementia there is the risk that they will get lost or run away' 'Patients can get lost quickly and do not find the way back to station again'
Helping staff	3.7 (2)	'Discharge of the transport service' 'It relieves the staff'
Faster recovery	1.8 (1)	'Because the recovery can progress quicker'
Social contact	1.8 (1)	'Also very important for social contacts'

4.1.2 Barriers that Patients Encounter in the Physical Environment

Staff members participating in the study reported issues that belong to several categories: orientation, physical obstacles, visual communication and other issues (Table 3). The majority of the respondents found orientation (wayfinding) to be the main issue that patients encounter. More than 40% of the respondents consider this the main obstacle to mobility in their clinic. Patients are not able to find their way easily, they can get lost and be late for therapies. This could be a consequence of poor visual communication (signage system) in the building, as it was specifically pointed out by nine respondents in two participating clinics. The most common attributes used to describe the rehabilitation clinics by the staff in three out of five participating were: 'large', 'labyrinthine', 'with a lot of add-ons' and having 'long paths'.

4.2 Patient Perspective

Patients were asked to identify the mobility issues they encountered in relation to the building design. They were also asked whether they encountered any physical obstacles when moving independently in the clinic.

Table 3 Most common barriers to mobility reported by the medical staff

Category	Prevalence % (n)	Comments made by questionnaire respondents
Orientation	40.8 (20)	'There are always difficulties with good wayfinding of patients in our house. Reasons: brain disease, bad signage system' 'Some patients have difficulties distinguishing the various wards and floors, since they are very similar' 'Patients often have difficulties to find their way around the winding clinic and find all the rooms in the back corners'
Dimensions/ physical obstacles	24.4 (12)	'Large house, not all corridors wheelchair accessible, heavy transit traffic in the corridors' 'It is always tight on the therapy corridor (many people/ chairs)' 'Up and downhill, very winding, a lot of add-ons…'
Visual communication	18.4 (9)	'Yes. The patients do not find the way to the therapies. Better labelling (colour,…) would be useful' 'Incorrect labelling for stations and treatment rooms'
No issues	10.2 (5)	'No, everything is well described. Elevators are available, handrails are there and wide corridors'
Other issues	6.1 (3)	'Elevator takes long time' 'Electric doors often malfunctioning'

Table 4 Most common barriers to mobility reported by the observed patients

Category	Prevalence % (n)	Comments made by questionnaire respondents
Orientation	23.5 (8)	'It is difficult to orientate, I always need to look left and right' 'Wayfinding is difficult. Everything seems chaotic to me' 'Since the rooms do not have a clear arrangement, the paths are unclear'
Dimensions	20.6 (7)	'It is a bit too tight to pass with walkers or wheelchairs' 'Too many patients in hallways, too narrow, unpleasant atmosphere' "Width of the therapy corridor (too narrow), all other corridors good"
Distance	17.6 (6)	'Long corridors, I am still weak and slow when driving the wheelchair' 'Therapies need to be more centralised'
Floor	14.7 (5)	'Uneven floor tiles, carpet flooring stops movement' 'There is a connecting corridor that is a slope. This can't be handled alone using wheelchair'
Other	14.7 (5)	'Wheelchair accessible walkways are missing' 'Not good for disabled. Too few elevators'
Physical obstacles	8.8 (3)	'There is too much stuff in the hallways' 'Mats in the entrance area (main entrance)'

The participating patients reported the wayfinding issues ($n = 8$), insufficient dimensions of spaces ($n = 7$) and the long distance between spaces ($n = 6$) as the main mobility issues they encountered in connection with the architectural design of the clinics. The clinics were described as having unclear paths, long distances between therapies and narrow corridors. Table 4 summarises the patient responses together with some of their descriptive comments. Only 26% of patients responded that they did face an issue with the building design during their stay in the clinic and 22% responded that they encountered some physical obstacle when moving independently in the rehabilitation clinic. The reasons could be that the patients answering the questionnaire were in later rehabilitation phases and, therefore, having less mobility issues or their unwillingness to report experiencing mobility issues. The shadowing data showed that more patients experienced mobility issues related to the physical environment on the observation day than it was reported in their questionnaires (56% of patients during observations compared to 48% in questionnaires).

5 Findings from the Observations

Ten patients from five clinics ($n = 50$) were included in the study. Each patient was shadowed over the course of one whole day (from 08:00 to 19:00 h). This resulted in around 550 h of observations in total. Any issue connected to the built environment during the day was noted down. The mobility issues were divided into five categories, previously reported as the most important in the patient and staff questionnaires. These five categories were defined as following: *Orientation (OR)*: Difficulties with finding the way to the therapy, mistaking the corridor or the floor (does not apply to patients visiting therapy for the first time). *Dimensions (DM)*: Not having enough space to pass or to park wheelchair/walker. *Distance (DI)*: Significant issues (needing help) with reaching a certain place. *Floor (FL)*: Difficulties related to the flooring, slopes, uneven floor, etc. *Physical objects (PO)*: Issues with objects on the way such as heavy doors, unused equipment in the corridors, etc.

Wheelchair users are a group that encounters the most obstacles, predominantly in the dimensions, orientation and floor categories (Table 5). Only 35% of the patients who could walk independently encountered problems, mainly in the wayfinding category. Patients using a walker encountered mobility issues predominantly related to the orientation and physical obstacles.

There is a moderate negative correlation between the level of mobility and the number of categories in which the patients have issues ($r = -0.472$, $p<0.001$), which indicates that the level of physical impairment is related to the higher number and larger variety of obstacles in the built environment.

The comparison of patients in different rehabilitation phases (Fig. 1) shows that the B phase patients (very low mobility) encounter the most obstacles in the built

Table 5 Issues with the built environment by mobility level ($n = 50$)

Mlobility level (l)	Total no. of patients	Obstacles in the built environment		Prevalence of the obstacles				
		No	Yes	OR	DM	DI	FL	PO
$l = 1$ (wheelchair)	$n = 13$	15% $n = 2$	85% $n = 11$	23% $n = 5$	32% $n = 7$	13% $n = 3$	23% $n = 5$	9% $n = 2$
$l = 2$ (walker)	$n = 20$	45% $n = 9$	55% $n = 11$	53% $n = 8$	13% $n = 2$	7% $n = 1$	$n = 0$	27% $n = 4$
$l = 3$ (independent walking)	$n = 17$	65% $n = 11$	35% $n = 6$	72% $n = 5$	14% $n = 1$	$n = 0$	$n = 0$	14% $n = 1$

phase B (n = 3) ▬▬▬▬▬▬▬▬▬▬▬▬ 100%

phase C (n = 30) ▬▬▬▬▬▬▬▬ 70%   30%

phase D (n = 17) ▬▬▬ 35%   65%

▬ patients that had issues with the built environment
▬ patients that did not have issues with the built environment

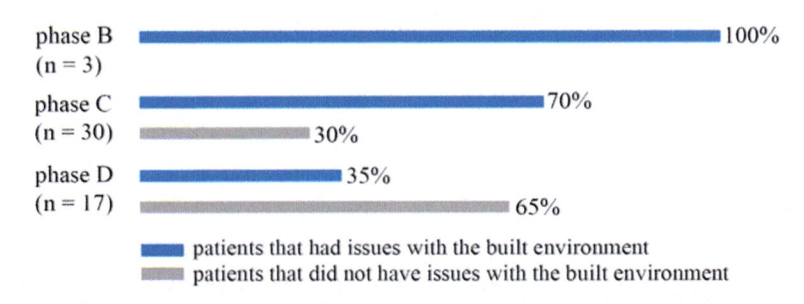

Fig. 1 Prevalence of patients' mobility issues in three rehabilitation phases

environment. The largest group of the sample belongs to the C phase and 70% of these patients did face a barrier in the physical environment on the day of the observation. Even in the group with the highest mobility (D phase), 35% of patients encountered problems with the built environment of the rehabilitation clinic. The wayfinding difficulties remain present in all the rehabilitation stages, regardless of the patient's mobility level.

6 Implications for Architectural Design

Patients (23, 5%), staff members (40, 8%) and shadowing data identify orientation as the most common issue related to the built environment of the rehabilitation clinics. This could be related to the patients' cognitive impairments after stroke, to the unclear spatial configuration of rehabilitation clinics or to the poor visual communication (signage), as pointed out by staff members (16, 4%). Besides orientation, the main barriers to mobility are insufficient dimensions of spaces (mostly corridors), large distance between spaces, issues with the floor surface and physical obstacles (objects blocking the way).

The study results indicate that the mobility issues patients face in the rehabilitation clinics are mostly related to the floor plan configuration and interior design of the rehabilitation clinics (Table 6).

Certain obstacles such as stairs or slopes in the floor can be a good training for the patients in later rehabilitation phases. Not every patient is able to overcome these barriers in the built environment. For this reason, the design of rehabilitation clinics should be in close connection to the rehabilitation phases. It is important to understand the needs of patients in each rehabilitation stage and offer an environment where every patient can feel autonomous and exercise mobility.

Small interventions, such as a clear signage design or a change of flooring could improve the problematic areas in the existing clinics. In order to design truly mobility supportive clinics, it is essential to start considering this goal in the early stages of architectural design by planning specifically designed wards for each rehabilitation phase. Patients in the B phase (where many are bed confined) should have their patient rooms closely connected to therapies and nurse stations for constant monitoring and easy wayfinding. Many patients get meals in their rooms, so only a small separate dining room could be planned. In the C phase, therapy rooms should be in close surroundings of patient rooms, reachable via the clear path. The patient should be able to go there alone or with minimal help. Separate

Design aspects/issues	OR	DM	DI	FL	PO
Floor plan configuration	•	•	•		•
Interior design	•			•	•
Signage system	•				

Table 6 Relationship between design aspects and the issues that patients encounter

dining room should be in the ward, so that the less mobile patients could go to the meals independently. The accommodation of the D phase patients should be hotel-like, where patient sleeping rooms are separate from all other activities. That way, they could train independent mobility when going to therapies and meals.

7 Discussion and Conclusion

This research study identified the most common physical barriers to mobility that stroke patients encounter in rehabilitation clinics. The findings show significant differences in experienced barriers between patients with different mobility levels.

Stroke patients in rehabilitation emphasise walking and mobility as important forms of physical activity (Luker et al. 2015). In contrast, several research studies demonstrate patients' predominant inactivity during the day. The study of walking and mobility of stroke patients after rehabilitation found that the physical environment factors influence the frequency of community walking, with the increased avoidance of environmental features that stroke survivors perceive as challenging (Robinson et al. 2013). The avoidance of barriers in the physical environment could also be one of the reasons for the patients' inactivity in the rehabilitation clinics. By posing less barriers, the building itself has the potential to actively participate in the rehabilitation process.

Rehabilitation clinics are a significant place of recovery and their design should be connected to the organisation of care. Physical and cognitive impairments of stroke patients need to be taken into account. The study results indicate that each rehabilitation stage should have specifically designed wards where every patient would be able to exercise mobility according to their physical abilities.

One limitation of the study is the small number of participants from each clinic. Additionally, only the questionnaires of the cognitively and physically able patients were available. The limitations of the methods used should be resolved in further research on the effects of the built environment on the independent mobility of patients. The next step in this research study is further data analysis to establish the set of design guidelines for mobility supportive rehabilitation clinics.

Acknowledgments This research study was funded by the European Social Fund (RL ESF Hochschule und Forschung 2014 bis 2020, no. 100235479). We also thank BDH-Klinik Hessisch Oldendorf, Aatalklinik, Gesundheitszentrum Glantal, BDH-Klinik Elzach and Schwarzwaldklinik Neurologie for their support and participation in the study.

References

Adamson J, Beswick A, Ebrahim S (2004) Is stroke the most common cause of disability? J Stroke Cerebrovasc Dis 13(4):171–177

Anåker A, Von Koch L, Sjöstrand C, Bernhardt J, Elf M (2017) A comparative study of patients' activities and interactions in a stroke unit before and after reconstruction—the significance of the built environment. PLoS ONE 12(7):1–12

De Wit L, Putman K, Dejaeger E, Baert I, Berman P, Bogaerts K et al (2005) Use of time by stroke patients: a comparison of four European rehabilitation centers. Stroke 36(9):1977–1983

Dobkin BH (2005) Rehabilitation after stroke. N Engl J Med 352(16):1677–1684

Langhorne P, Coupar F, Pollock A (2009) Motor recovery after stroke: a systematic review. Lancet Neurol 8:741–754

Luker J, Lynch E, Bernhardsson S, Bennett L, Bernhardt J (2015) Stroke survivors' experiences of physical rehabilitation: a systematic review of qualitative studies. Arch Phys Med Rehabil 96 (9):1698–1708

Robinson CA, Matsuda PN, Ciol MA, Shumway-Cook A (2013) Participation in community walking following stroke: the influence of self-perceived environmental barriers. Phys Ther 93 (5):620–627

Schönle PW (2000) Neurological rehabilitation in Germany. In: Christensen AL, Uzzell BP (eds) International handbook of neuropsychological rehabilitation. Critical issues in neuropsychology. Springer, Berlin

Skarin M, Sjöholm A, Nilsson ÅL, Nilsson M, Bernhardt J, Lindén T (2013) A mapping study on physical activity in stroke rehabilitation: establishing the baseline. J Rehabil Med 45(10): 997–1003

A Practical Tool for the Evaluation of Contrast

S. Danschutter and B. Deroisy

Abstract The provision of suitable contrast in the built environment not only contributes to a better accessibility and safety, but also improves wayfinding in buildings for all users, when applied well. Many standards on accessibility require a level of contrast for better visibility of different critical elements, such as signage, differences in floor level or the indication of treads on stairs or localisation of obstacles (furniture and sanitary fittings…). Standard descriptions are available illustrating how the contrast should be realised and where it should be provided. Unfortunately, many of these standards are difficult to put in practice and contain much other information besides the contrast requirement. This chapter describes the development of a tool, focussing on visual contrast and its use in the built environment. The tool has been developed to be easy to use by any building professionals and helps providing good contrasts in different particular situations which are integrated into the tool.

1 Introduction

Visual information is crucial for a pedestrian to interact with their immediate environment and to move around safely. Especially people with visual impairments may benefit from a better-designed environment. However, assessment methods proposed in different standards vary in contrast formula being used, type of applications and target values.

Therefore, the proposed tool offers some flexibility, by allowing to check and compare several existing standards and guidelines. How is contrast defined? Which applications are found in these documents? What are the metrics and criteria for acceptance? How can we translate these criteria to colour communication or colour

---

S. Danschutter (✉) · B. Deroisy
Belgian Building Research Insitute, Limelette, Belgium
e-mail: stefan.danschutter@bbri.be

B. Deroisy
e-mail: Bertrand.deroisy@bbri.be

classification systems such as Natural Colour System (NCS) or RAL Classic (Abk. Für Reichs-Ausschuss für Lieferbedingungen)? The purpose of the tool is to translate the information into understandable and usable information for people who are not familiar with the different notions regarding contrast used in standards and guidelines. To ensure that the tool would serve its purpose, we had regular contact with architects, specialised contractors and paint suppliers. The information obtained from this tool can be used to prescribe colours from building elements in specifications or to define requirements for building projects. This is also the phase of a building project, where the tool should be used.

Special attention was given to signage aspects, with a calculation module, allowing to determine the text size based on the research described in 'Guide to increasing accessibility in light and lighting' (CIE 2011).

2 The Calculation of Contrast

Before calculating contrast, it is important that the term is correctly defined. In EN 12665 (Bureau voor Normalisatie 2011, art. 3.1.5), contrast is stated as:

1. In the perceptual sense: An assessment of the difference in the appearance of two or more parts of a field seen simultaneously or successively (hence, brightness contrast, lightness contrast, colour contrast, simultaneous contrast, successive contrast...)
2. In the physical sense: Quantity intended to correlate with the perceived brightness contrast, usually defined by one of a number of formulae, which involve the luminances of the stimuli considered, for example: $\Delta L/L$ near the luminance threshold, or L_1/L_2 for much higher luminances.

These definitions suggest that there are many possible ways to define contrast. The perception of contrast is influenced by many parameters, so an accurate prediction is rather complicated (Van de Perre et al. 2016). Nevertheless, to approximate the brightness contrast, most standards and guidelines on the accessibility of buildings make use of contrast formula, which are characterised by the difference in the photometric quantity luminance (L) or even a difference in light reflectance value (LRV). The CIE-report (2011) is an exception. It describes an alternative concept of '*categorical colour perception*', where colours are divided into basic categories (red, orange, yellow, green–yellow, green...), which can result in colour contrast. The assumption is that colours will not be confused with each other when belonging to different basic colour categories. It is explicitly stated that the use of such basic colour categories is insufficient for people who have a deficiency in the perception of colour. It was decided not to use this theory in the development of the tool, as the method is rather complex and an important group of users is excluded (people with colour deficiency).

The luminance contrast was taken as the most robust metric. But different formulas for luminance contrast are proposed (Danschutter et al. 2010). An architect

Table 1 A review of some contrast formula and the associated acceptance criteria

Document	ISO 21542 (ISO 2011)	BS 8300 (BSI 2009)	DIN 32975 (DIN 2012)	INLB (CISSS 2017)	AS 1428.1 (Australian Standard 2001)
Contrast formula	[4]	[4]	[2a]	[1a]	[1a]
Criteria	15 points	15 points	40%	70%	[1a] on site
	30 points	20 points	70%		[5] 30%
	60 points	30 points			
		70 points			

can refer to national guidelines, where a certain formula is suggested (in Belgium the Weber formula is mostly used), or he can refer to sources where other contrast formulas are implemented. During a review, the following contrast formulas were found and thus integrated into the tool:

[1] Webers formula: [a] $(L_2 - L_1)/L_2$ or [b] $(LRV_2 - LRV_1)/LRV_2$
[2] Michelsons formula: [a] $(L_2 - L_1)/(L_2 + L_1)$ or [b] $(LRV_2 - LRV_1)/(LRV_2 + LRV_1)$
[3] Bowmans formula: [a] $(L_2 - L_1)/0.5 * (L_2 + L_1)$ or [b] $(LRV_2 - LRV_1)/0.5 * (LRV_2 + LRV_1)$
[4] Cooks formula: $LRV_2 - LRV_1$
[5] Bowman–Sapolinskis formula: $(250*|LRV_2 - LRV_1|)/(LRV_1 + LRV_2 + 25)$

L is the luminance (see above) and LRV is the light reflectance value as defined by BS 8493 (BSI 2008).

These formulas were found in a number of standards and guidelines as listed in Table 1. The use of these formulas requires some caution as some are based on 'light reflectance values' and 'luminances' values as input, while others should only be used with the 'light reflectance value' (see the list above). Although this would be desirable, it appears difficult to converge to a unique formula and unit for the evaluation of brightness contrast. However, this could be solvable, especially considering that all these formulas are approximate.

3 The Development of a Calculation Tool

The variety of definitions creates ambiguity when defining contrast. Therefore, the tool had to be clear in its definitions and documents it was referring to. On the other hand, building professionals can be confronted with other standards and guidelines, so a key feature of the tool is its flexibility. It was decided to create two levels:

1. A basic tool, checking compliance with the international standard ISO 21542 (ISO 2011) and its criteria for different applications: contrast on doors, contrast on stairs, contrast for TWSI (Tactile Walking Surface Indicators), contrast for signage... After choosing colours by its RAL or NCS code, the tools checks if the criterion that was set is met.
2. A more advanced tool, where users can choose a reference document with its contrast formula and acceptance criterion. After choosing an application from this document, the procedure remains the same. Select the first colour from a certain colour communication or classification system. The second colour can be chosen freely or restrained by the set criterion and contrast formula. It is then possible to check different standards, containing different contrast formulas and acceptance criteria.

Defining a difference in terms of LRV-values in specifications is interesting, but often not practical if you are used to work with colour classification or colour specification systems. Architects often specify the colours of the building elements with these systems. With this tool, it should be possible to find out if the chosen colours respond to the applicable contrast value as from preliminary design phases.

The ISO 21542 standard contains two important threshold values that can be used for different situations (the difference of $\Delta LRV \geq 15$ points is an exception and used for door hinges):

1. $\Delta LRV \geq 30$ points, for large surface areas (i.e. walls, floors, doors, ceiling) elements and components to facilitate orientation (i.e. handrails, switches and controls, tactile walking surface indicators, and visual indicators on glazed areas)
2. $\Delta LRV \geq 60$ points, for potential hazards and self-contrasting markings (i.e. visual indicator on steps) and text information (i.e. signage)

These situations are rather specific, but within the standard you often find more information on how the contrast should preferably be used (e.g. width of contrasting tread nosing on stairs, the use of contrast on doors, when to use contrast on TWSI...). This offers extra support on how to provide good contrast. A list of situations was created for the tool. When a selection is made, an acceptance criterion (ISO 21542) and more information on how to apply the contrast is displayed. Some examples of different situations are given in Table 2. For clarity, all situations are always illustrated with a figure, not necessarily coming from standards or guidelines, but illustrative of the situation at hand.

The basic version of the tool was presented to architects, paint suppliers and painters on a number of occasions. They gave feedback on how the tool could evolve and what information was necessary to use it.

For the more advanced tool, the available situations are dependent on the chosen document, with a description, illustration and criterion. The tool administrator can add situations and documents, in this way it can evolve and include experience from practice and infield measurements. The user interface for the basic version is shown in Fig. 1, the more advanced version can be found in Fig. 2. A licence was obtained

Table 2 Example of situations

Situation	Illustration		Criterion
Tactile walking surface indicator			≥ 30 points
Sanitary fittings			≥ 30 points
Joinery—door leaf			≥ 30 points
Signage			≥ 60 points

to copy crucial information from ISO 21542 and ISO 23599, but this was not the case for other standards. The more advanced tool is not freely available. Instead, a blank file was made that can be filled in by the user.

4 Important Considerations

The tool was developed to choose colours in advance, allowing specifiers to make a choice that gives sufficient contrast. It presupposes that sufficient light is available to view the contrast, it can also only be used for opaque, diffuse reflecting surfaces (most building elements). So glossy surfaces or light-emitting signage cannot be correctly evaluated. It is also no guarantee that the same contrast will be obtained on site, other factors such as humidity, discolouration, pollution, or other factors such

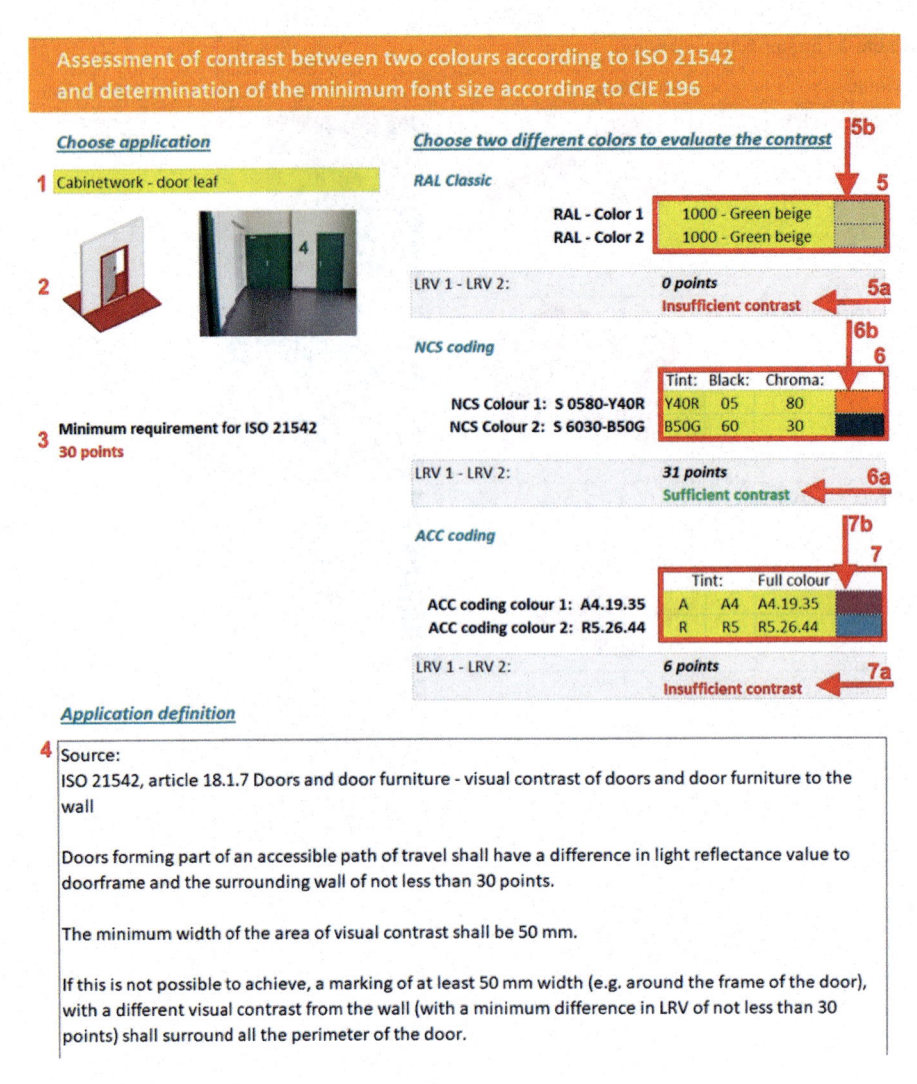

Fig. 1 Procedure using the tool—Version 1.0

[1] Choose an application – the list of applications is based on a review of ISO 21542, it does not guarantee that all situations where contrast is relevant are integrated in the tool.
[2] An illustration of the chosen application, showing how to add contrast. Illustrations where not taken from the standard, but they show how the contrast can be applied.
[3] A minimum contrast of 30 points is required for this application → LRV_1-$LRV_2 \geq 30$.
[4] A description on how the contrast should be provided for the chosen application. For instance, contrasting stair nosing should have certain dimensions and be placed on the riser and the going of the stair for optimal visibility.
[5] Option1: The user can chose 2 colours from het RAL Classic Colour communication system to verify if they give sufficient contrast (30 points). [5b] a representation of the chosen colours, in this case both colours are Green beige, so both cells are the same and the obtained contrast is insufficient (0 points) [5a].
[6] Option 2: The user can chose 2 colours form the NCS Colour Classification system to verify if they give sufficient contrast (30 points). Three drop downs (Tint, Black & Chroma) define a colour. [6b] a representation of the chosen colours in excel, in this case the obtained contrast is sufficient, S 0580-Y40R and S 6030-B50G give a difference in LRV of 31 points [6a].
[7] Option 3: Additional colour systems can be added to the spreadsheet by the tool administrator. This colour classification system is comparable with NCS and has also 3 drop downs: 2 for the tint and a third one for the full colour. Resulting in a representation of the chosen colour [7b] and an indication whether sufficient contrast is obtained [7a].
Additional colour systems can be added in the future.

Fig. 1 (continued)

as light distribution (shadows) can reduce the foreseen contrast. Following-up, the building process is required to obtain a good result on site. Good contrast could also be obtained with lighting conditions (light and dark areas) and/or colour differences, but such an approach is not dealt with in this tool.

5 Signage

Special attention was also given to the evaluation of signage. Good signage is not only related to the provision of sufficient contrast, but many other perceptual factors are involved. It's hard to control all these elements in a practical tool without creating excessive complexity. For instance, the viewing distance is based on the type of signage and the height of installation, railway timetables are viewed from a much larger distance than nameplates at a door. The user of the tool decides what distance should be used for this application. The information on signage is based on the CIE 196 report (CIE 2011; Sagawa and Kurakata 2013), which contains recommendations for the minimum letter size as a function of lighting conditions, distance of observation, and age of the observer. Other reports were also considered, like the research commissioned by ANEC 'New standard for the visual accessibility of signs and signage for people with low vision' (Lenoir et al. 2010) which contains information for the dimensioning of signage for people with low vision. But it was noticed that this results in much larger letters than the previous

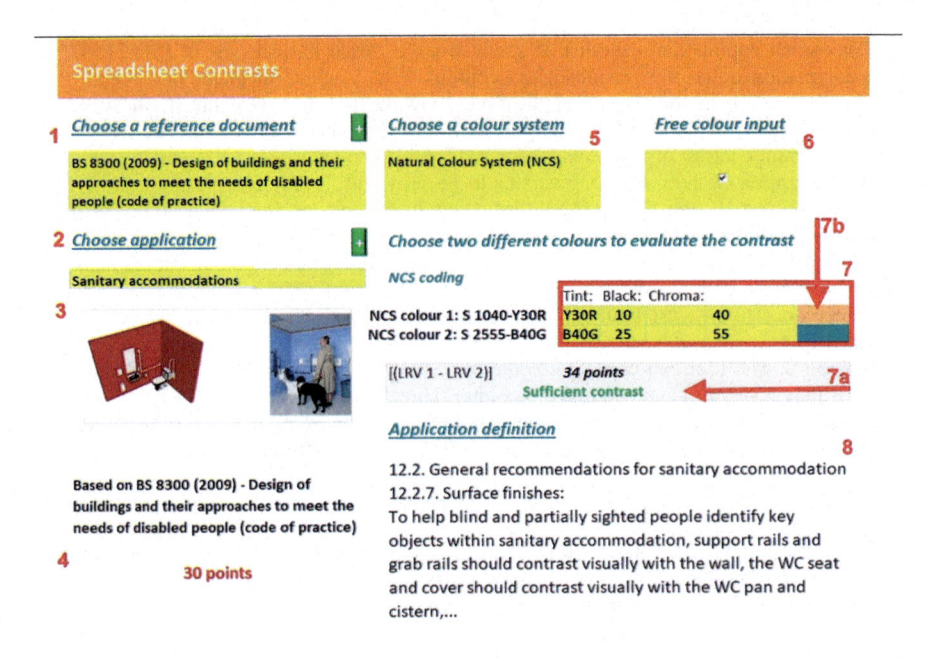

[1] Choose a reference document, several standards and guidelines are integrated in this version of het spreadsheet. Additional.
[2] A list of applications appears from which the user can chose, the list is based on a review from the chosen reference document. It does not guarantee that all situations where contrast is relevant are integrated in the tool.
[3] An illustration of the chosen application, showing how to add contrast. Illustrations where not taken from the standard, but they show how the contrast can be applied.
[4] A minimum contrast of 30 points is required for this application → $LRV_1-LRV_2 \geq 30$.
[5] A dropdown allows the user to choose from different colour communication or colour classification systems. The options for the colour picking [7] are dependent on the choice that was made here (in this case NCS).
Additional colour systems can be added in the future.
[6] This checkbox is selected in its standard position, both colours can be chosen freely, when not selected, the second colour choice will be restricted by the first colour, the contrast formula and the criterion that is applicable for the chose application and reference document.
[7] The drop downs for the chosen colour system are shown, in this case NCS [5], as within version 1.0, the two colours are picked. A representation of the two colours [7b] and an indication whether sufficient contrast is obtained [7a] is also added.
[8] A description on how the contrast should be provided for the chosen application and reference document.

Fig. 2 Procedure when using the tool—Version 1.1

one (observation as a function of age). The advanced version of the tool allows to adapt the method described in CIE 196 (CIE 2011), so it can be used for people with low vision (VA = 0.3 or lower). This method is also proposed in DIN 32975 (DIN 2012), by replacing the visual acuity with lower values, the text size of signs

Table 3 Letter size and type of signage according to different standards

Standard	Letter type	Letter size
ISO 21542	The font should be a sans serif font similar to Helvetica or Arial medium	The *letter height* depends on the reading distance. A letter height between 20 and 30 mm for each metre of viewing distance is preferred. The letter height should not be less than 15 mm
BS 8300	Any sans serif typeface with a relatively large x-height (lower case letter height should be used	For long viewing distances *x-height* of minimum 150 mm. For medium viewing distances an x-height of 50–100 mm and for short viewing distances an x-height of 15–25 mm should be provided. As a rule of thumb, a blind or partially sighted person is likely to be able to read text on a signboard when the x-height is approximately 5.7% of the viewing distance
DIN 32975	The use of sans serif font is advised + referring to CIE Guide 196 (CIE 2011)	The letter size [P] is based on the formula described in CIE Guide 196, while considering a visual acuity of 0.1 (20/200, 6/60 VA or people with low vision). Detailed information on letter choice and spacing can also be found in DIN 1450. The observation angle is also taken into account when determining the minimum font size (e.g. railway timetables)
INLB	Gives a few font types that can be used	The letter size is 1/30 of the viewing distance

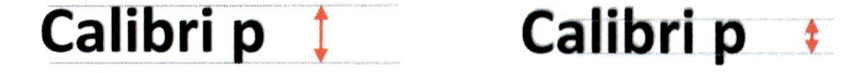

Calibri p ↕   Calibri p ↕

Fig. 3 Illustration of letter height (left) and x-height (right)

increases, DIN 32975 proposes a value of 0.1 as a reference for the visual acuity when dimensioning text (Table 3).

The information on signage is dispersed and often difficult to implement. Values for letter size are formulated in different ways, see Fig. 3. The creation of knowledge platform on the subjects of contrast, signage seems useful and could also handle questions of wayfinding in a broader sense (United States Sign Council Foundation 2017).

6 Conclusions

The different contrast formula and acceptance criteria in accessibility standards complicate the communication about contrasts. Most contrast formulas that are used in accessibility standards are approximate, so it should be possible to evolve towards one unified formula. On the other hand, the perception of contrast is influenced by many factors, all of which cannot be controlled precisely in the design phase. Our tool starts with the situation as it is today and offers support in the choice of colours providing adequate contrast for several precise situations, while respecting most used standards. It is a practical resource that should be used correctly within a global wayfinding approach. It could hopefully contribute to the discussion on how to better integrate accessibility aspects into the buildings and in the design process. The tool was released in May 2017 and can be downloaded from our website (http://www.toegankelijk.be/index.cfm?n01=projects&n02=Projecten_Projecten_Partners&n03=Tool).

References

Australian Standard (2001) 1428-1: Design for access and mobility, general requirements for access, new building works. Standards Australia, Sydney

BSI (2008) BS 8493—Light reflectance value (LRV) of a surface—method of test. British Standard Institution, London, UK

BSI (2009) BS 8300—Design of buildings and their approaches to meet the needs of disabled people—code of practice. British Standard Institution, London, UK

Bureau voor Normalisatie (2011) NBN EN 12665—Light and lighting—basic terms and criteria for specifying lighting requirements, p 53

CIE (2011) CIE 196—Guide to increasing accessibility in light and lighting—vision data and design considerations for better visibility and lighting for older people and people with disabilities. International Commission on Illumination, Vienna, Austria

CISSS (2017) Institut Nazareth and Louis Braille. http://www.inlb.qc.ca/grand-public/accessibilite-et-adaptation/amenagements-des-lieux/. Accessed 10 Mar 2017

Danschutter S, D'Herdt P, Deneyer A (2010) Eclairage et contraste pour les personnes malvoyantes, vol 3, no 12. WTCB-Dossier, Brussels, Belgium, pp 1–5

DIN (2012) DIN 32975—Gestaltung visueller Informationen im öffentlichen Raum zur barrierefreien Nutzung. Beuth Verlag, Berlin

ISO (2011) ISO 21542—Accessibility and usability of the built environment. International Organization for Standardization, Switzerland

Lenoir M, Den Brinker B, Kestelyn P, Leroy B, Jonia I, Walraedt S et al (2010) New standard for the visual accessibility of signs and signage for people with low vision. ANEC report, ANEC-DFA-2008-G-044-Annex 6rev

Sagawa K, Kurakata K (2013) Estimation of legible font size for elderly people—accessible design of characters in signs and displays and its standardization. Synthesiology 6(1):34–44

United States Sign Council Foundation (2017) www.usscfoundation.org. Accessed 17 Nov 2017

Van de Perre L, Hanselaer P, Scheir GH, Smet K, Ryckaert WR (2016) Contrast metrics evaluation. In: Proceedings of CIE 2016, Melbourne, Australia, 3–5 Mar 2016, pp 70–78

Part IV
Breaking Down Barriers Between People with Impairments and Those Without

Breaking Down Barriers Between Undergraduate Computing Students and Users with Disabilities

Jonathan Lazar

Abstract One of the subthemes of the 2018 CWUAAT is "Breaking down barriers between people with impairments and those without impairments." This chapter describes an innovative undergraduate class that has, over a 10-year period, broken down barriers between undergraduate computing students without disabilities and computer users with disabilities. The chapter discusses the need for teaching about ICT accessibility within the computing curriculum, and offers details on how to implement innovative approaches in an undergraduate class, including field trips, and one-to-one partnerships between students and computer users with disabilities outside of the university community.

1 Introduction

Most undergraduate students in the computing majors (computer science, information systems, and information technology) do not have personal experience in interacting with or designing technology for people with disabilities. Students often come in with stereotypes, preconceived notions, and incorrect assumptions. Trying to dispel these notions can often be challenging using only standard classroom techniques. This chapter describes the approaches used by the author over a 10-year period at Towson University, to connect undergraduate computing students without disabilities to the community of computer users with disabilities, breaking down barriers between these two populations.

It is important to note that these are not two discrete groups (undergraduate students and people with disabilities). There are usually students with disabilities on any given campus, but often, these students have been incorrectly convinced that

---

J. Lazar (✉)
Department of Computer and Information Sciences,
Towson University, Towson, MD, USA
e-mail: jlazar@towson.edu; jklhci@pennlaw.upenn.edu

J. Lazar
University of Pennsylvania Law School, Philadelphia, PA, USA

© Springer International Publishing AG, part of Springer Nature 2018
P. Langdon et al. (eds.), *Breaking Down Barriers*,
https://doi.org/10.1007/978-3-319-75028-6_15

the STEM (Science Technology Engineering and Mathematics) majors are not for them. Despite efforts for STEM education to be more inclusive, e.g. the AccessComputing and AccessEngineering projects (University of Washington 2017), the percentage of students with disabilities in the STEM majors continues to be low. This becomes what Dan Goldstein refers to as a "death spiral": Students without disabilities in the STEM fields do not know or interact with any people with disabilities, leading them to not consider people with disabilities in the designing of technologies. These inaccessible technologies are then utilized in STEM fields and in STEM education, further excluding people with disabilities from education and practice in these STEM careers (Lazar et al. 2015). We can help to stop this cycle of exclusion by connecting people with disabilities with students who will be designing the technologies of the future. In parallel, the author of this chapter has also been involved in initiatives to make professional organizations for computing more inclusive for people with disabilities (Lazar et al. 2017a).

2 The Need for Accessibility Content in the Curriculum

The lack of ICT accessibility content in the undergraduate computing curriculum was a problem that the author of this chapter first identified and wrote about more than 15 years ago (Lazar 2002). Happily, it is possible to report that there have been some improvements since then. Putnam et al. (2016) identify a number of universities that are now teaching about ICT accessibility, including prestigious universities, such as Harvard, MIT, the University of Washington and Cornell University. Unfortunately, the ICT accessibility content is often an elective, or a course added on towards the end of the undergraduate career, rather than integrated throughout the academic requirements. This "tacked on the end" approach limits the usefulness of learning these topics, since students may simply view accessibility as "optional," an "add-on" or something to do "later on." It has been well-established that adding accessibility after the fact, known as "retrofitting," adds to costs and complexity, making it unlikely that accessibility will actually take place (Wentz et al. 2011). When accessibility is included proactively, as a design specification, as a part of the initial design, the costs are considered to be low and the design is considered to be better. An individual in charge of accessibility for a state government has told the chapter author that for web accessibility, the difference between retrofitting after the fact, and proactively including accessibility in the design specifications, has a great impact on the costs. This individual has said that proactive accessibility adds only 1% to the budget for web development, whereas retroactive accessibility is estimated to cost around 7% of a website budget. So in the real world, there are financial incentives to address accessibility early on, and it is important that those same messages get across to undergraduate students, that accessibility should be integrated throughout the development process, rather than an add-on at the end of the development. The University of Dundee in Scotland is one of the few universities to take this "injection" approach to teaching accessibility, where it is included as a topic throughout the undergraduate curriculum (Waller et al. 2009). There has also been an organization called "Teach Access," founded by companies such as Microsoft, Google, Facebook, and Yahoo!, that focuses on getting universities to teach more content about ICT accessibility within computing curricula (TeachAccess 2017).

Unlike graduate students, who may be focused on a specific topic within accessibility and work on collaborations that cross semesters and even academic years, undergraduates are often taking multiple course topics, and projects must often wrap up within a semester time frame. This makes it harder to form long-term bonds and understandings between students and users with disabilities (Lazar 2011). Therefore, it is imperative to create a memorable, lasting experience for students, on the topic of interface design for people with disabilities.

3 Logistics and the Need to Leave the Campus

There are many logistical challenges with trying to introduce students to accessibility-related topics. Realistically, you cannot often do a proper job in communicating the topic if the students and the faculty member only stay on a university campus. The following sections detail why simply staying on campus will not meet the goal of fully introducing students to accessibility-related topics.

3.1 Limited Number of Technologies on Campus

A specific university is unlikely to have a full range of assistive technologies available for students to interact with. Many universities do have an office of Disability Student Services, which serves students (and perhaps faculty) with disabilities. Often these offices come under different names and different academic structures (some offices fall under student affairs, others fall under academic affairs). While such an office may have basic assistive technologies available (e.g., screen readers, magnifiers, and OCR scanning techniques), these offices are unlikely to have technologies not utilized in a classroom setting, for instance, point-of-sale terminals, voting machines, or large-scale Braille embossers.

3.2 Limited Number of People on Campus

You are unlikely to have a large number of, or a wide range of people with different disabilities, available on your campus, for students to interact with. If you have people with specific disabilities who are willing to engage with students and the administration, often, these individuals will receive a high number of requests for interaction, to serve in many roles, many committees, many research studies and may be overburdened (Dee and Hanson 2014).

3.3 Just Bringing People to Campus Isn't a Good Idea

It might seem that, if there aren't enough people with disabilities available on your campus for students to interact with, then you should just bring people to campus to meet with your students, right? There are multiple reasons why this isn't a good idea. First of all, transportation may be a challenge for some users with disabilities and the university may have some facilities that are inaccessible (Lazar et al. 2017b). Second, the learning is minimal when someone with a disability comes into a physical and technical environment that students are already familiar and comfortable with. Instead, it is important for students to see people with disabilities in their home and work settings, which are often maximized for accessibility, to see what is possible (with accessibility features that often may be lacking at the university). Third, performance on tasks will be maximized in the physical and technical environments which the users with disabilities have already optimized, allowing for students to see the potential capability of a user, rather than the barriers that may exist at a university (Lazar et al. 2017b). Fourth, if it is possible, seeing different environments utilized by different users, allows for students to understand that each individual is unique and may have different needs requiring different adaptations to physical and technical environments.

3.4 Before Understanding Technology, You Need to Understand Capability

Furthermore, if students only experience the technologies available on a specific campus, they will miss one major point: part of studying accessibility is understanding the *capabilities* of people with disabilities (Wobbrock et al. 2011). Often, students, especially those who don't have previous experience interacting with people with disabilities, have a limited view of what people with disabilities are capable of. Put another way, undergraduate students often say, "well, I know that Blind people can't do X," when they actually have no knowledge or experience of interacting with Blind people or knowing what they are or are not capable of. So, before you can teach students about specific technologies or design methods, it's important to break down those stereotypes, those barriers, those preconceived notions about the capabilities of people with disabilities. When you can break down those stereotypes, then students can more fully focus on designing for people with disabilities, without their stereotypes (their barriers) getting in the way.

4 The "Interface Design for Blind Users" Class

Over a 10-year period, a class has been offered at Towson University approximately once a year, informally called "Interface Design for Blind Users." (The formal name, "Universal Usability" was decided by a committee and really doesn't accurately represent the class content, since the class focuses strictly on Blind users.). This class is an elective for Information Systems and Information Technology majors, most of whom are in their senior year. While it would be ideal to offer the class, and the experiences, to freshman and sophomores, the current structure of the majors does not allow for such a scenario.

To meet some of the logistical challenges described in Sect. 3, the class is structured around a series of four field trips to local sites in the Baltimore area, which are involved with Blindness. It is important to note that the first two listed here (BISM and NFB) are private organizations, and the second pair (LBPH and MDTAP) are a part of state government.

BISM: *Blind Industries and Services of Maryland* is an organization that among other things, provides "Blindness adjustment" training for individuals to learn the full range of nonvisual techniques. Over a 6-to-9 month period, students in the training program at BISM learn Braille, assistive technology, job readiness, orientation and mobility, independent living, and woodshop. Some of the final requirements before completing the training program are to cook dinner from scratch (without the use of any mixes) for 40 people and to build a small piece of furniture using power tools. The stated purpose of the organization is to "positively change people's attitudes about Blindness," and when undergraduate students visit BISM, meet the students, and understand what Blind people are capable of, it certainly does change their attitude about Blindness.

NFB: *The National Federation of the Blind*, the largest organization of Blind people in the United States, has their national headquarters in Baltimore, Maryland. The International Braille and Technology Center at the headquarters is a large resource center containing one of almost every technology in the world for Blind people, including screen readers, magnifiers, portable devices, GPS, voting machines, braille displays and embossers, tactile graphic devices, and many other types of accessible technologies. This is the biggest Blindness technology center in the USA.

LBPH: *The Maryland Library for the Blind and Physically Handicapped* provides services for Marylanders with print-related disabilities, including those who have trouble seeing print, physically handling print or cognitively processing print. Books can be provided free of charge to qualified patrons in multiple formats, including large-print, Braille, and audio. There are also cultural and interest groups meeting at the library, including a technology user group, and there is a comfortable children's reading area in the library. The LBPH is affiliated with the US Library of Congress National Library Service (NLS) for the Blind and Physically Handicapped and is a part of the Maryland State Library.

MD TAP: *The Maryland Technology Assistance Program* provides a range of assistive technologies and equipment that can be loaned out for Marylanders with disabilities to try out, free of charge. In addition to a demonstration center with various assistive technologies and adaptive devices, Marylanders can borrow these devices for up to a few months, to determine if the device would meet their needs. MD TAP doesn't actually sell any items, it only demonstrates items, lends them out and helps provide low-interest loans to Marylanders with disabilities. MD TAP is a project under the Federal Assistive Technology Act of 2004, under which every US state receives funding to help promote the access to, and awareness of, assistive technology. The Maryland Technology Assistance Program is a part of the state Department of Disabilities.

The field trips have been a core requirement of the class, since the class was first created a decade ago. The course is offered once a week, usually from 2–4:40 PM in the afternoon. The field trips cannot require that students do anything outside of the scheduled class time or miss any other classes. Since most of the field trips are within 15–20 min of the campus, the students can leave the Towson University campus at 2 PM, arrive at the field trip site, typically the tours last from 2:45–4 PM, and then students immediately leave and return to the campus. This schedule balances two constraints: (1) students cannot miss any of their other scheduled classes and (2) most of the sites are only open for visiting during weekdays, and tours cannot be provided on nights or weekends. It is important to note three other logistics with the field trips: (1) students are responsible for providing their own transportation, (2) all students must sign a legal waiver, protecting the university, department, and professor in case there are any injuries or accidents, and (3) students are required to abide by a strict professional dress code for the field trips.

5 Projects in the Class and Breaking Down Barriers

Since the class was first offered in 2007, there were two related goals: field trips to give students the opportunity to meet people with disabilities and to get to know the service organizations better, and a separate project with the general goal for students to get hands-on experience with the accessibility of technologies. For the projects, over the years, the students have partnered with Federal agencies (the US Department of Agriculture), state agencies (evaluating the accessibility of Maryland State government websites), county agencies (the Baltimore County Public Library system), and even university offices (working with the Office of Technology Services at Towson University). In all of these projects, students either evaluated the existing level of accessibility, provided suggestions on how to improve accessibility or both. Perhaps the best example of a class project was the project in the 2014 class, where the professor created a partnership with the Baltimore County Public Library. Students evaluated current accessibility and came up with suggested improvements for accessibility. In the past, the library had not considered the needs of patrons with print-related disabilities, figuring that the Maryland Library for the

Blind and Physically Handicapped took on that role. However, as more library resources were moving to digital format rather than print (e.g., digital libraries, newspaper, magazine subscriptions online, etc.), the library saw the opportunity to focus on how they could serve people with print disabilities at local branches. At the library's request, the students focused on five distinct areas: (1) website accessibility and maintenance, (2) staff awareness and training, (3) physical environment of the library, (4) library offerings, including databases, materials, and equipment and (5) marketing materials (Lazar and Briggs 2015). More information about those findings is available in Lazar and Briggs (2015), and there is also a video of the final student presentations available (Towson University 2014).

In the Spring 2017 class, after the four field trips were completed, students made repeated requests to go back to these sites. They wanted to meet more Blind people and interact with them more. Based on those requests, the author of this chapter created a different approach to a project, focusing on creating meaningful one-to-one connections between students and Blind people in the community. But it wouldn't be enough to only focus on meeting people, because the class itself is a computing class, not a sociology class. The connections between people, therefore, had to be focused around a computing topic. It was decided that the connections between people would focus around the topic of what frustrates them as a Blind user, with technology.

The author of this chapter had previously done research about the topic of Blind user frustration with websites, having 100 Blind users fill out a series of time diaries, documenting the causes of their frustration, the solutions, and the corresponding time lost (Lazar et al. 2007). But the purpose of this class wasn't to do a research study, nor were the undergraduates sufficiently trained in research methodology for collecting valid data. Due to the thorough previous testing, the same time diary materials from 2007 were used (after being slightly updated), but not with a goal of research, but rather simply to be used for structuring the conversations. Since the research materials that were being used, had previously needed to be approved by the institutional review board (IRB) at the university, the IRB was contacted, simply to confirm that no IRB approval was needed, since this was an educational activity with no research goals. The IRB confirmed that indeed, as a non-research activity, no IRB approval was needed.

Each undergraduate student was partnered with a Blind individual in the local community (and it's important to note that while, in some semesters, there are Blind students as a part of the undergraduate class, this time there were not any Blind students in the class). These partnerships were formed through collaboration with three local chapters of the National Federation of the Blind, all of which were geographically close (10–20 min transit) to the university. Each student was encouraged to contact their partner and set up a time to informally meet. While a few students chose to meet for dinner, most of them met their partner for something informal, such as coffee or pizza. The meeting allowed the students and the Blind individual to talk one-on-one and get to know each other. The students were encouraged to ask their partner about what frustrates them, as a Blind user, with various technologies. After their face-to-face meetings, students sent their partners a short time diary to fill out, documenting the frustrations that they face with technology. The students were then expected to give a short presentation in the class, about the Blind person that they collaborated with, and about the frustrations that the individual faces with inaccessible technology.

In the class presentations, students told many interesting stories about the Blind people that they collaborated with, their life experiences, and how the students were now more committed to ensuring a world of fully accessible technology. One of the more interesting stories was how a student was supposed to meet his partner at a Panera restaurant, and when he got there, he saw someone with a white cane, and went over to introduce himself. It turns out, it wasn't his partner, it was another Blind individual, but the student started talking with this individual while waiting for his partner to arrive. When the student presented in class, he excitedly commented that he now had two Blind partners!

The course experience can be summed up by comments from students that appeared on the course evaluations. These comments have included the following:

> the class is very interesting to learn and a "must-take" for people who simply do not understand the world of the disabled', 'I learned a ton of valuable insights that helped me grow as an individual in society', '[the course was] extremely eye-opening, unlike any class you'll ever take!', 'Gives insight to why it is important to not forget about Blind people when it comes to technology', 'The ability to be able to go out and see a lot of what we could only read about before', 'I never interacted with a Blind person before this class, but now I am more comfortable interacting with [Blind People]' and 'I never took a class like this where I got to interact with what we were learning before, so this was a fresh way of learning and it really helped me understand people with disabilities better and gave me a new prospective that I probably wouldn't have had if we didn't take these field trips or meet the people that we did.

6 Summary

It is important to teach students about ICT accessibility. However, just reading about accessibility isn't sufficient (as one student mentioned in the course evaluations). To truly learn about ICT accessibility, it is necessary to experience different types of technology, different environments of usage and to get to know the users themselves. It is, therefore, necessary to get students out of the classroom and into the real world environment, interacting with various technologies unavailable at the university, and interacting with people who are not based at the university, learning about ICT in a hands-on, experiential approach. Having students meet with and collaborate with individuals with disabilities, not only helps students gain a better understanding of ICT accessibility, but it helps to break down the barriers between undergraduate computing students without disabilities and computer users with disabilities, leading to a more inclusive world of computing.

Acknowledgements The author of this chapter would like to acknowledge the time contributed by the employees at the field trip sites: MDTAP, NFB, BISM, and LBPH, to providing excellent educational experiences for the students. The author would also like to acknowledge the work of the partners in projects from previous semesters: the US Department of Agriculture, MD Department of Disabilities, the Baltimore County Public Library system, and the Office of Technology Services at Towson University. The author would also like to gratefully acknowledge the 27 partners from the National Federation of the Blind, who collaborated with students at Towson University during the Spring 2017 semester.

References

Dee M, Hanson VL (2014) A large user pool for accessibility research with representative users. In: Proceedings of the 16th international ACM SIGACCESS conference on computers and accessibility, Rochester, NY, US, 20–22 October 2014, pp 35–42

Lazar J (2002) Integrating accessibility into the information systems curriculum. In: Proceedings of the international association for computer information systems, pp 373–379

Lazar J (2011) Using community-based service projects to enhance undergraduate HCI education: 10 years of experience. In: CHI'11 extended abstracts on human factors in computing systems, Vancouver, BC, Canada, 7–12 May 2011, pp 581–588

Lazar J, Briggs I (2015) Improving services for patrons with print disabilities at public libraries. The Libr Q 85(2):172–184

Lazar J, Goldstein DF, Taylor A (2015) Ensuring digital accessibility through process and policy. Morgan Kaufmann/Elsevier, Waltham

Lazar J, Allen A, Kleinman J, Malarkey C (2007) What frustrates screen reader users on the web: a study of 100 blind users. Int J Hum Comput Interact 22(3):247–269

Lazar J, Churchill EF, Grossman T, Van der Veer G, Palanque P, Morris JS et al (2017a) Making the field of computing more inclusive. Commun ACM 60(3):50–59

Lazar J, Feng JH, Hochheiser H (2017b) Research methods in human-computer interaction, 2nd edn. Morgan Kaufmann/Elsevier, Cambridge

Putnam C, Dahman M, Rose E, Cheng J, Bradford G (2016) Best practices for teaching accessibility in university classrooms: cultivating awareness, understanding, and appreciation for diverse users. ACM Trans Accessible Comput (TACCESS) 8(4):13

TeachAccess (2017). http://teachaccess.org/. Accessed 15 Nov 2017

Towson University (2014) TU/BCPL presentation. https://www.youtube.com/watch?v=9BOIhKHQdo8&feature=youtu.be. Accessed 15 Nov 2017

University of Washington (2017) AccessComputing: the alliance for access to computing careers. https://www.washington.edu/accesscomputing/. Accessed 15 Nov 2017

Waller A, Hanson VL, Sloan D (2009) Including accessibility within and beyond undergraduate computing courses. In: Proceedings of the 11th international ACM SIGACCESS conference on computers and accessibility, Pittsburgh, PA, US, 28–28 Oct 2009, pp 155–162

Wentz B, Jaeger PT, Lazar J (2011) Retrofitting accessibility: The legal inequality of after-the-fact online access for persons with disabilities in the United States. First Monday 16(11)

Wobbrock JO, Kane SK, Gajos KZ, Harada S, Froehlich J (2011) Ability-based design: concept, principles and examples. ACM Trans Accessible Comput (TACCESS) 3(3):9

Improving Design Understanding of Inclusivity in Autonomous Vehicles: A Driver and Passenger *Taskscape* Approach

M. Strickfaden and P. M. Langdon

Abstract Recent developments in autonomous vehicle technology now make SAE Levels 3–5 vehicles (Walker Smith in SAE levels of driving automation. http://cyberlaw.stanford.edu/blog/2013/12/sae-levels-driving-automation, 2016) a realisable goal for transportation over the next 10 years. In particular, SAE Level 3 (conditional automation) automates the main aspects of driving including steering, accelerating and braking on the basis that the driver will frequently respond to a request to intervene. It is likely that in the coming 5 years Level 4 (high automation) will handle all aspects of driving even if a human driver does not intervene. It is also likely that autonomous vehicles will be available in various forms, including conventionally equipped contemporary Original Equipment Manufacturers' (OEMs) cars and public transport 'pods' with no conventional controls. Public perception of such developments has been sampled more frequently in the past 3 years and this reveals increasing awareness of the key technologies and positivity towards introduction. However, while attitudes appear to be changing rapidly, the nature of this awareness throughout the population is partial and opinions vary with methods of sampling. We examine data regarding the public's understanding of how autonomously capable vehicles could be used to benefit the inclusive population, including those with capability impairments; their carers, and those who require transportation to support dependent family members. We then use a driver and passenger *taskscape* approach for the analysis of the perceived benefits of use and barriers to use in these populations. This analysis is made in the context of existing transportation conditions and citizen's needs, and leads towards a tangible conceptual design criterion that may be implemented by design engineers.

M. Strickfaden (✉)
Department of Human Ecology, University of Alberta, Edmonton, AB, Canada
e-mail: megan.strickfaden@ualberta.ca

P. M. Langdon
Cambridge Engineering Design Centre, The University of Cambridge, Cambridge, UK
e-mail: pml24@eng.cam.ac.uk

© Springer International Publishing AG, part of Springer Nature 2018
P. Langdon et al. (eds.), *Breaking Down Barriers*,
https://doi.org/10.1007/978-3-319-75028-6_16

1 New Wave of Autonomous Vehicles

New vehicle technologies are making the development of affordable self-driving vehicles a reality. Considerable effort is being exerted by Original Equipment Manufacturers (OEMs) to incrementally add features that implement automation functionality. These features usually include adaptive cruise control; lane departure warning and lane keeping systems; automated emergency braking and avoidance; cross-lane warning; self-parking; stop and go traffic support; blind-spot detection; and cross-traffic monitoring. Currently, combinations of adaptive cruise control, automated emergency braking and stop and go traffic support will cover most of the longitudinal requirements of highway driving by controlling braking and acceleration, as demonstrated by a number of vehicles available on the market today, such as Tesla, Mercedes and BMW. If this is combined with lane departure detection and warning it provides the possibility of automated lane keeping. The next logical progression is towards the possibility of lateral acceleration control and hence steering in and out of a lane, for example in automated overtaking. Finally, advanced AI and engineering algorithms can be used in conjunction with sensor technologies such as Camera, Radar, Lidar and Ultrasonics, to recognize objects and features of the environment and process these as context for manouvering through a space that is represented by an internal model or map of the actual road displayed within a vehicle.

SAE Level 3 vehicles (conditional automation) automate the main aspects of driving including steering, accelerating and braking on the basis that the driver will respond to a request to intervene. However, they may only be able to operate under limited constrained conditions, such as motorways and require the driver to monitor the driving and intervene by engaging or disengaging the self-driving features. This means that such vehicles require conventional controls and driving position. Usually, driver behaviour monitoring is implemented to ensure attention, for example by requiring holding the steering wheel at set intervals such as 12 s (e.g. Mercedes S class), hand on wheel detection (e.g. Tesla) and eyes on road detection (e.g. Cadillac). In some cases, failure to comply leads to a stop.

SAE Level 4 vehicles use some of the technologies similar to Level 3 such as sensors, but the underlying architecture parameters (i.e. redundancy, accuracy, latency) are more stringent. The Level 4 vehicle is capable of managing a more dynamic drive over a wider range of less constrained conditions. It is proposed that they will operate even if the driver does not respond to a request from the vehicle to intervene. SAE Level 5 vehicles would manage all the driving that a human is capable of and, in principle, do not require driving controls (Fig. 1).

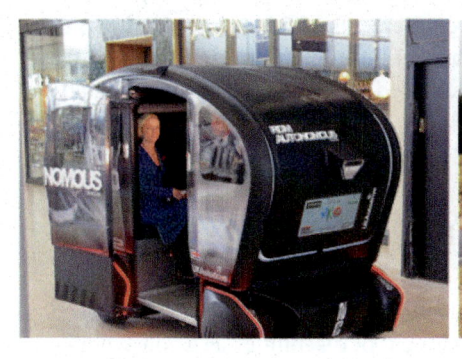

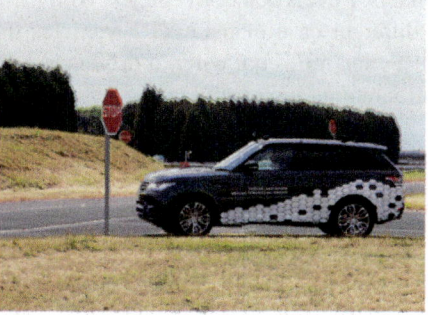

Fig. 1 Level 5 autonomous vehicles (left) prototype Level 3 vehicle (right)

2 Public Perception of Autonomous Vehicles

There are numerous detailed surveys of public perception of autonomous vehicles (e.g. Kyriakidis et al. 2015), such as: (1) The UCL Transport Institute report on Social and Behavioural Questions Associated with Automated Vehicles, (Cohen et al. 2017); (2) The UWE, Venturer Project: Understanding the Socioeconomic Adoption Scenarios for Autonomous Vehicles (Clark et al. 2016); and (3) The LSE/Goodyear THINKGOODMOBILITY survey 2016, Autonomous Vehicles: Negotiating a Place on the Road, (Tennant et al. 2016). A representative detailed survey of public perception of autonomous vehicles in the UK was carried out by *UK Autodrive* (2016), a government-funded consortium made up of major companies from the UK's automotive industry; manufacturers, research and development organisations and the supply chain. Partners include major OEMs, SMEs and a technology start-up; UK academia and major players from the legal and insurance worlds.

The *UK Autodrive* survey provides some clarity around how people are imagining the use of autonomous vehicles. Some of the key questions queried around how trustworthy autonomous vehicles might be including: vehicle safety and reliability; whether people would recommend self-driving vehicles to older loved ones or children; and, most importantly for this chapter, whether self-driving vehicles could be useful to assist people with impairments or disabilities. It is clear from the details of *UK Autodrive* public opinion survey that people believe that autonomous vehicles have the potential to be useful and be trustworthy, however, some people seem to be least trusting of using autonomous vehicles to transport children. What is most striking about the findings of the survey is that most people strongly agreed that autonomous vehicles have the potential to assist persons with impairments or disabilities. Based on our overview of Level 3, 4 and 5 vehicles and considering the challenges presented, the key question still open is: how can these vehicles be designed to consider people with impairments, older adults, carers and children?

That is, Levels 3 and 4 vehicles, with the requirements of driver intervention present a different case than Level 5 vehicles that present similar design needs to that of buses and trains but without drivers. As such, we further unpack the current status of autonomous inclusivity.

3 Future Autonomous Vehicle Users

A good basis for formulating the principles to assess the needs of inclusive populations; including persons who have impairment or disabilities as a consequence of ageing, temporary disablement resulting from injury or surgery, or other situations; and how needs may be met by autonomous vehicles, would be a survey of accurate national survey data that took into account the journeys and personas of users. The *IM Traveller Needs and UK Capability Study: Supporting the Realisation of Intelligent Mobility in the UK* (Wockatz and Schartau 2015), a recent survey of UK journeys and transportation usage with 10,000 respondents in the UK, enabled the formation of sampling categories of 'persona-journeys' (Fig. 2).

Table 1 shows that potential users are classified by their journey types, however, some of the categories are more relevant to inclusion than others, particularly when considering ageing and impairment. The user persona-journeys—including dependent passengers, local drivers and default motorists—illustrate three different types of drivers who could potentially benefit from more inclusive approaches towards autonomous vehicle design. *Dependent passengers* rely on personal mobility strategies such as walking and using a wheelchair/scooter, and rely on public transportation or assistance from friends/family. *Dependent passengers* are people who currently have either never driven or have lost their ability to drive due to the requirements made on them by current vehicles. Local drivers and default motorists make up the majority of drivers on the road in the UK who do leisure driving, drive others (e.g. grandchildren, friends) and commute. Local drivers and default motorists currently drive as needed; not always by choice, and clearly meet the requirements to drive current vehicles.

Most striking is that persons are divided into passengers and drivers based on the *IM Traveller Needs and UK Capability Study* user persona-journeys. When it comes to autonomous vehicles, it is useful to consider the differences and similarities between drivers and passengers, and to recognise the fluidity that might occur between the tasks embodied within each.

4 Driver and Passenger *Taskscape* Analysis

All people, regardless of ability, expect to be able to realise their dreams and live a certain life (Albercht 2003). For example, people may expect to walk to the local markets, commute across a city and/or drive to work. Each person assesses their

Attitudes towards trust of SDVs

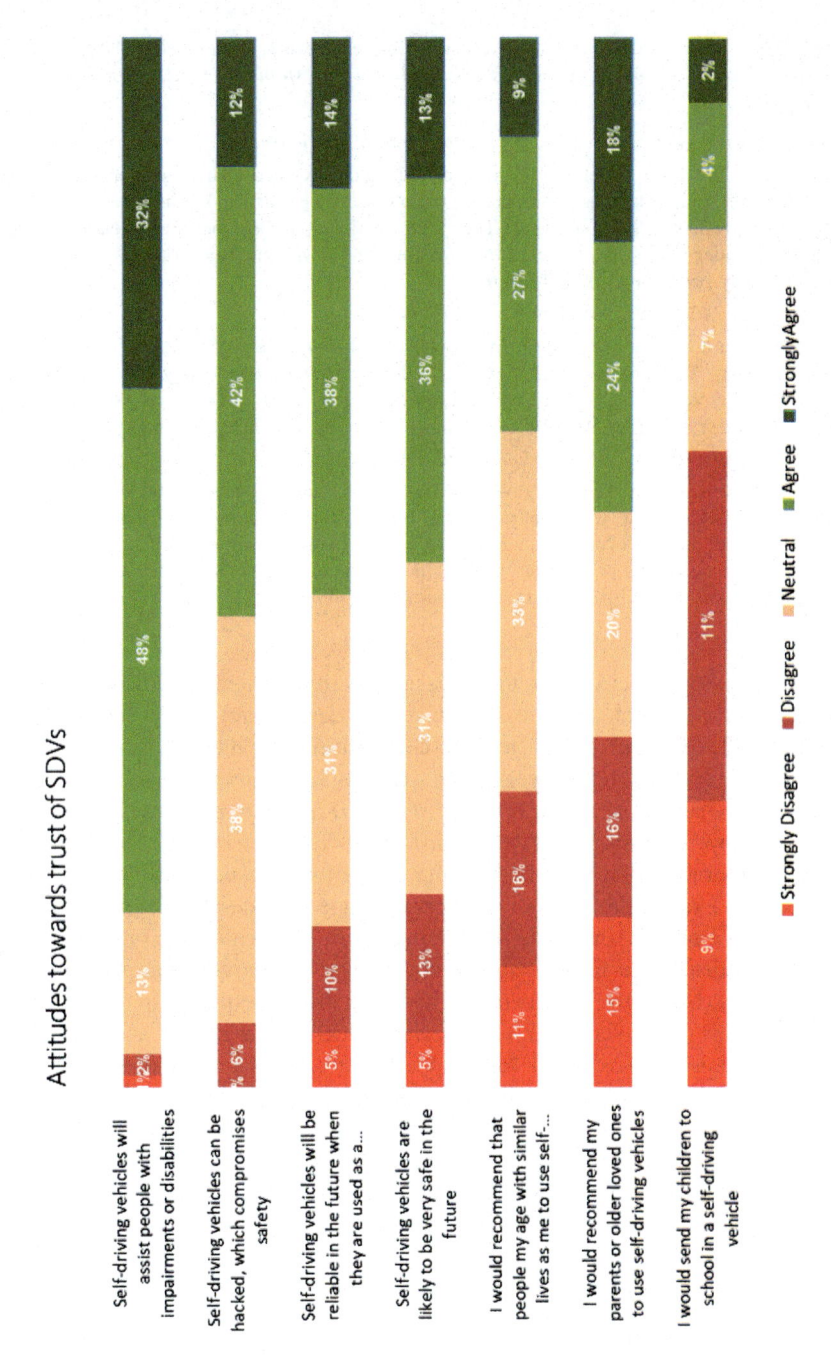

Statement	Strongly Disagree	Disagree	Neutral	Agree	Strongly Agree
Self-driving vehicles will assist people with impairments or disabilities	2%	5%	13%	48%	32%
Self-driving vehicles can be hacked, which compromises safety	–	6%	38%	42%	12%
Self-driving vehicles will be reliable in the future when they are used as a…	5%	10%	31%	38%	14%
Self-driving vehicles are likely to be very safe in the future	5%	13%	31%	36%	13%
I would recommend that people my age with similar lives as me to use self-…	11%	16%	33%	27%	9%
I would recommend my parents or older loved ones to use self-driving vehicles	15%	16%	20%	24%	18%
I would send my children to school in a self-driving vehicle	9%	11%	7%	4%	2%

Fig. 2 Summary attitudes towards trust of autonomous vehicles. Taken from the *UK Autodrive* (2016) public opinion survey

Table 1 User persona-journeys (top-level) as identified by the *IM Traveller Needs and UK Capability Study: Supporting the Realisation of Intelligent Mobility in the UK* (Wockatz and Schartau 2015)

Dependent passengers: 21% of UK population and 18% of journeys
It is a segment that is dependent on others to meet its mobility needs. This traveller type consists of a number of groups, such as young people (who typically get driven by their parents), elderly people and travellers with impairments. They take a majority of their journeys as car passengers and the remainder is typically covered by either bus or by walking, with journeys split representatively between work and leisure
Local drivers: 24% of UK population and 19% of journeys
Local Drivers are a more suburban or rural, typically older segment (70% aged 55 or over and 60% are retired). They are non-working (either retired or have chosen to stay at home) and their travel demand is very much focused on local journeys. They own cars but tend not to be heavy drivers (half drive less than 5000 miles per year)
Default motorists: 26% of UK population and 37% of journeys
This is a segment of very frequent travellers who live in smaller urban centres or suburbs of larger cities. They make a significant number of journeys for work (twice the UK average) and also make a high number of leisure journeys (15% more than UK average). The vast majority of their journeys are taken by private car, which is their 'default' mode of transport. This 'always on the road' segment makes up 46% of all car journeys in the UK

own abilities to participate in these desired activities and (to some degree or another) to what extent they are able to realise desires and societal expectations. Ingold (1993, p. 158) refers to the composition of these various activities throughout daily, weekly and yearly lives of people as *taskscapes* defined as: '... *any practical operation carried out by a skilled agent in an environment as part of his or her normal business of life... [and] an array of inter-related activities...*'.

Kirsh elaborates upon what he calls the '*task environment*' (Kirsh 1996, p. 417) as a means to examine the ways that people engage with designed things, stressing the importance of assessing tasks in isolation as well as within the broader general environment or context in order to reveal the layers of activity that people act out unconsciously. Naturally, each person's lives and the subsequent *task environments* and *taskscapes* vary across time, are dynamically performed, and are flexed depending upon changes in interests, opportunities, expectations and capabilities. The barriers to realising even simple tasks can relate to physical capabilities, designed things and environments, social constructions, financial situations, the time needed to accomplish a task and more.

Persons with impairments or disabilities clearly have a defined set of challenges with greater additional barriers to realising their *task environments* and *taskscapes*. For the purpose of discussion, imagine an older adult who has recently encountered a temporary disability such as a hip replacement. This older adult may have undergone rehabilitation whereby they learned to perform several new sequences or activities to become independent once again, including dressing, toileting and grooming. The older adult and society; including family and friends, have the expectation of performing daily tasks that provide independence and self-reliance in order to establish the individual's value as a productive person. Along with learning about a new corporeal potential, a person's potential is often augmented with technologies, equipment supplements, and modifications to surrounding environments. For instance, people are supported by wheelchairs, walkers or canes in order to engage in alternative or enhanced modes of mobility: *'Technology [is] seen as restoring our view of a complete and 'normal' human being.'* (Macdonald 2003, p. 187).

By supporting people with technologies, a person is transformed from a fragile and mortal self into someone with a higher capacity to complete a task, such as ambulating somewhere. Technologies, in the case of a wheelchair, for example become an extension of the body-self and are core aspects of supporting people's *task environment* and *taskscape*. One significant task within the category of mobility is 'getting somewhere' including; to engage in work or school, fetch groceries, do laundry, engage in entertainment and more. The idea of 'getting somewhere', as identified within the user persona-journeys, is easily identified into various categories including:

- Mobilise oneself or ambulating through walking or wheeling
- Being a passenger by taking public transportation (buses, metros, taxis)
- Being a passenger in or on another person's vehicle
- Being a driver by mobilising one's own vehicle

The tasks for driving and being a passenger are summarised as driving-related activities, non-driving-related activities (Pfleging and Schmidt 2015), and commonalities that cross each (Table 2).

When deconstructing the *taskscapes* involved with user persona-journeys around 'getting somewhere' it is clear that there are different tasks for driving and being a passenger. It is important to note that although transitioning between modes of mobility (e.g. walking–driving–walking or walking–cycling–metro–walking) are a significant part of a journey; and part of the *task environment* of the 'getting somewhere', these are not highlighted in this chapter. Through the deconstruction of the driver and passenger *taskscapes*, various tasks are identified that allow for an alternative approach towards thinking about the capabilities of people when designing more inclusive autonomous vehicles.

Table 2 Summary of driver and passenger *taskscapes*

Driving-related activities	Commonalities	Non-driving related activities
Steering	Mobility	Entertainment
Braking	Safety	Climate control
Accelerating	Seating	Luggage and storage
Gear selection	Cabin configuration	Pleasure
Cognition	Navigation	Enjoyment
Awareness	Information	Sleeping
	Communications	Eating
	Driving joy	

5 Case Study

Considering passengers and drivers within their corresponding *taskscapes* of driving-related and non-driving-related activities in relation to the three levels of autonomous vehicles currently available results in a case study that points towards a need to elaborate upon how to create a more inclusive product. Our case study is derived from ethnographies that include observations and interviews with persons with disabilities (e.g. visually impaired, wheelchair users) and older adults (e.g. all levels of capability including persons with dementia) about their lived experiences (e.g. Devlieger and Strickfaden 2012; Strickfaden and Vildieu 2014; Strickfaden 2016). One common theme throughout the ethnographies is that people wish to mobilise themselves as independently as possible regardless of their capabilities or need to depend on others. Typical considerations are illustrated through this quote from a visually impaired man interviewed about his mobility:

> Mobility depends on how a city is adapted but I can tell you that it's easier to do things on your own because when you're with your parents or with friends they don't necessarily know what to do. When you are with people in a taxi they know what to do, they know where to take you and it is way faster.

Classic *dependent passengers* are parents with children; children with ageing parents; children or youths that need to get somewhere safely; older adults who need medical treatments, services or groceries; and people with impairments or disabilities who wish to be independent (go to work, get groceries, etc.). For these passengers, it is clear that Level 3 and 4 vehicles are dimensions of the same thing, although they have the potential for design variations. To begin with, these vehicles require human interventions of intermittent driving, which are likely inappropriate unless dependent passengers are also drivers.

The benefits of having a driver in the vehicle are many. First, there may always be situations where drivers are required to intervene or at least direct an autonomous car to the strategy it needs to take such as in order to break the rules of the road in special circumstances such as when there are roadworks. Second, having a driver in a vehicle means it is much like in a bus or taxi where the driver can assist a passenger when needed, for example to stow their gear and drive the vehicle when prompted. Level 3 or 4 vehicle drivers may also provide reassurances, options and choices, such as finding special routes to cut down on walking, or other beneficial information. According to another man with a visual impairment:

> Drivers also help, you know. Taxi, well the taxi depends on what kind of taxi you have because if you don't know where you're going or if you're going to a train station; which can be quite complicated, you ask the taxi driver if they can take you to the reception or the help desk for disabled.

The main difference between the Level 3 and 4 vehicles is that Level 4 vehicles involve less frequent driver assist (as few as once or twice per drive), which means that because the vehicle is likely to request fewer driving interventions it is conceivable that the driver of the vehicle can support the dependent passenger in the role of a caregiver instead of merely as a driver. That is, during autonomous driving the driver may be rotated/slide to one side and face the passenger/s and thus engage in deeper levels of sociality, whereas the Level 3 driver will always need to be available to drive the vehicle and therefore will be facing forward and correspondingly less available to assist dependent passengers.

On the surface, Level 5 vehicles seem to be geared towards *dependent passengers,* who are not drivers because the vehicle can be entrusted to do everything including handling emergencies and navigation options. The challenges for the *dependent passenger* are that there will be no driver to assist with aspects relating to the passenger *taskscape,* such as vehicle entry and exits, navigation, safety and even general mobility issues. Even so, older adults might prefer a Level 5 vehicle if they need little assistance; parents might be less likely to have their children ride independently, or children might be less likely to have a parent with dementia ride independently. Design considerations may still reflect the impairment related needs, as identified by a visually impaired woman interviewed about orientation:

> I have residual vision. So here for example I see window—I mean residual vision means I see colours very slightly, I see light shadow so windows will help me to find my orientation, will help me to know where I am.

Local drivers and default motorist are extremely heterogeneous with wide variations in age and ability. *Local drivers* are retirees that are elective workers that drive by choice but may have pressures from their children, spouses or friends. As demographics evolve there will likely be more and more older people in this category. *Local drivers* have come to rely on cars because they are there, yet as they age their abilities will continue to worsen which means that autonomous cars have the potential to provide significant support. *Local drivers* may be concerned with route choices because they are accustomed to driving. They may also have a higher proportion of appointments related to ageing; such as pickups and drop-offs related to childcare (grandchildren) and may avoid multi-modal mobility options due to their decreased abilities.

Default motorists; much like *local drivers*, grow out of a culture of driving. They often live in suburban areas and need to commute into urban areas. *Default motorists* may also use a car rather than multi-modal transport options as they may have disabilities and wish to simplify their mobility. Along with commuting, the default driver likely uses the car for leisure and other activities simply because they have it.

Differences between *local drivers* and *default motorists* may relate to route navigation and choice of driving timings. *Local drivers* may go on longer trips to visit friends and family, doing this in a more ad hoc way at various times, because they have the opportunity to choose. Whereas *default motorists* may have fewer choices because they are led by work schedules and other external forces. *Local drivers* and *default motorists* are drivers who can also be passengers (but may not prefer this). In the case of autonomous vehicles, these drivers have greater flexibility than dependent passengers because they have the option of engaging in intermittent driving.

In all situations for *dependent passengers, local drivers and default motorists*, autonomous vehicles need to have options with inclusive configurations to accommodate people with various abilities, impairments or disabilities. For instance, Levels 3, 4 and 5 vehicles require: (1) No step entries, including pivot seats and handholds for ease of entry; (2) Space to stow gear including luggage, walkers, wheelchairs, guide dogs; (3) Navigational and communication options to interface with the vehicle in a variety of modally different ways across disability. Variations between the vehicle levels should include: alternative reconfigurable seating in Levels 3 and 4 for drivers to engage with passengers as desired (e.g. Level 3 may have a fixed seat for driving while Level 4 may have a pivot seat).

6 Discussion

With the goal of developing autonomous vehicles into realisable technologies that can be implemented in the next 10 years, it is necessary to improve design understanding of inclusivity in autonomous vehicles. The aim of inclusive design is to move people from marginal positions where they are not participating or cannot participate at all to places where they can participate. An initial strategy for making autonomous vehicles more inclusive may be to consider designing specialised vehicle variants for different taskscapes, needs and capabilities. These specialised variants could include (but are not limited to) autonomous vehicles geared towards working persons (e.g. getting to work, working while in the vehicle), leisure driving (e.g. scenic tours, driving as a sport), children (e.g. getting to school or a grandparents home), the seated clientele (e.g. persons who use wheelchairs or other assistive devices) and persons who are visually impaired (e.g. alternative modes of communicating between vehicle and passenger/s).

6.1 Assistance and Adaptation

If autonomous vehicles are to be considered broadly assistive to all it is critical to develop a means to accommodate people with various impairments and disabilities. It is clear from our analysis that Level 5 vehicles have the potential to cater to totally dependent passengers, while Level 4 vehicles have the potential to extend mobility by having the vehicle do sections of fatiguing long-distance driving. Furthermore, Level 4 vehicles presumably could be adapted to accommodate persons with higher levels or specific impairments. If Level 3 and 4 vehicles are adapted adequately, it is possible that persons with visual impairments, for example may even be able to use these vehicles independently of assistance. Visual information may be configured to the advantage of the specific user, in terms of visual field, brightness or colour information. Multi-modal human–machine interfaces can provide enhanced redundancy in display and controls using vocal, auditory, haptic and physical functional areas by creating specific user profiles. Equally, a physically or cognitively impaired driver may benefit from reconfigured controls that are supported by boosting or adapting other modalities. Although these adaptations might be modest, the effect on reduced workload and independence has the potential to be large.

6.2 Training and Licencing

As a consequence of reconsidering the design of autonomous vehicles with a view to moving towards a more inclusive approach, it is also possible to reconsider the future of the drivers' licences. Because autonomy raises the possibility of reducing the demand on the driver, it is possible that not all drivers will need to have full licences in order to manage the intermittent driving required in Level 3 and 4 vehicles. Obtaining a restricted or reduced drivers licence may be assessed and based on capabilities, which opens up different possibilities for different people. Different licence ratings, for example may mean that two people with complementary yet restricted driver licences could meet the driving requirement that takes them individually from a Level 4 to collectively a Level 3 with consequent enhancement of their independence. These design and licence opportunities are a modest beginning to reimagining the future of autonomous vehicles (Table 3).

Table 3 Conceptual design criteria for Levels 3, 4 and 5 autonomous vehicles based on our analysis of the passenger and driver *taskscape*

Level	Description	Requirements	Key functions	Constraints
3	Relatively conventional human–machine interfaces: driving controls, entertainment and cabin ergonomics	Entry/exit Storage Training for intermittent driving	Communication interface/s Orientation	Fixed seat and controls within drivers grasp
4	May have minimised human–machine interfaces with inclusive dimensions and features: focus on cabin ergonomics for impairment	Entry/exit Storage Moveable or assistive seat	Communication interface/s Orientation	Requests for occasional intervention by 'driver'
5	Potential for totally dependent passengers No conventional controls—hidden emergency or maintenance controls	Entry/exit (critical) Assistive lifts Storage Safety	Destination and route Orientation Payment options Facilities for pickup/drop-off Emergency calls	Potentially no driver

7 Conclusions

The aim of this chapter was to raise design awareness and propose opportunities around the multi-dimensionality of impairments and what it means to be independent in relation to autonomous vehicles. By investigating public perception through the driver and passenger *taskscape*, guidance is given towards design solutions that can be nuanced between the three types of autonomous vehicles currently being tested. To date, car design has generally evolved in such a way that vehicle design has leaned towards a more universal design approach, where one size is meant to fit all. One risk with vehicle automation, therefore, is that if it is predicated on an approach where diversity of drivers and passengers are too narrowly defined inclusivity may not be realised. Through the passenger and driver *taskscape* insights are gained on how Levels 3 and 4 can be focused on design towards drivers whereas Level 5 can be focused on design towards passengers. Designers and engineers are encouraged to consider inclusivity as a means to realising autonomous vehicles as a viable technological solution for a range of users with varying capabilities.

Acknowledgements This work includes material partly funded by UK EPSRC/JLR TASCC and UK Autodrive.

References

Albercht G (2003) Disability values, representations and realities. In: Devlieger P, Rusch F, Pfeiffer D (eds) Rethinking disability: the emergence of new definitions, concepts and communities. Garant, Antwerpen

Clark B, Parkhurst G, Ricci M (2016) Understanding the socioeconomic adoption scenarios for autonomous vehicles: a literature review. University of the West of England, Bristol, UK

Cohen T, Jones P, Cavoli C (2017) Social and behavioural questions associated with automated vehicles: final report scoping study. UCL Transport Institute, Department for Transport, London, UK

Devlieger P, Strickfaden M (2012) Reversing the {im}material sense of a non-place: the impact of blindness on the Brussels metro. Space Cult 15(2):224–238

Ingold T (1993) The temporality of the landscape. World Archaeol 25(2):152–174

Kirsh D (1996) Adapting the environment instead of oneself. Adapt Behav 4(3/4):415–452

Kyriakidis M, Happee R, De Winter JCF (2015) Public opinion on automated driving: results of an international questionnaire among 5000 respondents. Transp Res Part F Traffic Psychol Behav 32:127–140

Macdonald A (2003) Humanizing technology. In: Clarkson J, Coleman R, Keates S, Lebbon C (eds) Inclusive design: design for the whole population. Springer, Berlin

Pfleging B, Schmidt AL (2015) (Non-)driving-related activities in the car: defining driver activities for manual and automated driving. In: Workshop on experiencing autonomous vehicles: crossing the boundaries between a drive and a ride. CHI'15, Seoul, Korea, 18–23 Apr 2015

Strickfaden M (2016) In focus: blind photographers challenge visual expectations. In: Devlieger P, Miranda-Galarza B, Brown S, Strickfaden M (eds) Rethinking disability: world perspectives in culture and society. Garant Publishers, Antwerpen

Strickfaden M, Vildieu A (2014) On the quest for better communication through tactile images. J Aesthetic Educ (JAE) 48(2):105–122

Tennant C, Howard S, Franks B, Bauer MW, Stares S (2016) THINKGOOD MOBILITY survey. In: Autonomous vehicles: negotiating a place on the road. A study on how drivers feel about interacting with autonomous vehicles on the road. LSE Consulting, London School of Economics and Political Science, City University of London, UK

UK Autodrive (2017) www.ukautodrive.com/. Accessed 15 Nov 2017

Walker Smith B (2016) SAE levels of driving automation. Update 2: 2016 version of SAE J3016. CIS, the Center for Internet and Society. http://cyberlaw.stanford.edu/blog/2013/12/sae-levels-driving-automation. Accessed 15 Nov 2017

Wockatz P, Schartau P (2015) IM traveller needs and UK capability study: supporting the realisation of intelligent mobility in the UK. Transport Systems Catapult, Milton Keynes, UK. https://ts.catapult.org.uk/wp-content/uploads/2016/04/Traveller-Needs-Study-1.pdf. Accessed 15 Nov 2017

The Role of Inclusive Design in Improving People's Access to Treatment for Back Pain

Y. Liu, T. Dickerson, S. D. Waller, P. Waddingham
and P. J. Clarkson

Abstract Inclusive Design is usually applied to consumer products and services; here we investigate if it can be applied to healthcare delivery services. *Methods*: A case study approach was used by applying Inclusive Design methods to a telephone 'Physio-Direct' service for patients with back pain. Online surveys and interviews with healthcare professionals were used to gather insight into the delivery of back pain care and to construct a task analysis of the patient care journey. The task analysis was used to estimate the service demand made on patients' capabilities. Finally, an exclusion calculator was used to estimate the proportion of a population excluded from the service. *Results*: The surveys ($n = 30$) and interviews ($n = 4$) showed that communication difficulties, patients' reduced capability, service misconceptions and difficulties in obtaining information were the main barriers, which prevented patients from accessing the service. Some tasks placed a high demand on the patients' capabilities. These included telephone assessment, waiting for a telephone response, memorising the verbal advice, understanding the posted exercise leaflets and doing the exercises. It was estimated that at least 15% of the British population are excluded from the 'Physio-Direct' service. *Conclusion*: Inclusive Design methods were applied to the 'Physio-Direct' service and demand on its users identified ways in which the service could be improved. This suggests that Inclusive Design may be a useful tool in improving healthcare service delivery.

Y. Liu (✉) · T. Dickerson · S. D. Waller · P. J. Clarkson
Department of Engineering, Cambridge Engineering Design Centre,
University of Cambridge, Cambridge, UK
e-mail: yl528@cam.ac.uk

T. Dickerson
e-mail: tld23@cam.ac.uk

S. D. Waller
e-mail: sam.waller@eng.cam.ac.uk

P. J. Clarkson
e-mail: pjc10@eng.cam.ac.uk

P. Waddingham
Cambridgeshire Community Services NHS Trust, Cambridge, UK
e-mail: paula.waddingham@nhs.net

1 Introduction

We investigate if Inclusive Design can be applied to healthcare delivery services through its application to a back pain service case study.

1.1 Inclusive Design

Inclusive Design can be defined as: (i) 'the design of mainstream products and/or services that are accessible to, and usable by, people with the widest range of abilities within the widest range of situations without the need for special adaptation or design' (British Standards Institute 2005), (ii) ensuring that the demand made on an individual in a given environment does not exceed their capability to respond (Clarkson and Coleman 2013).

The Inclusive Design approach is a user-centred approach to design, where the fundamental premise is that accessible and usable products and services can only be developed by first knowing the intended users (Keates and Clarkson 2003). By estimating the system demand on users' capabilities along their care journey, it is easier to identify patients' capability-related needs in accessing the service.

1.2 Back Pain

In the UK, 2.5 million people suffer from back pain (Schultz and Gatchel 2006); it is the second most common reason why patients seek medical advice. Up to 9% of the UK population visits a GP because of back pain every year. Treatments cost the NHS £480 million per year (McClean et al. 2015) and 10 million working days are lost because of back problems (Batchelor 2015). Patients with back pain may also suffer from disability; low back pain is the largest single cause of loss of disability-adjusted life years in England (Murray et al. 2013). A lack of understanding of back pain (Lustick 2002) and the difficulties associated with accessing treatment are exacerbating the problem. In many cases, with better information and active self-care, back pain can be managed by people themselves (May 2010).

The 'Physio-Direct' service is a self-management physiotherapy pathway. Patients with back pain can make a telephone call to a physiotherapist for assessment and advice, and be sent information on self-management or referral to other appropriate services (Taylor et al. 2002). This service aims to offer timely assessment and treatment, thus avoiding long waiting times and preventing patients' back pain from worsening in the early stages. However, the self-referral by patients to telephone assessment is limited and most referrals still come from GPs; hence many patients who could use the service may not be aware of it. In addition, those who are aware of the service may not be able to make the best use of it (Foster et al. 2011).

1.3 Patients' Capabilities

A person's capabilities affect their ability to access health services. Inclusive Design categorises people's capabilities into sensor abilities (vision and hearing), motor abilities (mobility, dexterity and reach and stretch) and cognitive abilities (communication and thinking) (Clarkson et al. 2007; Schifferstein and Hekkert 2008). There are two main factors that cause a change in a person's capabilities, age-related change and medically related conditions. People with back pain may have a lower level of capability due to age-related decline, e.g. in hearing or vision.

1.4 Care Journeys (Pathways)

'Care journey' or 'care pathway' are terms used to describe the process of healthcare service delivery. A patient's 'care journey' refers to the process that he or she goes through in order to receive the care. Care pathway is the process from an organisational perspective and may take the form of a management plan that provides a sequence and timing of actions necessary to achieve a standard care process and optimal efficiency for clinicians (Panella et al. 2003).

In this work, care journeys describe the process that patients use in accessing the 'Physio-Direct' service. Here, we define the care journey using tasks, such as making a telephone call, engaging in a telephone consultation and self-managing one's care through exercise leaflets or referrals to other services. Each task can be defined in more detail: for instance, making a call can be divided into finding the number, picking up the phone, dialling the number and waiting for a response. Patients' care journeys can be defined through this structured task analysis approach which is amenable to subsequent exclusion analysis.

1.5 Inclusive Design and Patients' Access to the 'Physio-Direct' Service

Any service makes some demands on patients, and they have to have sufficient capabilities in order to access the service (Fig. 1). If the demands from the 'Physio-Direct' service exceed the capabilities of the patients then exclusion or difficulty in using the service will arise. Taking the task of making a telephone call as an example, if the patient with back pain also has poor hearing, he or she may not able to hear and answer the questions. In this case, this patient is excluded from the 'Physio-Direct' service.

Fig. 1 Interaction context-demand and capabilities (Persad et al. 2007). The example is a physical product but this applies equally to services. Reproduced from www.inclusivedesigntoolkit.com with permission

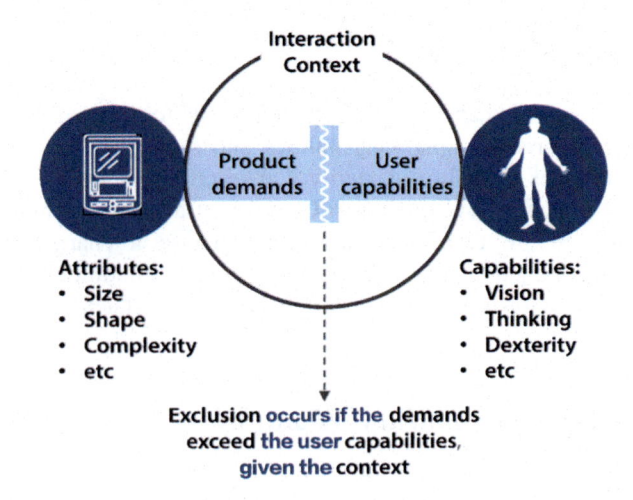

1.6 The Research Gap

A patient must have the capabilities to access the 'Physio-Direct' service as a prerequisite for them to use the service. There are few studies about how Inclusive Design can be used to improve healthcare service delivery. One study applied Inclusive Design to patient experience, but it was more focused on getting to the services rather than the services themselves (Beniuk et al. 2011). No research was found investigating if Inclusive Design can be applied to healthcare service delivery.

2 Methods and Results

We investigated the case study using mixed methods, including qualitative research (online survey and semi-structured interviews), task analysis and quantitative analysis (exclusion calculation) to gain insight into patients' needs regarding access to the 'Physio-Direct' service.

2.1 Online Survey

The survey aimed to gather insight into healthcare professionals' experiences of diagnosing and delivering back pain treatment, and assisted in recruiting some physiotherapists for further in-depth interviews.

Design: The online survey was designed to investigate: telephone assessment and related services, i.e. self-referral and GP services. It was developed from contributions by physiotherapists, a senior research fellow from Cambridgeshire Community Services NHS and findings from a literature review. For ease of completion, most items were closed questions with some open questions for more details; the questions could be completed in about 5 minutes.

Sampling strategy: The online survey (Qualtrics survey) link was disseminated to physiotherapist leads and advertised in the Trust Community Service Cascade. It was also disseminated by sending the invitation through LinkedIn (a professional social media network) and email. The survey was time limited and had to be returned within 2 weeks and a further reminder was circulated after 1 week.

Results: 30 physiotherapists responded to the survey. 77% of the respondents had over 5 years' work experience within the back pain services, and 57% had been directly involved in the telephone assessments. The physiotherapists considered challenges for patients accessing the 'Physio-Direct' service are: patients do not know the availability of the service, are not sure how to describe their symptoms to physiotherapists and cannot understand the instructions given to them. As for physiotherapists themselves, the top three challenges are the difficulties in building rapport, hearing patients and understanding patients.

2.2 Interviews

Interviews with physiotherapists were used to identify the clinical pathway and patient journey for back pain treatment.

Design: The same topics were discussed as in the online survey, i.e. self-referral, telephone assessment and GP services.

Sampling strategy: Convenience sampling of physiotherapists with experience or knowledge of delivering telephone services for back pain.

Results: Four physiotherapists were interviewed; two were face-to-face and two by telephone. Each interview took about 30 min and was audio-recorded and transcribed verbatim. Framework analysis was used to allow data to be themed and categorised. Besides the communication challenge identified by the online survey, patients' reduced capability, their misconception regarding the survey, and the difficulty for them to obtain the correct information or self-referral were discussed during the interview. Some suggestions were also proposed by the interviewees. One physiotherapist said, 'sending booklets that have pictures would describe things better (to patients)'. Two interviewees mentioned Skype and the use of video calls to help describe the symptoms and see patients' facial expressions. The importance of patients' direct contact with the service and not via their GP was emphasised by a senior physiotherapist. The key topics associated with patients' challenges and related suggestions from interviewees are shown in Fig. 2.

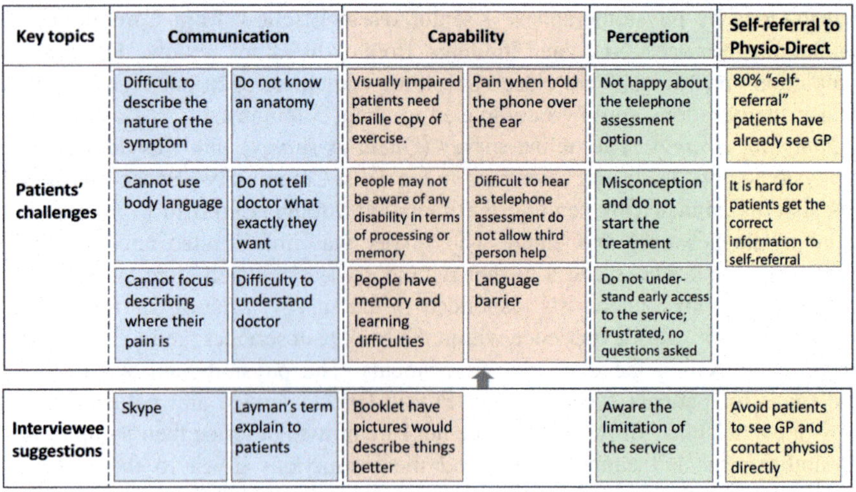

Key topics	Communication		Capability		Perception	Self-referral to Physio-Direct
Patients' challenges	Difficult to describe the nature of the symptom	Do not know an anatomy	Visually impaired patients need braille copy of exercise.	Pain when hold the phone over the ear	Not happy about the telephone assessment option	80% "self-referral" patients have already see GP
	Cannot use body language	Do not tell doctor what exactly they want	People may not be aware of any disability in terms of processing or memory	Difficult to hear as telephone assessment do not allow third person help	Misconception and do not start the treatment	It is hard for patients get the correct information to self-referral
	Cannot focus describing where their pain is	Difficulty to understand doctor	People have memory and learning difficulties	Language barrier	Do not understand early access to the service; frustrated, no questions asked	
Interviewee suggestions	Skype	Layman's term explain to patients	Booklet have pictures would describe things better		Aware the limitation of the service	Avoid patients to see GP and contact physios directly

Fig. 2 Key points identified from the interviewees

2.3 Exclusion Analysis

Data from the interviews and online survey were used to set a scenario for the exclusion analysis. Task analysis was used to understand the demands that the service places on patients, and an Inclusive Design tool was used to estimate the proportion of the population who might be excluded from using the service.

2.3.1 Estimate Demand of 'Physio-Direct' Service on Patients

It was important to define the scope and analyse a representative patient journey of accessing the 'Physio-Direct' service, see Table 1. As different patients may have different tasks along their journeys, it was impossible to cover all the possibilities. In addition, typical tasks (activities) that a patient is likely to do along the care journey are identified in Fig. 3. The physiotherapist could offer other care options to the patient, but this work only focused on patients self-managing back pain with written advice and the exercise leaflet. Based on each specified task, the demand that the 'Physio-Direct' service places on patients' capabilities could be estimated.

Specifically, the demand of every task was rated by predefined scales. These scales were constructed based on the questions in the Disability Follow-up to the Family Resources Survey, which was performed to help plan the welfare support for disabled people (Grundy et al. 1999; Waller et al. 2009, 2013). Examples of assessing hearing and long-term memory demand scales are shown in Fig. 4. Higher demand on peoples' capabilities causes higher scale ratings, and the symbol '>' off scale means it is excessive for a mainstream service.

Table 1 Peter: the patient scenario

Service name	'Physio-Direct' service of Cambridge city
User goal being assessed	The service's demand on user's capability when user makes a telephone call, performs telephone assessment and does exercise to self-manage back pain
User scenario	*Background*: Peter, 45 years old, works in an office. He lives independently by himself and is able to see the GP. One day, he woke up with a very stiff back and could not even tie his shoelaces. Things did not improve after 2 weeks, so he had to ask for leave. He called NHS direct and was told that there is a 'Physio-Direct' service available to Cambridge residents from 1–5 pm on weekdays *Telephone assessment*: Peter telephoned the service and waited for a response for about 15 min, which made his neck stiff. The physiotherapist answered the call and checked his personal information. Peter was not sure how to describe his symptoms. He could not find a way to get comfortable, either standing or sitting. Peter was worried that his pain would affect his work, so he asked some questions and the physiotherapist gave him immediate advice and the written advice and leaflets were sent after the call *Read leaflets and Do exercise*: Peter received the letter after 2 days. He opened and read it, including a summary of treatment and an exercise leaflet. Peter read the leaflet and did exercise to self-manage his back pain

Make a call
- Read number
- Pick up phone and dial number
- Wait for response

Telephone consultation
- Check personal info by physio
- Describe symptoms
- Receive verbal advice
- End call

Self-management with exercise leaflet
- Receive the letter
- Read and open letter
- Read leaflet and do exercise

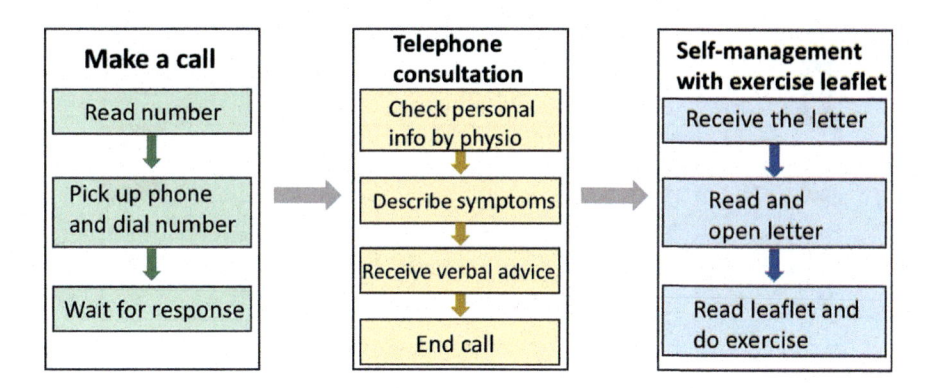

Fig. 3 The tasks of a representative patients' care journey

With the predefined scales, the demand for every task was then evaluated. For example, the task of receiving verbal advice makes demands on patients' hearing, cognitive ability (concentration, memory and speech comprehension) and motor ability (stretch, dexterity and forward). The demand of this task on patients' hearing capability is close to 8 on the scale, i.e. 'use telephone without special adaptations for hearing impairment', so it is rated scale 8; while as for the demand on patients' memory, to remember all the advice is harder than 12 on the scale, i.e. 'remember

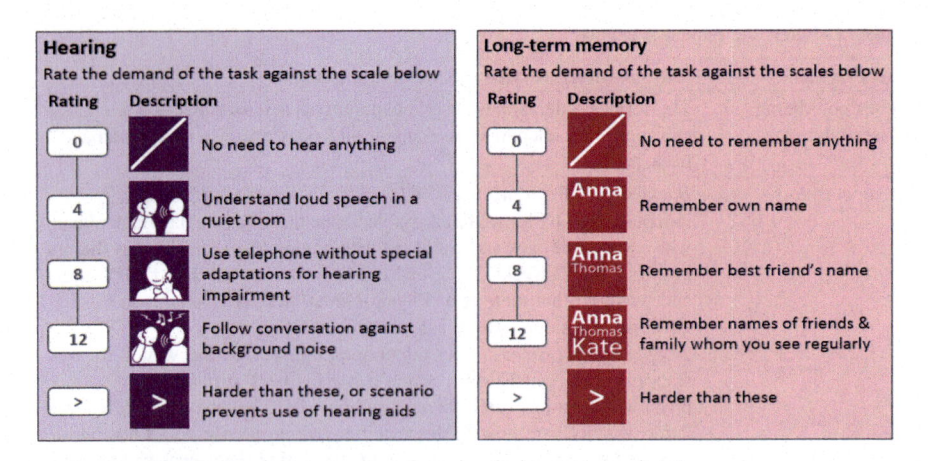

Fig. 4 The standard of measuring hearing (left) and long-term memory (right). Adapted from http://calc.inclusivedesigntoolkit.com with permission

Table 2 Demand on every task of the service (based on Peter's scenario in Table 1)

Task No.	1	2	3	4	5	6	7	8	9	10
Task name / Capability	Read number	Pick up phone and dial number	wait for response	Check personal info by physio	Describe symptoms	Receive verbal advice	End call	Receive the letter	Read and open letter	Read leaflet and do exercise
Vision	12	10	0	0	0	0	4	12	12	>
Hearing	0	0	8	8	8	8	0	0	0	0
Concentration	12	12	12	12	12	12	12	4	12	>
Memory	12	12	12	12	12	>	12	4	12	12
Literacy	4	4	0	0	0	0	0	4	12	>
Speech Comp.	0	0	4	8	12	12	0	0	0	0
Speaking	0	0	0	8	12	12	0	0	0	0
Strength	0	4	4	4	4	4	0	0	0	0
Dexterity	0	4	0	0	0	12	4	0	0	0
Forward/Up	0	8	>	8	8	8	6	0	0	12
Down	0	0	0	0	0	0	4	0	0	12
Strength	0	0	0	0	0	0	0	1	1	0
Dexterity	0	0	0	0	0	0	0	6	8	0
Forward/Up	0	0	0	0	0	0	0	0	4	12
Down	0	0	0	0	0	0	0	8	0	12
Walking	0	0	0	0	0	0	0	0	0	2
Stairs	0	0	0	0	0	0	0	0	0	0
Standing	0	0	0	0	0	0	0	0	0	8

names of friends and family whom you see regularly', so it is rated '>' off scale. The detailed rating results are listed in Table 2.

There are 5 capabilities of 3 tasks along the patients' care journey that were rated as '>' off scale (marked in red). These tasks place excessive demand on patients'

Table 3 The tasks that place excessively high demand on patient's capabilities

Task name	Wait for response	Receive verbal advice	Read leaflet and do exercise
Capability	Forward	Memory	Vision, concentration and literacy
Reasons rating '>'	Waiting on hold for about 15 min to get through the service is challenging	Patients may not be able to remember all the oral advice	1. It is difficult for patients to understand some diagrams within the leaflet, e.g. missing movement pictures (Vision and literacy) 2. Patients are not sure whether they do the exercise in a correct way (concentration)
Suggestions	Give things to do during the hold period: provide care information; minutes countdown; reminder for people who do not keep holding the phone	What patients can do before receiving a written letter? Other options should be provided such as email information or giving a patient information website link	1. The diagrams should show the steps of every movement. The instruction of every movement should be unambiguous 2. Patients may need an assistant check whether they are doing the exercise correctly

capabilities, which implies patients will need extra support. The reasons for the ratings and corresponding suggestions are shown in Table 3.

2.3.2 Estimate the Proportion of the Excluded British Population (Quantitative Analysis)

The 'Exclusion Calculator' produced by the University of Cambridge Engineering Design Centre represents a large database of British users with a range of disabilities and quantified information regarding the use of a product according to their disability. The original population data is also from the Disability Follow-up to the Family Resources Survey (Grundy et al. 1999), which estimates the proportion of the British population who are unable to use a service because of the demands that it places on the users' capabilities. A basic version of this calculator is freely available at http://calc.inclusivedesigntoolkit.com.

In this work, the 'Exclusion Calculator' was used to estimate the exclusion population based on the rated demand scales of the possible user scenario, i.e. Peter (Tables 1 and 2). Overall, about 15% of British people who are in a similar scenario as Peter could be excluded from the 'Physio-Direct' service. If the back pain was more severe and limiting, then the exclusion would be larger. Among all the service's tasks, it is estimated that the largest percentage of the population is excluded from 'read leaflet and do exercise' (Table 4), namely 13.5%.

3 Discussion

Inclusive Design could potentially help understand patients' capability-related needs and make the service more inclusive and hence increase uptake. This is because when designing a healthcare service, care providers often tend to assume patients can do some 'simple' tasks such as make a call and remember medical advice. In fact, some tasks are beyond some patients' capabilities. An example is the task, 'read leaflet and do exercise', which causes the largest percentage of the population to be excluded from the care journey (Table 4). Figure 5 shows two movements from the back pain exercise leaflet of NHS. Exercise No. 6 has two sub-pictures with the steps of movement, which are relatively easy for patients to follow; while Exercise No. 7 does not show how to start the movement, so patients may become confused by the picture and not gain any benefit from the exercise. However, if we could understand these capability-related needs when we design the service, e.g. making the exercise diagrams clearer, patients would be less likely to be excluded from the service.

Table 4 The exclusion of every task

Task name	Read number	Pick up phone and dial number	Wait for response	Check personal info by physio	Describe symptoms	Receive verbal advice	End call	Receive the letter	Read and open letter	Read leaflet &do exercise	Overall demands
Exclusion (%)	7.2%	8.1%	8.4%	8.0%	8.2%	10.4%	7.2%	10.8%	9.9%	13.5%	15.2%
Vision only (%)	4.1%	2.6%	0.0%	0.0%	0.0%	0.0%	1.0%	4.1%	4.1%	4.1%	4.1%
Hearing only (%)	0.0%	0.0%	2.3%	2.3%	2.3%	2.3%	0.0%	0.0%	0.0%	0.0%	2.3%
Thinking only (%)	4.4%	4.4%	4.5%	4.9%	5.3%	5.3%	4.2%	1.5%	4.6%	4.6%	5.5%
Reach & dex only (%)	0.0%	3.2%	3.9%	2.8%	2.8%	6.2%	3.3%	8.2%	4.8%	9.5%	11.1%
Mobility only (%)	0.0%	0.0%	0.0%	0.0%	0.0%	0.0%	0.0%	0.0%	0.0%	6.0%	6.0%

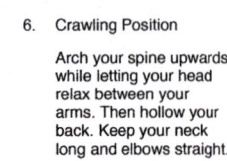

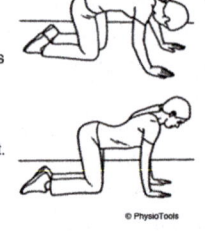

6. Crawling Position

    Arch your spine upwards while letting your head relax between your arms. Then hollow your back. Keep your neck long and elbows straight.

7. Lying face down, leaning on your forearms.

    Arch the small of your back, and press your pelvis and stomach to the floor. Bend your back upwards, keeping your arms on the floor. If your leg symptoms increase, stop.

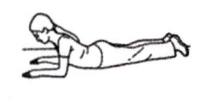

Fig. 5 Example movements from low back pain exercise booklet of NHS. Copyright permission from the Cambridgeshire Community Services NHS Trust

The Inclusive Design approach to estimate service demand on patients' capability required us to have a clear map of the service delivery, understanding the tasks of the users' care journey. Therefore, we were able to identify gaps in the healthcare service during the process of mapping patients' care journey. For example, it was easy to miss the gap after the telephone assessment and before patients received written advice, when patients could forget the verbal advice. During this waiting period, some other options, such as giving a patient information for a website link or emailing information, could be offered to help patients control their pain. Estimating the demands of every task within the service more rigorously would help to provide a better understanding of patients' needs.

Overall, Inclusive Design has the potential to improve the 'Physio-Direct' service by estimating the service's demand on patients and identifying whether there are challenges for the patients.

4 Conclusions

In this work, Inclusive Design is used to understand the 'Physio-Direct' service delivery by understanding the service system demand on its patients' capabilities along their care journey. An online survey and interviews were used to help understand the patients' journeys in accessing the 'Physio-Direct' service and identifying the advantages and limitations of the service. The accessibility of the 'Physio-Direct' service was evaluated through task analysis and exclusion calculation. The tasks that place a higher demand on patients' capabilities were identified and the proportion of the British population potentially excluded was estimated.

This work has demonstrated that the application of Inclusive Design to health services is possible and that the tools applied can make a useful contribution to understanding service provision and hence service improvement.

As for the limitations of this work, it is based on a single case study and a limited subset of Inclusive Design tools were applied. The population database used has not been updated for about 20 years, although it remains the most holistic source of data about people's capabilities. In addition, the number of interviewees was relatively low because of the difficulty in recruiting physiotherapists due to their high clinical workload and limited availability. Although this research was more focused on understanding the barriers to patients' back pain self-management from the perspective of healthcare professionals, inputting first-hand data directly from patients was equally important. Further research can focus on how we can implement improvements to the 'Physio-Direct' service demands on patients while maintaining the quality of service and this could be achieved by interviewing users of the service.

Acknowledgements This research has been reviewed and approved by Research Ethnics Committee of the Department of Engineering, University of Cambridge. The authors would like to acknowledge Dr. Andrew Bateman, Stephen Wilson and their colleagues at Cambridgeshire

Community Services NHS Trust for their help and support in developing research; and all the physiotherapists who participated in the interview and survey. The work was partly supported by the NIHR CLAHRC East of England based at Cambridge and Peterborough NHS Foundation Trust. The Excel version of Exclusion Calculator 2.0, as part of the ID-3 Inclusive Design Consortium run by the Centre for Business Innovation, was used in this research.

References

Batchelor T (2015) EXCLUSIVE: millions of working days lost to back pain—and it costs us £1 BILLION a year. http://www.express.co.uk/news/uk/583948/back-pain-experts. Accessed 23 Nov 2017

Beniuk C, Ward J, Clarkson PJ (2011) Applying inclusive design principles in the assessment of healthcare services. In: Proceedings of conference on design 4 health, Sheffield, UK, 13–15th July 2011, pp 22–36

British Standards Institute (2005) BS 7000-6:2005: design management systems. Managing inclusive design. Guide, BSI, UK

Clarkson PJ, Coleman R (2013) History of inclusive design in the UK. Appl Ergonomics 46:233–324

Clarkson PJ, Coleman R, Hosking I, Waller S (2007) Inclusive design toolkit. Engineering Design Centre. http://www.inclusivedesigntoolkit.com. Accessed 13 Nov 2017

Foster NE, Williams B, Grove S, Gamlin J, Salisbury C (2011) The evidence for and against 'PhysioDirect' telephone assessment and advice services. Physiotherapy 97:78–82

Grundy E, Ahlburg D, Ali M, Breeze E, Sloggett A (1999) Disability in Great Britain: results from the 1996/7 disability follow-up to the family resources survey. DSS research report no. 94, HMSO, London, UK

Keates S, Clarkson PJ (2003) Countering design exclusion. Springer, London, UK

Lustick B (2002) Common back pain misunderstandings. Back Be Nimble Newsletter

May S (2010) Self-management of chronic low back pain and osteoarthritis. Nat Rev Rheumatol 6:199–209

McClean S, Brilleman S, Wye L (2015) What is the perceived impact of Alexander technique lessons on health status, costs and pain management in the real life setting of an English hospital? The results of a mixed methods evaluation of an Alexander technique service for those with chronic back pain. BMC Health Serv Res 15:293

Murray CJL, Richards MA, Newton JN, Fenton KA, Anderson HR, Atkinson C et al (2013) UK health performance: findings of the global burden of disease study 2010. Lancet 381:997–1020

Panella M, Marchisi S, Di Stanisla F (2003) Reducing clinical variations with clinical pathways: do pathways work? Int J Qual Health Care 15:509–521

Persad U, Langdon P, Clarkson PJ (2007) Characterising user capabilities to support inclusive design evaluation. Univ Access Inf Soc 6(2):119–135

Schifferstein H, Hekkert P (2008) Product experience. Elsevier Science, Netherlands

Schultz IZ, Gatchel RJ (2006) Handbook of complex occupational disability claims: early risk identification, intervention, and prevention. Springer Science and Business Media, Berlin

Taylor S, Ellis I, Gallagher M (2002) Patient satisfaction with a new physiotherapy telephone service for back pain patients. Physiotherapy 88:645–657

Waller SD, Langdon PM, Clarkson PJ (2009) Using disability data to estimate design exclusion. Univ Access Inf Soc 9:195–207

Waller SD, Bradley MD, Langdon PM, Clarkson PJ (2013) Visualising the number of people who cannot perform tasks related to product interactions. Univ Access Inf Soc 12:263–278

Inclusivity Considerations for Fully Autonomous Vehicle User Interfaces

T. Amanatidis, P. M. Langdon and P. J. Clarkson

Abstract Autonomous vehicles could become an important part of the mobility solution for members of society previously excluded from driving. This paper presents the results of an interview study on users' needs and expectations of fully autonomous vehicles, and specifically on the inclusivity considerations that emerged. Six drivers and two individuals that are currently excluded from driving participated in this study. The main finding was that conventional multimodal interfaces would indeed enable a broader range of users to operate these vehicles. However, fundamental considerations such as the accessibility of displays and easy ingress/egress were of equal importance. We hope the emerging recommendations would form part of an inclusive set of user requirements to be taken into account by industry and academia when designing fully autonomous vehicle user interfaces.

1 Introduction

Autonomous vehicles could provide currently excluded individuals a means of transportation previously unavailable to them (Jeon et al. 2016). Yet, this inclusion is dependent on eliminating the dependency of automobiles on their current user interface, i.e. by replacing traditional automotive controls. An inclusively designed user interface is needed, designed to take into consideration the diverse range of needs of different members of society (Clarkson et al. 2013; Langdon et al. 2015).

'Level 5' or 'fully autonomous' vehicles do not require any user interaction to operate, other than selecting a destination and giving feedback on location and

---

T. Amanatidis (✉) · P. M. Langdon · P. J. Clarkson
Department of Engineering, Cambridge Engineering Design Centre,
University of Cambridge, Cambridge, UK
e-mail: ta323@cam.ac.uk

P. M. Langdon
e-mail: pml24@eng.cam.ac.uk

P. J. Clarkson
e-mail: pjc10@eng.cam.ac.uk

progress (SAE International 2016). As such, the user may be disconnected for the entirety of the journey, allowing for no knowledge of driving and almost no situational awareness (Stanton et al. 2007; Endsley 2016). As such, vehicles in this highest level of automation could be designed without a steering wheel or pedals, creating new possibilities in interface design. Users of these vehicles may not need a driving licence or otherwise be excluded from driving due to age, capability loss or cultural norms. Fully autonomous vehicles could thus provide the freedom of the automobile to members of society that were previously excluded (Jeon et al. 2016).

2 Related Work

This section presents related work regarding inclusively designed and developed user interfaces for fully autonomous vehicles.

2.1 Travellers' Needs and Public Introduction of Driverless Vehicles

The intelligent mobility: Traveller needs and UK capability study (Catapult Transport Systems 2015) surveyed over 10,000 members of the public, experts and transportation companies in order to understand the transportation needs of different members of the public, including what needs can be satisfied by intelligent mobility. The study identified five groups of traveller types, all with different needs and expectations, as per Table 1.

The study also identified two groups of users who would immediately benefit from the shift described above: the progressive metropolites and the dependent passengers—young, elderly or people with impairments who usually do not hold a

Table 1 The five traveller types as identified in the traveller needs study (Catapult Transport Systems 2015)

Traveller type	Description
Progressive metropolites	Living in the heart of the city, typified by the technology-savvy young professional, with significant amounts of personal and business travel. Want to reduce their transport footprint
Default motorists	High mileage drivers, with a mix of those who enjoy driving and many for whom it is a functional choice
Dependent passengers	Dependent on others for their mobility needs, representing a mix of students, elderly and those with impairments
Urban riders	City dwellers, who travel less frequently than the progressive metropolites, making use of public transport available to them
Local drivers	Mainly retirees or stay at home parents, making low mileage local journeys

driver's licence. The goal of this study is to gain insight into the needs and expectations of the latter category of users: dependent passengers.

It is, however, worth noting that the specifics of public introduction of autonomous vehicles are still unknown and perspectives vary substantially. For example, a meta-study by Clark et al. (2016) found expert predictions for autonomous vehicle mass adoption vary from <5 years to never, reported public adoption from 30 to 95% and expected cost from less than $2000 to over $30,000.

2.2 User Experience of Autonomous Vehicles

We argue that fully autonomous vehicle interfaces should be designed using principles of inclusive design (Clarkson et al. 2013; Langdon et al. 2015). As autonomous vehicles are not popular yet, Jeon et al. (2016) believe that there is a window of opportunity to develop inclusive interfaces as early as possible to avoid a potential 'automation divide'. Jeon et al. (2016) recommend three 'themes' for autonomous vehicle interfaces to adapt to the above considerations: an office theme, a playful theme and an inclusive/ergonomic theme. These themes are worth considering as they could guide our development towards multiple dedicated interfaces rather than one unifying design.

When designing a vehicle interface, it is important to consider the type of journey (Meschtscherjakov et al. 2014). Krome et al. (2016) performed a contextual inquiry study on future commuting journeys in autonomous vehicles. Instead of a Wizard of Oz techniques, as found in Large et al. (2016), researchers took on the driving task themselves to simulate an autonomous vehicle. This allowed passengers to focus on his task of choice such as gaming, working or reading, in an attempt to relieve the stress of the commute. Three contextual observations can be yielded from this study:

(a) The to-work and to-home commutes are different. In the former, users were usually quiet or bored, in the latter more upbeat and planning their evening.
(b) Almost any change in environment (e.g. entering a motorway) or speed (e.g. traffic) resulted in a change in activity, such as using a smartphone.
(c) Standstill is the most annoying driving situation and a design challenge.

2.3 Expected Baseline User Interface for 2017–2020

The ultimate goal of automation is to have a 'system that can permanently perform all the driving tasks without the driver having to monitor the system' (Robert Bosch GmbH 2014). Yet dependent passengers must be able to interact with the system too, and automotive designers must start developing a way for them to do so before 2020 when the first autonomous vehicle prototypes are predicted to hit the roads.

Given the previous experience of automotive user interface designers with touchscreens, we can deduce that the first, basic, autonomous vehicle interfaces will be touchscreen based, either in the users' devices or integrated in the vehicle. However, there are concerns regarding the inclusivity of such interface layouts, and as a result, a number of research projects such as Amanatidis et al. (2017b) are investigating complementary and alternative solutions.

3 Research Design

3.1 Purpose and Methods of Study

A wider interview study was performed with the purpose to obtain insight into the needs and expectations of fully autonomous vehicle users (Amanatidis et al. 2017a). Two participants, one visually impaired and one with restricted mobility, were also interviewed. This paper collates and presents the findings from these two individuals as well as findings from all participants that related to inclusivity. Qualitative tools (based on Field and Hole 2002; Purchase 2012; Ritchie et al. 2013; Stanton et al. 2013) were considered, and the format of interviews was selected.

3.2 Participants and Interview Structure

Initially, seven participants were interviewed. They were selected to cover all five categories of traveller identified by the UK travellers needs survey (Catapult Transport Systems 2015) as described in Table 1. One of these participants was visually impaired and did not hold a driving licence; all other participants were drivers. Upon discussion between the research team, one further interview of a dependent passenger was conducted: this participant was a wheelchair user but did hold a driving licence. Thus, a total of eight participants were interviewed; four of which were male and four were female. Ages ranged from 25 to 63 years old, with a mean age of 38 years old. The sample of users was inclusive: this was ensured by having a good representation in the dependent passenger category. The interviews were conducted in person or on Skype. No monetary reward was given for participating in this study. The interview process consisted of three parts:

1. Background questions on age, education, employment, familiarity with autonomous vehicles or any other associated experience.
2. A showing of the YouTube video 'A first drive' by the Google (2014) self-driving car project, which showed people of different ages, including a visually impaired individual, using and describing some of their experiences with a Google self-driving vehicle prototype.

3. The main interview consisted of eight questions, see Amanatidis et al. (2017a), with follow-ups depending on participants' responses. One of these questions was directly related to inclusivity: 'In the video shown, some of the users were elderly, impaired or otherwise excluded from driving. What aspects of the Google prototype do you like? What changes if any would you make to better cater for and include a broader range of users?'

3.3 Apparatus and Interview Analysis

The interviews were recorded using an HTC One M8 smartphone and then transcribed. Both recordings and transcripts were anonymised. As a qualitative study, the analysis of the collected data for the interview study was based on the methods recommended by Ritchie et al. (2013, Chaps. 10 and 11). As such, transcripts were analysed using Nvivo 11 software (Wikipedia 2017). Subsequently, the researcher classified the answers in nodes and analysed the contents of each node by order of references count, identifying findings and compiling the results.

4 Results and Discussion

As discussed previously in this paper, the user interface to be developed should be inclusively designed. While not all questions of this interview study focused specifically on inclusivity, some findings do relate to accessibility of the interface to individuals that currently cannot drive. These findings are discussed in this section.

Autonomous vehicles have the potential to liberate the mobility of dependent passengers in all but the cities with the best public transportation systems. For them, the most envisaged scenario is for autonomous vehicles to be used for the majority of journeys: '*I can't drive legally because of my vision. So for me, a self-driving vehicle would be tremendous*' (Interview 3) and '*I would use it for my daily life to move everywhere*' (Interview 8). These high-usage patterns result in dependent passengers interviewed to mostly prefer privately owning autonomous vehicles rather than using them as a mobility service. Therefore, an inclusively design interface should take these usage patterns into account. Other inclusivity considerations relate to the interior of the vehicle and feedback media used, depending on the type and extent of impairment.

One of the participants interviewed was a dependent passenger with reduced eyesight. For them, it was important to have the ability to access interface information both visually and verbally. In terms of the visual interface, they wished the screen(s) to be adjustable in terms of angle, distance and could ideally be held in their hands. Moreover, in terms of accessibility settings, they expressed the wish to be able to adjust the brightness, colour, contrast, font size and zoom in and out, in order to be able to see clearly. In terms of advantages of autonomous vehicles, some users mentioned they would allow them to rethink where they currently lived and what non-work activities they participated in. This was particularly the case with a dependent passenger who was restricted to housing which was on the bus route that led to their place of work.

> It has a lot to do with my vision. Most cars that I see now, the interface the information dials are set at a specific angle and a specific distance. Unless you can see at that exact distance, then you're missing out on a lot of information. Also being able to change the colour is important, because different angles, different lights and also different visual requirements for people might mean that the manufacturer's preferred scheme is just unreadable.
>
> (Interview 3)

Whether inclusive design of autonomous vehicles should extend to include wheelchair users is a question in itself. However, some projects such as UK Autodrive (2017) have adopted a wheelchair friendly design. One participant of this study was a dependent passenger with reduced mobility, using either a manual or electric wheelchair. They wanted to have easy access to the vehicles, through a folding or a solid ramp for their manual and electric wheelchair, respectively. This request seemed to emerge from poor experiences with taxis and taxi drivers, occasionally having to cross into their personal space to physically help them into their vehicle. Finally, they also wanted the ability to charge the batteries of their electric wheelchair if possible.

> Me personally, I would like a ramp so you can get in in your chair without having to transfer to a normal seat. That's an important facility. […] I think that a ramp that works with enough space for a wheelchair to safely be secured in a car, is enough for my condition and for many people that I can think of.
>
> (Interview 8)

Other participants contributed with information from their own experiences from relatives or friends. One user warned that autonomous vehicles, being mentioned as a great hope for mobility of the elderly might cause the opposite effect, because the elderly cannot operate or do not feel comfortable operating an autonomous vehicle (Interview 5). However, one user thought the Google pods looked like '*a wheelchair but it can protect you from the wind, the rain and the sun*'; therefore, the user felt '*reluctant to use it. I will feel people may see me differently. They might say: "Oh, you're using a wheelchair"*' (Interview 1). Another area of discussion with some participants was the 'digital-have nots'; specifically, lack of smartphones was mentioned as a bottleneck of adoption (Interview 3). Finally, one user pointed out that autonomous vehicles would bring mobility to new groups of users from a costing perspective (Interview 2). This could be true in low-income inner cities.

Overall, requests from dependent passengers seemed to broadly fall into two categories: reduce their reliance on others and increase their feeling of being safe and in control of their experience. As such, the main design recommendations that seem to arise for fully autonomous vehicle interfaces are as follows:

1. Design multimodal interfaces, to both order/call and control vehicles.
2. Visual displays should be adjustable in brightness, contrast and angle.
3. Automate the ordering/calling, ingress/egress and control processes.
4. Provide facilities to store, fix and charge mobility aids, e.g. wheelchairs.
5. Promote in-vehicle safety mechanisms and processes for all users.

5 Conclusions

In conclusion, this study resulted in a number of novel and important insights regarding inclusivity aspects of autonomous vehicle user interfaces, based on the needs and expectations of users themselves. The main finding was that multimodal interfaces were necessary but not sufficient to address the needs of dependent passengers. A number of these users mentioned more fundamental considerations such as accessibility of the display and easy ingress and egress as equally important to consider. Furthermore, the participants' answers seemed to fall mainly into two categories: reducing their reliance on others and increasing their feeling of being safe. As such, a number of recommendations emerged for designers of inclusive fully autonomous vehicle interfaces. We hope these recommendations would form part of a user requirements specification that would be used by further academic and industrial research alike in order to improve the design of future fully autonomous vehicle interfaces and include a broader range of members of society.

References

Amanatidis T, Langdon P, Clarkson PJ (2017a) Needs and expectations for fully autonomous vehicle user interfaces. In: Manuscript submitted for publication in proceedings of human-robot interaction conference, Chicago, IL, US, Mar 2018
Amanatidis T, Langdon P, Clarkson PJ (2017b) Toward an "equal-footing" human-robot interaction for fully autonomous vehicles. In: Chen J (ed) Advances in human factors in robots and unmanned systems, Springer, pp 313–319
Catapult Transport Systems (2015) Intelligent mobility: traveller needs and UK capability study. Catapult Transportation Systems. https://ts.catapult.org.uk/current-projects/traveller-needs-uk-capability-study/. Accessed 13 Nov 2017
Clark B, Parkhurst G, Ricci M (2016) Understanding the socioeconomic adoption scenarios for autonomous vehicles: a literature review. Project report, University of the West of England, Bristol, UK. http://eprints.uwe.ac.uk/29134. Accessed 13 Nov 2017
Clarkson PJ, Coleman R, Keates S, Lebbon C (2013) Inclusive design: design for the whole population. Springer Science & Business Media
Endsley MR (2016) Designing for situation awareness: an approach to user-centered design, 2nd edn. CRC Press
Field A, Hole H (2002) How to design and report experiments. SAGE
Google (2014) Self-driving car project. A first drive. https://www.youtube.com/watch?v=CqSDWoAhvLU. Accessed 5 Dec 2017

Jeon M, Politis I, Shladover SE, Sutter C, Terken JMB, Poppinga B (2016) Towards life-long mobility: accessible transportation with automation. In: Adjunct proceedings of the 8th international conference on automotive user interfaces and interactive vehicular applications, AutomotiveUI'16, Ann Arbor, MI, US, pp 203–208, 24–26 October 2016

Krome S, Walz SP, Greuter S (2016) Contextual inquiry of future commuting in autonomous cars. In: Proceedings of CHI'16 conference on human factors in computing systems, San Jose, CA, US, pp 3122–3128, 7–12 May 2016

Langdon P, Johnson D, Huppert F, Clarkson PJ (2015) A framework for collecting inclusive design data for the UK population. Appl Ergon 46(Part B):318–324 (Special Issue: Inclusive Design)

Large DR, Burnett G, Anyasodo B, Skrypchuk L (2016) Assessing cognitive demand during natural language interactions with a digital driving assistant. In: Proceedings of the 8th international conference on automotive user interfaces and interactive vehicular applications, Automotive'UI 16, Ann Arbor, MI, US, pp 67–742, 4–26 October 2016

Meschtscherjakov A, Ratan R, Tscheligi M, McCall R, Szostak D, Politis I et al (2014) 2nd workshop on user experience of autonomous driving. In: Adjunct proceedings of the 6th international conference on automotive user interfaces and interactive vehicular applications, AutomotiveUI'14, Seattle, WA, US, pp 1–3, 17–19 September 2014

Purchase, HC (2012) Experimental human-computer interaction: a practical guide with visual examples. Cambridge University Press

Ritchie J, Lewis J, McNaughton-Nicholls C, Ormston R (2013) Qualitative research practice: a guide for social science students and researchers. SAGE

Robert Bosch GmbH (2014) Automotive handbook, 9th edn, Wiley

SAE International (2016) SAE J3016: taxonomy and definitions for terms related to driving automation systems for on-road motor vehicles. SAE International

Stanton N, Young MS, Walker GH (2007) The psychology of driving automation: a discussion with professor Don Norman. Int J Veh Des 45:289–306

Stanton N, Salmon PM, Rafferty LA (2013) Human factors methods: a practical guide for engineering and design. Ashgate Publishing Ltd.

UK Autodrive (2017) The UK autodrive project. http://www.ukautodrive.com/. Accessed 21 June 2017

Wikipedia (2017) Nvivo. Encyclopedia Article. https://en.wikipedia.org/wiki/NVivo. Accessed 5 Dec 2017

At Home in the Hospital and Hospitalised at Home: Exploring Experiences of Cancer Care Environments

P. Jellema, M. Annemans and A. Heylighen

Abstract Contemporary cancer care takes place within a healthcare system catering for a highly mobile demographic. This study aimed to better understand how patients experience the cancer care environment (CCE) and the role of spatial aspects therein. We explore the effectiveness of photovoice in discussing this experience over time and the extent to which image production helps emphasise the role of spatial aspects. Three patients were interviewed over the course of 6 weeks. Experiences of the CCE turned out to change over time and across space as repeated travel to the hospital and transitions within the hospital resulted in new impressions and routines. Participants describe the dynamic and linked makeup of the CCE, suggesting a concatenation of places over time. The photovoice method blurs the boundary between researcher and participant, allowing features of the CCE to come to the fore that would otherwise not be considered. Over time, the hospital becomes 'a second home' to some, facilitating more than medical consultations and treatments only. A particular challenge for hospital design is therefore to improve the initial experience. Simultaneously, the home environment becomes a place of medical care at a distance. Caution is required when transforming the home into such a place as patients can feel insecure and distant from the watchful eye of the specialists.

1 Introduction

Architecture is increasingly recognised to impact on people's well-being and quality of life (Sternberg 2009; Jencks 2012). Furthermore, there is a growing understanding of, and supporting evidence for, the role architectural design plays in

P. Jellema (✉) · M. Annemans · A. Heylighen
Department of Architecture, Research[x]Design, KU Leuven, Leuven, Belgium
e-mail: pleuntje.jellema@kuleuven.be

M. Annemans
e-mail: margo.annemans@kuleuven.be

A. Heylighen
e-mail: ann.heylighen@kuleuven.be

the creation of 'wholesome' healthcare environments. Especially in cancer care facilities, where people are confronted with stress and anxiety, exploiting architecture's potential is highly relevant. Examples such as the UK-based Maggie's Cancer Care Centres demonstrate that high-quality architecture is not an expensive luxury but the context responsible for quality of life and well-being. The buildings convey an encouraging and supportive message to all who enter. Studies suggest that designing buildings with people's emotional needs in mind can lift their spirits and support the care offered on multiple levels (Annemans et al. 2012; Van der Linden et al. 2015): by generating a feeling of identification; by affording different uses and atmospheres; and ultimately, by supporting social interaction between its users and those around them, without forcing it upon them. However, distinct differences exist between the Maggie's Centres, offering psychosocial support, and the cancer care environments (CCEs) that focus primarily on medical care. This study starts from the observation that the experience of people affected by cancer is not sufficiently taken into account in the design of environments where treatments and consultations take place.

This raises the question how people can be supported in expressing their experience of these environments. Using participant-made photographs within interviews has helped researchers to reveal experiences that are difficult to express or too abstract (Frith and Harcourt 2007; Radley 2010). It is additionally found to benefit the relationship between the researcher and a patient participant (Radley 2010). Namely, within community-based participatory research, photovoice has been used to identify spatial aspects of experience, often at the scale of a neighbourhood (Wang and Burris 1997). Using photovoice explicitly to integrate participant agency into the research procedure is less common where it concerns user experience of a particular health care environment. In part, this may be context-related, where taking photographs is not common or may be considered inappropriate due to privacy concerns.

In this study, we explore to what extent photovoice can be used to engage people affected by cancer in investigating how spatial aspects affect their experience while also taking into account the sensitive nature of the CCE as a context to conduct research in. Ultimately, our aim is to gain a better understanding of how people affected by cancer experience the CCE and the role of spatial aspects in this experience.

2 Context

In care practice, considerable efforts are made to avoid an institutional atmosphere and create CCEs that express hospitality. This trend can be observed in hospitals and oncology wards, in cancer care centres, in accommodations of peer support groups and palliative care centres. However, realising a hospitable CCE is not straightforward, for either the care organisations or architects. Since stress and anxiety are context- and person-specific, designing for people affected by cancer requires taking into consideration their particular concerns, wishes and experiences (Annemans et al. 2012; Huisman et al. 2012). In studies about the impact of the built environment on people's well-being and quality of life, these are hardly addressed. Research in evidence-based design predominantly examines the effects of isolated aspects, e.g. daylight, a view on green (Ulrich 1984) on people's primary clinical reactions, without addressing their opinions, ideas and views (Malkin 2006). Moreover, by focussing on a single aspect (Rubin et al. 1998), these studies fail to consider the outcomes holistically (Huisman et al. 2012), and invariably conclude that the findings cannot readily inform the design of care facilities (Kirkeby 2015; Lawson and Parnell 2015).

3 Method

Through the use of ethnographic methods, this study attempts to identify common threads in how the CCE is experienced by cancer patients and spatial aspects that play a role in that experience. By combining photovoice with semi-structured interviews, we see knowledge as created in interaction between the researcher and the participants (Guba and Lincoln 1994). Due to the exploratory nature of the study, participants who met predetermined selection criteria were approached through convenience sampling. We explore how the CCE is experienced by the following research participants:

Lisa, a 37-year-old female, was diagnosed with cancer, underwent an amputation followed by 6 months of chemotherapy. At the time of the interviews, she was receiving radiotherapy. She lives with her husband, a daughter of 12 years old and numerous pets.

Helen, a 57-year-old female, underwent an operation, chemotherapy and radiotherapy. At the time of meeting, she was receiving adjuvant therapy and rehabilitation physiotherapy. She was treated in a regional hospital, which offered radiotherapy through a collaboration with another hospital. While on holiday, she went to yet another hospital. She lives with her husband and a pet dog.

Walter, a 67-year-old male, has been confronted with different types of cancer over the past few years. Most of his cancer care has taken place in the same hospital as Lisa, although different campus buildings feature in his accounts. He received chemo, both as an in- and as an outpatient. He also underwent multiple radiotherapy treatments. He and his wife recently downsized to an apartment.

Participants agreed to be interviewed at their home. Before commencing, they were made fully aware of the aims of the study, the researchers involved and how the data were going to be collected and saved. An informed consent form was presented and signed and practicalities regarding the study were discussed. The form included supplementary information, a copy of which was left with the participant. The interview was audio-recorded and structured according to a topic list.

After this interview, the participants were asked to visually document their experiences of the CCE during (one of) their next appointments. To take photos, they were offered the choice of borrowing a device or using their own. A selection of the photos was emailed to the first author in preparation of a follow-up interview. This process was repeated two more times with Helen and Lisa. For various reasons, Walter was not able to take photographs. Our findings are based on an in-depth study of Lisa and Helen's material supplemented with the analysis of Walter's interview material.

Interviews were transcribed *verbatim* interspersing the text with photographs when these were being discussed. The analysis of interview transcriptions was done following the guidelines of the QUAGOL method based on the constant comparative method of grounded theory (Dierckx de Casterlé et al. 2012). The anonymity of the participants was ensured throughout (e.g. by anonymising photos and using pseudonyms in dissemination). Although the hospitals are not named within the study, it is impossible to guarantee their anonymity as the infrastructure is recorded in some of the photographs.

4 Experiencing the Cancer Care Environment

Through participants' verbal description and visual depiction of their experience over time, and its intertwinement with emotional and social aspects, their exposure to the CCE becomes clearer. How their experiences change over time and across space offers insight into the CCE as a dynamic and linked entity. Our focus is on the participants' experience as long-term outpatients even though their treatment has included a hospital stay at some point.

4.1 Home, Transit and Hospital

Gaining a sense of the 'places of importance' that the CCE is comprised of, from the participants' perspective, meant asking questions about what locations and movements were involved. A pattern emerges of cancer care taking place in different locations: a sequence of spaces and places that merge in and out of the individual's experience. As participants go through a course of treatment, different spatial aspects take on prominence. In both photographs and interviews, the hospital, home and other places have roles to play. All three participants find a sense of safety and comfort important. Sometimes this leads to the hospital being spoken about as a 'second home'. At the same time, by being asked to document their experience of the CCE, participants are able to put forward the idea that the home environment is, in its own way, also part of the CCE. To avoid confusion regarding this definition results will be discussed referring to the hospital and the home.

The hospital is rarely talked about as being one place or building. It consists of different places, and places within places. An initial experience of a particular setting or destination will linger in one's memory, be built upon and referred back to. The size, colours, furnishings and amenities contribute to the general atmosphere. Participants indicate their sensitivity towards the lighting, temperature, acoustics, odours and ventilation. The atmosphere is regularly compared to their idea, or image, of a 'typical hospital' (Fig. 1). It is also affected by the cadence, i.e. the busyness or occupancy of the space at a particular moment, and by challenging indoor routes or difficulties understanding the wayfinding signage. A period of cancer treatments is characterised by a string of initial impressions as they are directed to spaces for the first time. A sequence of spaces is the result. Some are left behind, while others are returned to repeatedly.

> Because of that bad experience... and because of the bad news that you received there ... I really... yeah, that took a very long time before I was brave enough to go in there again.
>
> (Interview Lisa)

As participants become accustomed to the place, there is then attention for what the environment has to offer and affords. Art in the hospital is a welcome distraction, as is the perceived connection with outdoor nature. Furniture is important, as well as being able to get a drink, or take in information about treatments or support-related services. Walter and his wife find it convenient that they know where they can find a blanket when necessary. Lisa wants to be able to use personal devices for entertainment and household-related activities. She likes the curtains that she can close around her while receiving chemotherapy treatments (although Walter claims no one uses these because the remaining space is too cramped). Lisa also appreciates jigsaw puzzles that are provided in the radiotherapy waiting areas.

Some actions only become possible when one feels sufficiently at ease. Helen considers the gym a good place for people to take off their wig (Fig. 2): in that setting it was necessary (hot and sweaty) and possible (generally supportive) to do that.

> It's a really big step to enter into that confrontation with other people. If you can do that there, then afterwards it will be easier with family and friends. So, that's a place to do that.
>
> (Interview Helen)

Fig. 1 Helen accepts this type of space with mixed feelings: *'really hospital-like'*

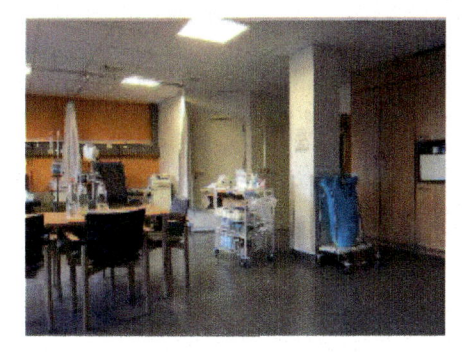

Fig. 2 Helen describes a gym space with green mats: *'happy colours, a great space'*

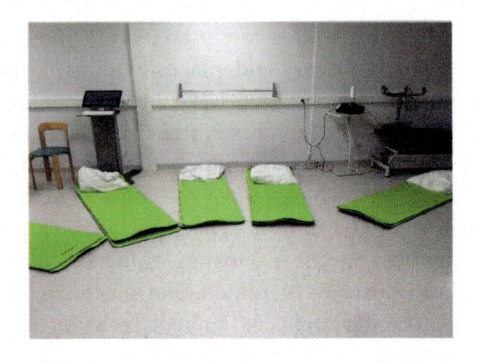

Participants eventually lay claim on (a piece of) the hospital. Lisa calls the oncology outpatient centre her 'second home'. She emphasises the transition between the typical hospital environment and 'her world' on the other side of the door where she receives chemotherapy. It is as though the door says 'welcome' by automatically opening, outwards, towards her:

> It's like a boundary you have to step over. And when those doors open … It's like… they come towards me those doors, as though they say 'welcome, come in, come into this world'.
>
> (Interview Lisa)

Different phases of treatment occur in different places, and as participants become more accustomed to a place and route, their needs and expectations evolve. Spatial aspects can be identified at different scales. The atmosphere at the time of the initial diagnosis sticks in one's memory. Key features of the environment get intertwined with other memories of the experience. A string of initial impressions and memories of the CCE are formed throughout the period of treatment. The environment is experienced as being supportive when patients can show initiative or exert some control there.

Experiences of transit, both within hospital buildings and on the way to the hospital, are described by all participants. The spatial aspects that become apparent in these experiences are intricately linked to changes over time. Throughout a period of treatment an awareness of time is apparent at different 'scales'. First, participants recount a personal motion through the period of illness and treatment. Second, the temporal comes up in the (repeated) experience of single hospital visits. How often one has been to a place makes a difference. Different types of treatment require different rhythms in terms of the regularity of hospital visits. As familiarity with a space increases initial feelings of fear and stress are replaced with a sense of safety and routine. When the general experience of a place is positive it is perceived as reliable and stable. Walter, looking back on at least 112 separate hospital visits for cancer care, summarises it as follows:

> The hospital for me is always… Yeah, it's there. I don't have any problems with it. I don't know how better to say that. Yes, we go to the clinic. I know my way 'round there.
>
> (Interview Walter)

Negative aspects of routines also surface. For example, Lisa describes being infuriated each time she has to pass by an ashtray outside the entrance to the oncology wing.

The convenience of 'being nearby', particularly in relation to the repetitive nature of hospital visits, contrasts with long distances walked within the hospital. There is an explicit appreciation for designated parking areas, near to entrances, allowing easy access. Appreciation (or frustration) is most often expressed about aspects of spatial organisation that relate to convenience and privacy. The participants notice when their interests and limitations are acknowledged (or not). As the route and place become more familiar, new habits emerge. Going 'there' and home again is described as happening in a certain way. Especially for Lisa, stopping for coffee became a cherished habit (Fig. 3). Both Lisa and Walter were usually accompanied by significant others. Helen was more independent in this respect.

The importance and comfort of the home is emphasised in relation to repeated travel to the hospital. It is generally a supportive environment. Family members and pets play a role in this (Fig. 4). The sofa is an important place to rest. Lying in bed seems to make one feel even sicker (both in the hospital and at home). Helen prefers having people visit her at home rather than in the hospital. Lisa refers to her home as 'her cocoon':

> Here you can hang around, lie down and do whatever you like. If I'd go somewhere I'd have to wear something other than my pyjamas. Or at home I'd take off the headscarf every now and then. Somewhere else I wouldn't do that. Here in my cocoon I always feel [takes deep breath]…

(Interview Lisa)

Fig. 3 Lisa and her husband stop for coffee: *'Our moment of relaxation'*

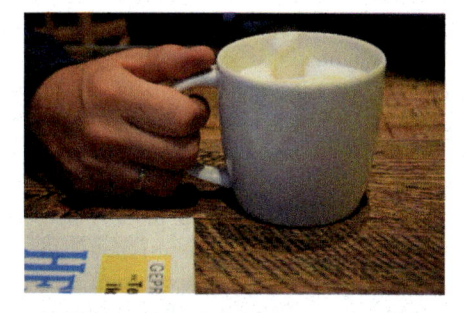

Fig. 4 Lisa talking about the dog: *'At home, my consolation when I'm alone'*

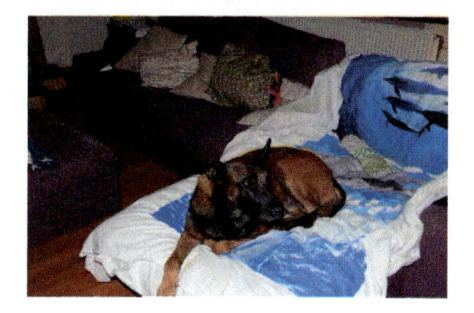

However, Helen describes the home as also a place of feeling unsure and invisible. Her days there were some of the worst. She would feel incredibly ill and not know what medication to take. She associates a particular corner in the living room with these bad days. Walter and his wife recently moved from a large home that was becoming too much to deal with.

4.2 As a Result of Treatment

How the CCE is experienced, and the role of spatial aspects therein, turns out to be considerably affected by the cancer treatment. First, *the changing body* interferes with routines and takes one by surprise. Feeling sick, tired or changed in terms of appearance, or sensory perception has people relate differently to their environment (sometimes suddenly) than if they were relying on a more healthy body. One clear example is the distance one can walk before needing to rest. Walter describes a situation after being in hospital for a 5-day chemo treatment:

> My wife was coming to pick me up. Me and my suitcase. And then I do find the oncology department really far to go on foot. In fact I find it a bit far. With my suitcase, after packing everything I was fine. But then on the way it was like being knocked with a hammer. Just so tired, tired, tired.
>
> (Interview Walter)

The changing body as a result of illness or medical procedures can result in feelings of helplessness. Helen describes a situation where a fellow patient had been warned to stay away from young children and pregnant women due to the radioactive medication she had been given. Subsequently, she had an appointment with a gynaecologist and found waiting in a room with pregnant women confronting and difficult. Lisa was challenged by the complete lack of privacy when she was in a full waiting room while really wanting a private moment to cry.

The second theme relates to *social interactions,* with staff, family and fellow patients. The hospital plays a role in facilitating these interactions. At the same time, it is described as a place where the participants are confronted with other patients, a type of interaction that is forced and uncomfortable. Lisa points out that talking to healthcare support staff was only possible after explicitly requesting an appointment. She also found access to fellow patients limited and mostly activity-based. Opportunities to connect with people in a similar situation were scheduled occasions and not always available at a time and place that suited her. Walter's partner played a key role in supporting social interactions. Helen seemed to connect with fellow patients more spontaneously. She appreciated sharing a room, emphasising that she had more in common with that roommate than with a friend who visited while she was receiving chemotherapy. She describes the way conversations start based on small gestures and non-verbal contact when the space allowed for a certain proximity:

> You saw the other man glancing over, he looked, nodded, hello sir and then I thought yeah, a comment, you know something you say as a joke about what he did and then our conversation was launched ... Partly that is about who I am but it's also a space for that. You're sitting close to each other the whole time and you can read a book or you can do what you like, it's the same. But sometimes it's fun to say something.
>
> (Interview Helen)

Additionally, participants touch on the topic of shame and stigma. They point out difficulties around communicating about cancer both with people who are familiar and with people who are unfamiliar to them. Consider the account of patients putting on a wig to cross a parking lot to then arrive in the gym where they promptly remove it. Helen talks about avoiding eye contact with an acquaintance on her way to having her breast amputated because she finds this experience more challenging to talk about than when she previously had surgery. There is, therefore, a need for physical barriers for privacy and discretion. At the same time, stigma and shame can be obstacles to interaction, requiring tactfully designed settings to bridge gaps and break barriers.

5 Discussion and Conclusion

Our study confirms the value of photovoice as a suitable method to extricate spatial aspects from people's personal experiences even in sensitive contexts. The act of documenting their experience with photographs blurs the boundary between researcher and participant. Participants willing to adopt photovoice may not be representative of all cancer patients. However, by documenting their experience with photos, participants made visible a CCE that exceeds the hospital boundaries. Further research is necessary to explore the extent of the differing descriptions of the CCE based on the perspectives of other users, healthcare providers and CCE designers.

Awaiting this exploration, our analysis of the interviews and photos shows participants' experience changing over time and across space as repeated travel between the home and hospital, and transitions within the hospital result in new impressions and routines. Photovoice allowed the researchers to question what spaces are considered part of the CCE. This aspect of the findings would likely not have come forward without this visual method that allowed participants to bring topics and their own focus to the interviews. Additional findings relate to how the body, changing as a result of treatment, affects perception and experience of the environment. Social interactions are affected by cancer demanding that the CCE takes issues of shame into account.

We recognise that the initial experience of cancer is one where all sense of normality is temporarily lost (Vollmer and Koppen 2010). A supportive hospital environment can help regain some of this and become through routine—as it was for Lisa—like a 'second home'. Much in this analysis is brought together in the idea of *normalisation*. The types of activities that participants valued during their hospital visits point towards regaining a sense of normalcy in their life. The environment can afford the opportunity to choose (furniture/seating type), initiate (closing curtains, taking coffee) and take some control or ownership (knowing where to find blankets) instead of users being fully reliant on others. Cresswell (2004) finds that a focus on place can act to normalise and naturalise identity through a shared geographical location. Identity can be constructed through the shared experience of place rather than (or instead of) a stigmatising feature that the people coming together in that place have in common. If we relate this to the success of the Maggie's Centres, there is evidence that architecture's potential is also in supporting a collective experience (Van der Linden et al. 2015), possibly alleviating some of the current stresses around confrontation and facilitating informal interactions.

This study supports previous findings with reference to the hospital being conceived as a type of 'home'. In looking closely at contesting meanings associated with hospital spaces Kellett and Collins (2009, p. 114) find that the 'uneasy relationship between home and hospital' is at the heart of a battle. Their study discusses the domestication of the hospital by examining ways in which a hospital space may be (re)constructed as 'home' by those occupying it. Although it is unusual to associate 'home' with an institutional building, it is fitting to consider the concept of home as a polar opposite to the typical hospital (Kellett and Collins 2009). Participants use these archetypical concepts to compare and evaluate their experience of spaces. At the same time, it is in referencing one's particular 'home' that personality, taste and other personal features result in diverse responses.

In terms of implications for hospital design, we see a particular challenge to improve the initial experience. There may be options to de-medicalise a consultation environment, creating a pleasant atmosphere to enter into. Designing hospitality is key, with clear signage, sufficient seating options and thoughtful attention to privacy needs for those receiving difficult news. This supports Vollmer and Koppen's (2010) conclusion in their design research in which they emphasised the need to architecturally link medical and psychosocial care for outpatient cancer care.

Our findings suggest that patients could be further supported by a *diversification* of activities offered within the hospital. Participants indicated an interest in aspects of the environment that offer or support distraction, (social) contact, information, relaxation and other daily activities. What one expects and needs in the hospital is influenced by the home and household situation—in terms of the location and distance to where the cancer care takes place, but also in relation to other household members and their availability to offer practical and emotional support. Again, this points towards a desire to have psychosocial care and support integrated with medical care. Healthcare professionals tend to see psychosocial care and medical care (treatments, etc.) as separate while participants in this study suggested, that in their experience these are (expected to be) fully integrated.

Lastly, it became necessary to see participants' homes as links in a concatenation of places that together form an individual's experience of the CCE. Increasingly, chemotherapy treatments are becoming available which can be self-administered at home (Bloom et al. 2015). For example, in Belgium, 12 pilot projects for 'home hospitalisation' were recently approved, six specifically for cancer care (De Block 2017). Our findings suggest that this indeed forms an extension of contemporary cancer care, whereby the home is transformed to a place of medical care. However, caution is required, as the patient can feel insecure and far removed from the watchful eye of the medical specialists.

Acknowledgements We are grateful to the three participants who generously gave of their time and energy for this study. This project was realised with the support of *Kom op tegen Kanker* (Suzanne Duchesne Fund) and Research Fund KU Leuven (PDM/16/092).

References

Annemans M, Van Audenhove C, Vermolen H, Heylighen A (2012) What makes an environment healing? In: Brassett J, McDonnell J, Malpas M (eds) Out of control, proceedings of 8th international design and emotion conference London 2012, Central Saint Martins College of Art & Design, London, UK, 11–14 Sept 2012
Bloom M, Markovitz S, Silverman S, Yost C (2015) Ten trends transforming cancer care and their effects on space planning for academic medical centers. HERD 8(2):85–94
Cresswell T (2004) Place: a short introduction. Blackwell Pub, Malden, MA, US
De Block M (2017) Twaalf pilootprojecten rond thuishospitalisatie in de startblokken [Press report 09/03/2017]. www.deblock.belgium.be. Accessed 18 Aug 2017
Dierckx de Casterlé B, Gastmans C, Bryon E, Denier Y (2012) QUAGOL: A guide for qualitative data analysis. Int J Nurs Stud 49(3):360–371
Frith H, Harcourt D (2007) Using photographs to capture women's experiences of chemotherapy. Qual Health Res 17(10):1340–1350
Guba EG, Lincoln YS (1994) Competing paradigms in qualitative research. In: Denzin NK, Lincoln YS (eds) Handbook of qualitative research, Sage, pp 105–117
Huisman E, Morales E, van Hoof J, Kort HSM (2012) Healing environment. Build Environ 58:70–80
Jencks C (2012) Can architecture affect your health? ArtEZ Press, Arnhem
Kellett P, Collins P (2009) At home in hospital? Competing constructions of hospital environments. ArchNet-IJAR 3(1):101–116
Kirkeby IM (2015) Accessible knowledge—Knowledge on accessibility. J Civ Eng Archit 9(5):534–546
Lawson B, Parnell R (2015) Quality of place and wellbeing. In: Stephen Clift S, Camic PM (eds) Oxford textbook of creative arts, health, and wellbeing, Oxford University Press, pp 299–308
Malkin J (2006) Healing environments as the century mark. In: Wagenaar C (ed) The architecture of hospitals. NAi Publishers, Rotterdam, The Netherlands, pp 259–265
Radley A (2010) What people do with pictures. Vis Stud 25(3):268–279
Rubin HR, Owens AJ, Golden G (1998) An investigation to determine whether the built environment affects patients' medical outcomes. The Center for Health Design, Martinez, US
Sternberg EM (2009) Healing spaces: the science of place and well-being. Belknap Press of Harvard University Press, Cambridge, MA, US
Ulrich RS (1984) View through a window may influence recovery from surgery. Science 224 (4647):417–419

Van der Linden V, Annemans M, Heylighen A (2015) You'd want an energy from a building. In: Proceedings of the 3rd European conference on design4health 2015, Sheffield Hallam University, UK, 13–16 July 2015

Vollmer T, Koppen G (2010) Architectuur als tweede lichaam. Layout 11, Stimuleringsfonds Creatieve Industrie, pp 1–16

Wang C, Burris MA (1997) Photovoice: concept, methodology, and use for participatory needs assessment. Health Edu Behav 24(3):369–387

Do Exergames Motivate Seniors to Exercise? Computer Graphics Impact

R. Alyami and H. Wei

Abstract Sedentary lifestyle is a serious problem which affects health. Sufficient physical activities help to maintain ability to manage daily lives. This can be a challenge. Exergames has become a possible stimulator to encourage especially seniors away from sedentary lifestyle. This paper, from a graphic interface point of view, investigates the impact of Microsoft Kinect-based exergames on seniors' motivation to exercise. The exergames include three different graphics user interfaces. Information from NHS recommended motions for seniors was adopted in the development of the games. These games induced a conduction of experiment and interviews with participants from Southampton Age UK. The experiment results showed that different graphics interfaces do have an impact on seniors' motivation to exercise.

1 Introduction

As people get older, they tend to become less and less physically active. Seniors are also the most vulnerable and more likely to contract diseases or experience health problems. This is also the time when they start losing interest in doing any kind of physical activities, as indicated by the study performed by Buman et al. (2010). It has also been proven time and again that a lack of physical activity can have a detrimental effect on one's health. On average, 30 min of moderate physical activity daily is recommended in order to obtain significant health benefits (Pate et al. 1995). Recent statistics show that the dangers associated with sedentary behaviour have been steadily increasing each year affecting people of all ages. According to the British Heart Foundation (2015) in England, sedentary levels are highest in those aged 16–24 years or aged 65 and over. Similarly, in Scotland, senior people (aged 65 and over) tend to be most sedentary both during weekdays (6.5–7.5 h) and weekends (6.7–7.6 h per day). Sedentary behaviour increases the risk of high blood pressure, anxiety, depression, certain cancers, type 2 diabetes and many other health problems.

R. Alyami (✉) · H. Wei
Department of Computer Science, University of Reading, Reading, UK
e-mail: r.y.alyami@pgr.reading.ac.uk

In order to prevent seniors from leading such sedentary lifestyles and to promote awareness of healthy living, it is important to first understand the barriers that restrict them from performing physical activities and the motivations that influence them to be physically more active along with the challenges of introducing them to Kinect.

There are difficulties associated with designing an exergame for seniors such as the needs to be satisfied by such games and technologies, and the motivational drivers required to be addressed whenever designing a game. Thus, there is a need to understand how seniors interact with technology, and it is necessary to investigate seniors' challenges in interacting with Kinect.

A decrease in physical activity plays a role in the onset of a multitude of health issues, such as hypertension, depression, cancer and type 2 diabetes, with cognitive, physical and sensory abilities lessening with age and ailments (British Heart Foundation 2015). Accordingly, much emphasis and attention has been placed on and directed towards how physical activity can be more regular and beneficial.

It has been recognised that technology may be valuable in giving vulnerable populations a greater degree of independence. However, such populations are not always open to trying and regularly using such technologies, with many factors established both as drivers and barriers to the implementation of these tools. Some drivers to technology use include design, ease of use, perceived usefulness and independent living. On the other hand, a lack of interest, a lack of awareness, complicated design, limited usefulness and some disabilities can hinder the application of these devices. Senior people face obstacles, particularly in regard to physical ailments, and the pain and suffering associated with these may consequently hinder feelings of happiness and enjoyment of movement. Hence, several enterprises have formulated technological devices that can track, monitor and facilitate physical activity.

This paper paid close attention to the concerns held by the seniors with regard to the use of motion-based technologies and game-based rehabilitation. Game formulation and assessment were carried out in consideration to different game aspects offered by Kinect. Other elements have been addressed to improve levels of physical activity amongst the seniors in a number of works, including those by Pate et al. (1995), Yim and Graham (2007), Buman et al. (2010), Mueller et al. (2010), Thin and Poole (2010) and Crounse (2014). This paper investigates exergames' ability to motivate seniors to exercise and if different graphics interfaces and scenarios would have an impact on seniors' motivation to exercise. The main goal was to motivate them to exercise and improve their mobility level.

2 Methodology

Observation, focus group, interviews and questionnaire were the general approach to this experiment to analyse the body movement and collect feedback to improve the game. Numerous researches were considered to understand the main problem

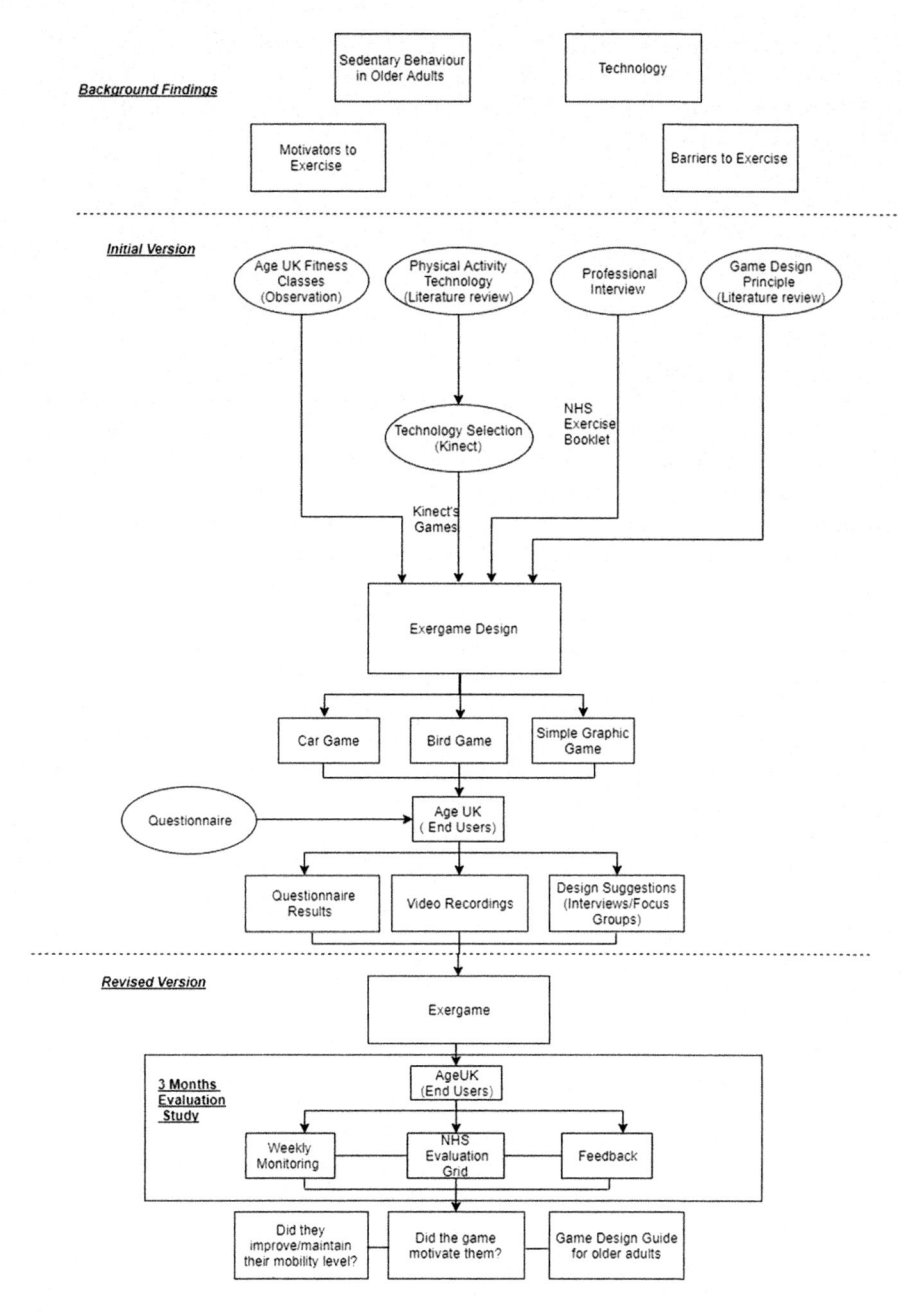

Fig. 1 Research model

with exercising amongst the senior population and the latest health technology. The next step was to approach Age UK to observe seniors and their lifestyles. However, professional physiotherapist also needed to be approached to understand seniors' obstacles from a different perspective.

The diagram in Fig. 1 is a guide model developed based on focus group, interviews, questionnaire and literature review, structuring and illustrating the flow of this research starting from collecting information needed from previous research and finding the gap to design and plan the next study.

This experiment was conducted at Age UK in Southampton. Age UK offered a room within their facility, which was more accessible for seniors, thus making it easier to recruit participants.

In consideration of both research and Age UK, three different specially designed exergames were developed to study the impact of different graphics interfaces on seniors' motivation to exercise. The results of this study and the feedback will help to improve a future study. The next study will allow participants to use the game for 3 months. They will be professionally evaluated by the researcher, who has been trained by professionals to use an NHS evaluation grid to monitor participants' mobility levels every 4 weeks.

2.1 Input from Professional

The authors interviewed a physiotherapist to update their previous research. Key information was obtained in order to develop efficient exercise games that address some of seniors' barriers and motivation. The following information was gathered: the most important types of exercises for seniors and their preference for the exercise movement, the right amount of time to exercise and if there were any exercise movements that suited all seniors with different conditions. All the information contributed towards designing and building the games.

2.2 Motion Selection

A couple of motions (spine twists whilst standing or sitting down on a chair), chosen from NHS booklets for home exercises (www.laterlifetraining.co.uk/llt-home-exercise-booklets/), were integrated in the exergame development (Fig. 2).

According to Belward (2015), ageing can affect bone structure and muscles causing pain and decreasing the range of motion in the shoulders, spine and hips. Therefore, the selected exercises, spine twists, were important in developing and maintaining flexibility in the upper body, offsetting the effects of a normal decline in joint flexibility and helping participants to remain active and independent. Taking into consideration seniors with mobility impairment, this exercise was amenable to an exergame design. An important reason for the motions selection is

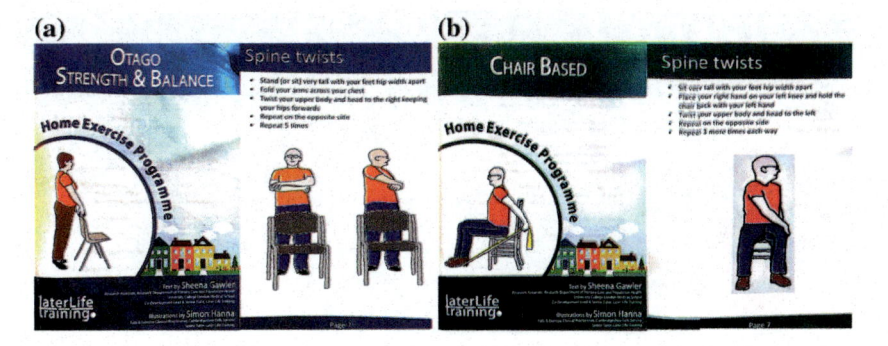

Fig. 2 NHS exercises booklet **a** Otago home exercise booklet illustration **b** Chair based exercise booklet ilustration. Reproduced with permission from Later Life Training Ltd, 24 Nov 2017. Further information on these exercises can be found at https://www.laterlifetraining.co.uk/llt-home-exercise-booklets/

Kinect's ability to detect most of the NHS booklet motions. Kinect has two tracking modes, the default mode and the seated mode. The default mode can detect 20 skeletal joints in both upper and lower body. However, the seated mode can only detect ten skeletal joints all in the upper body. Therefore, motions like 'March in the chair' could not be chosen to use for this study, as this study was dedicated for both standing and seated seniors.

2.3 Games Design

Exergame refers to the video games that are played with the help of a physical exertion. It is considered as a technology-driven physical activity, which encourages the users to be more physically active.

Microsoft Kinect was the chosen motion sensor to be used in this research, as it allows users to interact intuitively and without any intermediary device, such as a controller. It allows users to exercise freely without any attachment to their body.

Based on the selected motions, three different specially designed games were developed to test if the graphics interfaces can affect seniors' desire to play the exergame. These games designs were emanated from the research model in Fig. 1. The main idea of the games was to enable seniors to twist their upper body left and right and repeat it at least five times in order to develop/maintain upper body flexibility.

To determine if different scenarios had a different impact on motivating participants to exercise, three games with three different scenarios were developed. In the first scenario, an inanimate character was used as the main character whilst the second scenario used an animate one. However, the third scenario used a block, a simple object without any decorations. Each scenario had its own distinct setting and atmosphere but they all shared the same gameplay. The goal was to reach the finish line in less than a minute, whilst controlling the game by body motion. The rule was to avoid whatever obstacles appeared on the way to the finishing line whilst enjoying the music played, see Fig. 3.

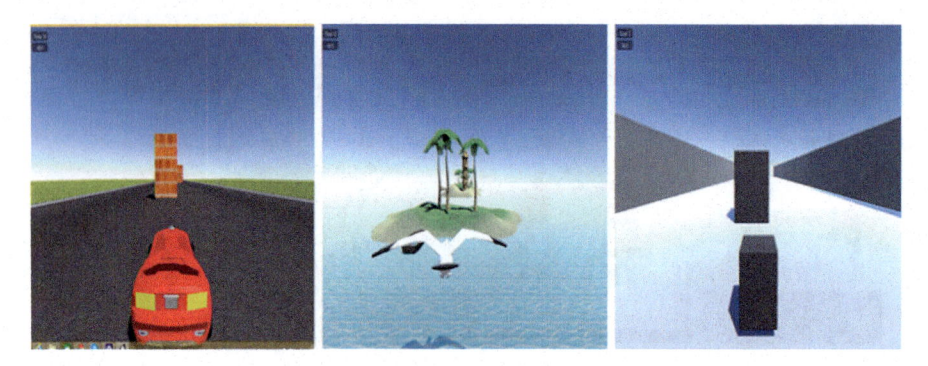

Fig. 3 The three different graphics interfaces for the exergames

This study aimed to help to examine if the graphics interfaces affected seniors' motivation to play and if the participants were interested in playing. The games were finalised, they passed the lab test successfully and they were thus taken outside the lab and were trialled amongst seniors.

3 Experiment

The interview with the professional physiotherapist helped to develop an understanding of how seniors react to different exercises, in terms of what their preferences were and what kind of exercises were most effective. Seniors, who had got involved in Age UK, had already attended exercise classes and had learned what kind of exercises they should have been doing and how, were identified as the main target audience. An ethical approval was obtained to involve seniors in this research.

However, few criteria had to be applied to the participants to be recruited in this experiment. They had to have attended Age UK fitness classes, be 60+ years of age, had to have had normal or corrected vision (e.g. with eyeglasses or contact lenses) and the ability to understand verbal explanations and written information in English.

The main reason for specifically targeting this group was that the classes run by Age UK, designed for seniors, were not always available and may even have been cancelled. Seniors were left to perform their daily routine of physical activity in their own homes without any instruction or assistance, leading some to potentially lose motivation and not following up after the classes had ended, thus becoming less active.

Each participant took a maximum of 5 min to complete the game. After that, they were asked to complete a questionnaire based on the overall gameplay, ease of use, how comfortable the player was and if the game was physically challenging. When all participants had completed the game and the questionnaire, there was a

20 min session to collect the questionnaires and delve further into the group's ideas, suggestions, improvements and recommendations for future iterations of the exergame. The following questions were asked to guide the discussion:

- Do you think it was helpful to use Kinect to play the game?
- Did you find it easy, or difficult, to simultaneously play the game and perform the exercises?
- Please explain what you particularly liked, and/or disliked, about the game.
- Would you change or recommend any improvements to the game?

The exergames provided game mechanics that aimed to keep the seniors motivated to keep performing physical activities, which they had learnt at Age UK classes, in their own time. This research aimed to help seniors to avoid being dependent on externally provided physical activity classes. However, the aim of developing the preliminary exergame was to investigate if different graphics Kinect-based exergames would affect seniors' motivation to exercise.

4 Results and Discussion

In total, 15 people, five male and ten female, who were retirees in the age range of 65–95 years, participated in this experiment. All of them attended Age UK exercise classes at least once a month. The mobility of the majority of them was good, and they did not need to use a wheelchair. Only three participants needed a cane to help them walk.

The results showed that the group was naturally divided into two groups: one used a computer at least once a month and the other never. None of them had ever used the Kinect sensor before.

It was expected that none of the participants would prefer the block game because of the simple and plain graphics. Surprisingly, a couple of them preferred the block game where the graphics were unattractive and simple. It reminded them of the old-school game, and it was simple and easy to play. However, the majority of the participants favoured the bird game. They thought it was visually attractive and gave them the feeling of being free. The different graphics interfaces not only affected their motivation but also their reactions. Although the game's motions were all the same, the reaction to the different graphics interfaces differed as was shown in the video recordings. When the participants were more concentrating on the game, i.e. in the car and the block game, their body movement towards the obstacles was faster whereas in the bird game, they felt more relaxed and effortlessly performed the exercise. One participant said, '*I liked the car game more than the bird because it's more difficult*' even though all the games were the same difficulty.

According to the Age UK exercise instructor, the different reaction to the games was beneficial for seniors. The instructor tries to make the seniors aware of their surroundings and have quick reaction to help to cope with the real-life demands, for example, people needing to be more aware of their surroundings when crossing the street. The participant interviews revealed that they did prefer one game over the other, which impacted on their motivation to exercise.

5 Conclusions

Our hypothesis was that exergames would help seniors to avoid sedentary lifestyles. This paper explored, through a case study, how users' motivation to exercise could be affected by different graphics interfaces and scenarios in Kinect-based exergames.

A guide model was established to assist the exergames design and development process. Three different graphical games interfaces were produced, and they were used in an experiment conducted with seniors in Age UK, Southampton.

The study was motivated by the challenges the seniors have. We analysed how the different graphics interfaces impacted participants' motivation. It was clear that different game designs not only had an impact on users' motivation but also on their body movement reaction, which researchers and developers should take into consideration in the future studies.

It was shown from the questionnaire that seniors were motivated to exercise using exergames. It was anticipated that users' mobility level would improve with the continuous use of this specially designed game. It was notable that all the exercise movements in the games were recommended by the NHS.

Acknowledgements The research is funded by Saudi Arabia Ministry of Higher Education and the University of Taif. The authors wish to thank Faustina Hwang, Southampton Age UK that arranged exergames experiment sessions and allowed us to interact with the participants.

References

Belward SA (2015) Interviewed by Raneem Alyami on personal interview. 3 November 2015
British Heart Foundation (2015) Physical activity statistics 2015. https://www.bhf.org.uk/research/heart-statistics/heart-statistics-publications/physical-activity-statistics-2015. Accessed on 30 Sept 2015
Buman MP, Yasova LD, Giacobbi PR (2010) Descriptive and narrative reports of barriers and motivators to physical activity in sedentary older adults. Psychol Sport Exerc 11(3):223–230
Crounse B (2014) Microsoft kinect sensor applications in health and medicine. Health Blog. https://blogs.msdn.microsoft.com/healthblog/2014/01/10/microsoft-kinect-sensor-applications-in-health-and-medicine/. Accessed on 25 Aug 2015
Mueller F, Gibbs MR, Vetere F (2010) Towards understanding how to design for social play in exertion games. Pers Ubiquit Comput 14(5):417–424

Pate RR, Pratt M, Blair SN, Haskell WL, Macera CA, Bouchard C (1995) Physical activity and public health: a recommendation from the centers for disease control and prevention and the American College of Sports Medicine. JAMA 273(5):402–407

Thin AG, Poole N (2010) Dance-based exergaming: User experience design implications for maximizing health benefits based on exercise intensity and perceived enjoyment. Trans edutainment IV:189–199. Springer, Berlin, Heidelberg

Yim J, Graham TC (2007) Using games to increase exercise motivation. In: Proceedings of the 2007 conference on future play, 3, Toronto, ON, Canada, 15–17 November 2007, pp 166–173

Part V
Breaking Down Barriers Between Research and Policy-making

On Becoming a Cyborg: A Reflection on Articulation Work, Embodiment, Agency and Ableism

Jennifer Ann Rode

Abstract This article auto-ethnographically explores my experiences over the course of several years as I transitioned from able-bodied, to frequent cane user, who used a scooter to attend academic conferences, to a user of robotic telepresence. I discuss the different affordances that those technologies allow, issues of embodiment, articulation work, agency and ableism. The telepresence robot did not 'fix me' as is often implicated in the medical model of disability (Thomson in Extraordinary bodies: figuring physical disability in American culture and literature. Columbia University Press, NY, 1997), or augment my experience to make it more palatable to the able-bodied majority. Instead, it allowed me to make conscious trade-offs between the affordances of my corporeal body and an emergent cyborg-self in the context of a degenerative autoimmune disease. Thus, in writing this article, it is my intention to improve the social acceptance of the disabled cyborg person, and through improved design, I aim to afford disabled persons choices.

1 Introduction

For three beautiful days during Ubicomp one fall, I could walk at a brisk pace for 6 hours at a time. Or rather, I learned to accept being a new form of one. I could nimbly weave through crowds, and I could look people in the eye. I became a cyborg. My flesh body was in Philadelphia, whereas my "other body" was in Seattle, and my mind was somewhere in between, or neither. Scooters, wheelchairs and canes were replaced by this other embodiment, I felt free. This essay auto-ethnographically reflects on my experiences using a telepresence robot. I have used this approach because reflexivity is critical to understanding this experience, and it allows me to address my experiences in ways that a positivist approach would not. In doing so, I hope to address issues of embodiment, articulation work, agency

---

J. A. Rode (✉)
University College London, London, UK
e-mail: j.rode@ucl.ac.uk

and ableism with the intention of improving the social acceptance of the cyborg, and its design to afford disabled persons' choices.

2 Method

In this paper, I will auto-ethnographically discuss my experiences since September 2014 with telepresence robots. The way an anthropologist represents oneself is a significant issue in applying anthropologic methods (Geertz 1988). One needs to simultaneously give oneself authority and credibility by illustrating you were really there, but at the same time accurately representing the culture of the people you are studying. Much debate exists on the benefits of 'objective' distant realists accounts, as compared to reflexive accounts where the role of the author is discussed (Geertz 1988). Elsewhere in my work, I have argued for the importance of reflexive practice in ethnography studies of technology use (Rode 2011). Auto-ethnography is an anthropological method that tries to resolve these tensions; it is a practice which Van Maanen (1988, p. 106) describes as a 'wet term signalling the cultural study of one's own people'. Often this is done to give authentic voice to marginalised groups, whose voices may have previously been tempered through anthropological tales told by academics from dominant groups (Duncan 2008; Ellis et al. 2010). Here, I write about myself as representative of an emergent group of disabled persons embracing this potentially transformative technology. Disability experience is central to critical disabilities studies and auto-ethnography in particular is a common technique (Smith and Sparkes 2008; Richards 2008). In this way, through my own experiences, I aim to study an emergent culture of disabled telepresence users.

My first experience with a telepresence robot was borrowing a Suitable Technologies' Beam system to remotely attend the Ubicomp Conference in Seattle. Afterwards, I purchased my own telepresence robot which I placed in my lab in the US and later the UK. I will discuss my own usage experiences in the context of my disability, as well as my colleagues using my robot to visit me.

I purchased my own robot using funds generously provided by the American National Science Foundation. I felt the robot allowed me to socially construct a different experience of my disability. I have called into the office using the robot on days I did not feel well enough to leave the sofa; I have also found myself in the office, and yet sending the robot down the hall to talk to a colleague. Yet, the telepresence robot did not 'fix me' or augment my experience to make it more palatable to the able-bodied majority. I do not condone a medical model of disability. Instead, it allowed me to make conscious trade-offs between the affordances of my corporeal body and my increased awareness of my cyborg-self in the context of a degenerative autoimmune disease. I am using Haraway's (1991) feminist STS definition of cyborg, "a creature simultaneously animal and machine, who populate worlds" rather than the AI community's usage of the term. Haraway (1991) argues, we have all always been cyborgs, and focuses on dissolving our notions that human (and animal) bodies exist and develop in some way separate from technology.

Certainly, this applies to those of us who are disabled with our accessibility apparatuses. Canes, scooters, reading glasses, and telepresence robots become extensions of ourselves. In this way society creates an artificial boundary between able bodied and disabled. The dissolution her framework offers for the separateness of the human/machine hybrid can be similarly applied to ability as well. Haraway's theoretical framework is appropriate for examining disability in that it allows us to explore the notion of "disabled" as an artificial construct imbued with charged meanings and discriminations in our society amongst a range of differently abled cyborg identities. Thus, in this paper I have embraced and explored my identity as a human-computer hybrid; a cyborg. In exploring this boundary, I have learned to take an activist stance on my (dis)ability.

My disability results in profound fatigue, difficulty walking and painful breathing during flares, while at other times I appear wholly able-bodied. The transition between these two states can be gradual or can occur suddenly. Thus, I am simultaneously negotiating my changing experiences as a cyborg and as a person with a disability in concert with one another.

All Beam interactions were documented in short session observation notes or 'jottings' in ethnographic parlance (Emerson et al. 1995), supplemented with screenshots of the Beam User Interface. The session observations were extended to provide ethnographic field notes, following each session. The data were open coded to explore telepresence use in light of existing human–computer interaction (HCI) interaction theory. I employed an abductive, qualitative analysis across iterative coding cycles (Emerson et al. 1995) to explore issues such as embodiment, articulation work, agency and ableism. My analysis ended when I reached theoretical saturation—that is when no new information on usage practice was revealed by further analysis.

3 System Description

The Beam Telepresence system consists of a video screen mounted on a 5-foot shaft connected to wheels (Fig. 1). As the person who is connecting remotely, I can then drive the Beam as I like and my image is displayed on the video screen. Local attendees can move the Beam only by physically pushing it.

The Beam user and local attendees can hear each other due to a microphone and speaker. The Beam has two cameras: one at near eye level for communication and another which is lit and pointed down at the ground to aid with navigation. The user interface allows one to monitor these two cameras, plus the camera on your own computer (see Fig. 2). One can drive with a touchpad (my preference) through a mouse, or USB Microsoft Xbox controller can be used. To aid navigation one can plot a planned course in the lower navigation window, so that you can determine your path which is especially helpful on turns.

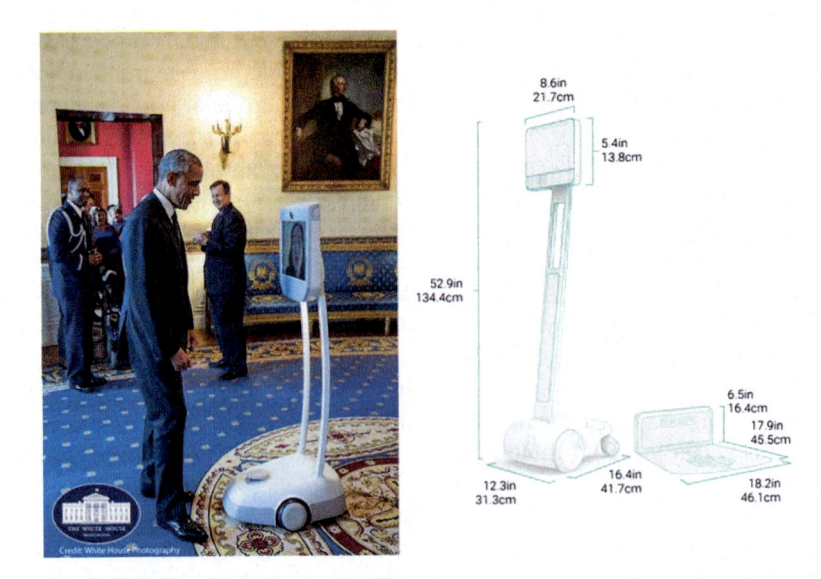

Fig. 1 (left) Photo of former U.S. President Obama with disability rights activist Alice Wong. *Photo credit* Pete Souza in his capacity as chief official white house photographer. Diagram with sizes of Beam system and docking station (right). *Photo credit* Suitable Technologies

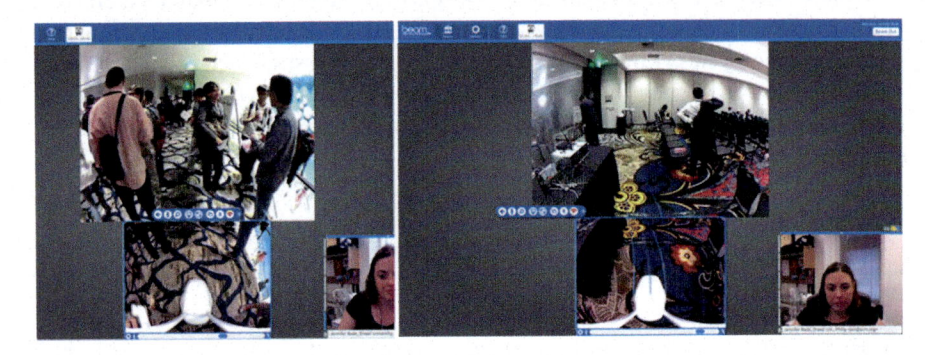

Fig. 2 (left) The view from my computer consisting of three windows, described counterclockwise from the top. The large window is the communication camera view. The smaller window is the navigation camera. Finally, the partial window is for monitoring your own camera. I moved it partially off screen, though later learned it could be minimised. (right) Here navigation tracking is turned on in the lower navigation window so that you can see your current planned course. This is especially helpful on turns. *Photo credits* Author

4 Findings

4.1 In the Beginning… of 'Bots and Beings'

On my first day as a telepresence robot, I felt a bit like a celebrity hounded by paparazzi, as I searched for the room with the first conference session with the aid of a hotel map. Some asked me for a photo, but others took one without permission leaving me feeling objectified and violated. This is akin to Thomson's (1997) discussions of the disabled persons often being a dehumanised object of curiosity. Scores of people photographed me. My disabled body was a spectacle.

On entering the room for my session, a senior colleague, Jane, came up and helpfully attempted to direct me to the 'blue box', a robot seating zone in the back of the room. This area had been designated such that we robots did not tower over the seated fully human attendees. After the spectacle of my arrival, it was reassuring to come across someone whom I knew. It made me feel grounded and cut through the surreal nature of my experience. It left me feeling that this far of space was connected to people with whom I had once had embodied experiences.

I saw a dear friend, Lawrence, and excused myself, though Jane was concerned that I might not be able to find the 'blue box', which was admittedly hard to see in comparison to the very gaudy carpet. Lawrence promised he would indeed help me find the blue box. Again, people were watching and snapping photos. I was a spectacle, but really, I just wanted to talk to a dear friend. Lawrence, gently explained that I was 'shouting' and estimated likely speaking at a volume that could be heard from 3 metres away. I blushed, ashamed of my faux pas, as I learned to regulate my new-found voice in a world where I could not truly hear myself. Finally, I achieved a 'reasonably private' conversation, and we got to catch up. It was lovely to see him, but as he requested and took a selfie with me, I recognised how the lack of a greeting hug momentarily made me aware of my dual body.

Finally, as the session was about to start, I moved to the 'blue box', and encountered another cyborg for the first time (Fig. 3). I had trouble recognising my colleague, and folks were fascinated by two robots having a conversation, and more photos ensued. Later, as I encountered another cyborg, I jotted:

> Neither J nor I could tell the other was moving so as we approached one another we bumped. It was kind of funny, but awkward. The whole conversation was strained. We do not know each other well, but suddenly had this shared experience and forced intimacy of being 'bots' amongst the 'beings'.

(Fieldnotes)

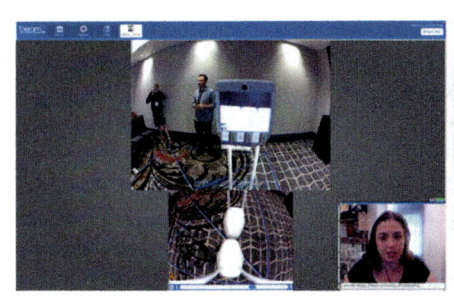

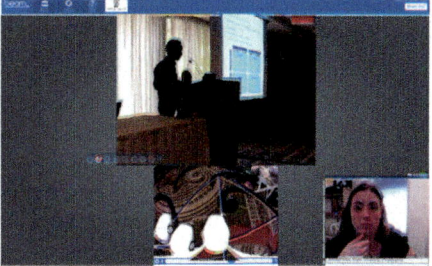

Fig. 3 (left) Meeting another 'bot'. Note it is wholly unclear to whom I am talking. Also, note the man photographing this encounter without consent. (right) The 'blue box' with three Beams watching the speaker. Note the oblique angle rendering the slides impossible to read and the speaker entirely in shadow. *Photo credits* Author

As I became more adept at the articulation work (Gerson and Star 1986) of manipulating my robot body, I had control of my voice and movements, and it became a part of me. I became a cyborg, but I began to recognise my new self with both limitations and new-found abilities.

I could zip about from place to place, and talk to colleagues without the walk tiring me and fatigue making my arguments less crisp.

I could look someone in the eye, rather than peering up at them from a scooter or wheelchair. Since most conversations at my conferences, especially receptions and coffee breaks, occur standing, this was profoundly empowering.

Still getting from floor to floor was problematic. Elevators act as Faraday cages, causing Wi-Fi signals to be dropped between floors. Ideally, one's elevator mates will wait for my Wi-Fi to reconnect, so I can drive myself off the elevator and onto the new floor. This is a very considerate thing to do, but often one's elevator mates might only place one's robot self on the correct floor facing a wall. Then, one 'wakes up' uncertain of whether you are on the correct floor. Of course, less considerate (or more oblivious) souls may not let one out of the elevator at all, or perhaps place my robot self on a floor at random by accident or out of malice. In a way, it is an improvement over clutching the elevator railings for dear life, hoping that the bounce that able-bodied peoples' knees can take does not cause you to topple over. It certainly beats crawling up or down stairs on one's hand or knees when overcome with fatigue and pain, but at least that makes disability visible and allows for advocacy. However, with my robot self, there is the fear of becoming trapped in an elevator and that fear is a new form of invisible disability. Fear of losing one's robot self, and getting that dreaded email, '*Subject: [Beam] Jennifer Rode's Beam has run out of battery*; *Jennifer Rode's Beam has run out of battery*; *Jennifer Rode's Beam shut down due to low battery*'.

Suddenly, one's robot self, one's agency, is cut off. You are stranded elsewhere, unable to return until you rescue your robot body to be recharged. This means asking a 'local' to fetch your robot 'corpse', and drag it back to a docking station to be recharged. This is worse than sitting in the hallway of a conference with a busted scooter waiting for the repairman, because without battery you become invisible. It is worse than having to crawl up or down a flight of stairs when the only elevator is broken, or on to a conference stage to give a talk when they forgot your ramp. At that moment, all of a sudden crawling does not seem so bad, because at least you can see and be seen.

Sure, in some future incarnation, one can hack the Beam to ensure there is signal in the elevator, and able-bodied people using the Beam have this same trouble. However, in this moment I question the design decision that led to this possibility, a sense of privilege and ableism embedded in its design. My dependence on my robot self is different from able-bodied folks. I send my Beam to where I cannot be; it is not about convenience, a temporary disability, or an issue with a visa that may one day be resolved. It is the portal through which I access the world. I am a cyborg, and it is part of my sense of self. Thus, perhaps for me and others with disability, stable access to one's robotic body is more crucial and lack of it fraught with more psychological baggage. Telepresence designers in their design decisions need to recognise this in order not to privilege the needs of the casual able-bodied convenience user.

4.2 Embodiment and Handless Feeling

I have no hands as a robot. I can attach things to my body—a Wi-Fi signal booster, or a basket to carry things. However, I cannot I knock at a door the way a physically present able-bodied person would. In the beginning, I would stand helpless at the door and hope someone inside would open it. Later, as I gained control of my robot self I would peer about, swinging my robot body in a circle to look for someone to ask for help. In the years since the conference, I have mostly perfected what I call the *whole-body robot knock*. One throws one body against the door as gently as possible, to best mimic a corporal knock. Usually, it works. Though occasionally one's hand slips on the controls, or perhaps my arthritis acts up and I startle the room's occupants. That seems rude and unfortunate, but I do not have hands. Even a gentle knock will startle someone who is not familiar with the whole-body robot knock. So even now, I still find myself standing helplessly by doors, waiting.

Once I make my hopefully not grand entrance, there is the question of greetings. I cannot shake hands or hug when greeting someone. So, greetings seem cold. On occasion, I've made very gentle contact with someone—knocking them gently. You see just as Vertesi (2008) discusses, 'Seeing Like a Rover', you can feel as a Beam. When I hit something, intentional or otherwise, the bottom of the robot stops abruptly, but the camera seated at the top of the robot, my portal to the world, continues forward until the centre of gravity jerks it back. When this jostling of the camera occurs unintentionally and my attention is wholly immersed in my virtual presence, I find myself jerking my head back as the camera goes far too close to a door or other object and the hairs on my arms bristle. It is not painful, but the experience of hitting something remotely is none the less embodied. Consequently, there are opportunities to play with this seamful interaction (Chalmers and Galani 2004), this sense of *handless feeling*.

Dourish (2001, p. 3) discusses *embodied interaction* as the site where humans interact with computer systems which 'occupy our world, a world of physical and social reality, and that exploit this fact in how they interact with us'. Dourish's theory well predated robotic telepresence, but can be extended to remove the duality between computer and human, and by extension the Cartesian duality between body and mind. Thus, *handless feeling* is a way I have developed to allow for embodied interaction by re-appropriating the technology in ways that I am sure the designers did not entirely intend.

Further, one can have an active embodied physical presence in this other space, especially as my telepresence robot has no proximity sensor or safety override to slow it down as I approach an object or person. Experimentation ensued; what could I do? I learned that with maximum speed, momentum and a little skill, I could push a chair across a room. Thus, when talking to a close friend or colleague who says something playful, I have the option of gently nudging them, the way one might faux box someone. There is then a realisation that one could be violent, even if it is only intentionally running over toes. By extension, a greeting could become embodied; gently coming into contact with another can create a mediated sense of physical intimacy.

On a more recent occasion in the last year, the video signal on my robot was lagging somewhat, such that my projected human movements on camera became a bit jerky, though my robot self was standing stationary. We were waiting for an event to start, and a well-meaning colleague proceeded to tease me for several minutes while by performing a jerky robot movement much to the amusement of her onlookers. These were increasingly close to the camera, and violating my sense of personal space, or should I say *cyborg space*. At some point, I felt a bit objectified, mocked for my robot self and technical limitations, and she just was uncomfortably close. After briefly considering whether I had adequate bandwidth to safely do so, I decided to assert myself. I very carefully and gingerly moved my robot self, *very* quickly to what I believe to be about two inches forward, and then abruptly stopped, abruptly invading her personal space. My colleague jumped back with a shriek of frightened surprise, and then joined the rest of my colleagues on both sides of the camera and laughed heartily. I might have limitations as my robot self, but I still have agency and in doing so I reasserted my humanity.

4.3 Agency, Embodiment and Comings and Goings

One aspect of life as a cyborg with limited agency is with regard to the circumstances under which you enter the room. On my second occasion using the Beam, I arrived in the room where Beams were docked. The room was also the headquarters for the conference staff, and thus was secure and large enough to store a half-dozen Beams. I entered the room to discover that I had crashed a birthday party for one of my senior colleagues. They had just rolled a wheeled cart with a cake which was quite literally blocking my exit from the room. There was a mixture of shock, laughter and uncertainty. I felt extraordinarily rude crashing the party; after all, I was not invited, and everyone else were senior members of the Ubicomp programme committee. Still, telepresence requires adapting as social norms are overturned inadvertently, so after an awkward moment I jokingly offered to take a 'Beam selfie' with him. I joined the party singing Happy Birthday. The guest of honour cut the cake, and going with the obvious joke I was immediately offered a piece, which I politely declined. I felt rude not being able to accept, but we laughed. Once they moved the cake cart to serve, I made my polite excuses and left.

This conversation as to whether I would like cake momentarily made me realise that while my senses of touch and sight extended to my experiences in Seattle, my senses of taste and smell were still rooted firmly in Philadelphia. I felt momentary torn, embodied in neither place. I love cake, yet I could not smell the vanilla frosting. Nor could I take a bite of cake that looked truly delicious. Consequently, my sense of immersion shattered. Further, while it was truly funny to remark on my inability to eat, and it was well-intended levity attempting to smooth an awkward social situation; nonetheless, it was commentary on my disability. I was handless, and I could not eat. I was other. Again, while my physical disabilities were augmented with this new technology, I encountered new disabilities by choosing this alternate cyborg form. This is in line with Herring et al.'s (2016) research that discusses how even able-bodied persons in telepresence robots are treated as somewhat disabled. In that way, I was not that different from an able-bodied person using a telepresence robot. While at the same time realising that I was oversensitive, I also recognised some new form of corporeal ableism at the core of this interaction. Yet, while I cannot become able-bodied, I recognise my new-found ability by selecting whether to attend an event in person or as a cyborg is in essence to select the suite of disability features I wish to present to the world.

I, similarly, had little control on when I left a social interaction. On one occasion, I was being interviewed about my experience using a telepresence robot, and mid-interview my Wi-Fi connection dropped. Suddenly, I was transported from my embodied world in Seattle, back to Philadelphia. When talking to the reporter, I had borrowed a colleague's robot as mine was having technical difficulty. In my hurry to get back to the interview, I logged back into the wrong robot. Consequently, rather than reappearing in the robot right next to the reporter, I logged into one back in the conference chair's room. As I rolled back to the reporter, I startled her. The poor woman shrieked audibly and commented that I startled her. I felt like I was playing one of those role-playing video games where I had to visit my corpse to restart the game.

Again, this reminded me of the fragility of this form of communication as a complement for my disability. I was dependent on the Internet and ultimately on a link that lacked any tangible form. This fragility made me feel intensely vulnerable, as it mediated my presence at an academic conference, where interpersonal networking is crucial for my professional status and ultimately the perception of my reliability as a colleague.

5 Conclusions

In this essay, I have reflected on my initial experiences using telepresence. I have engaged in a tremendous amount of articulation work to try to make this tool work for me. In some ways, the technology affords me significant newly found freedoms and in others is profoundly restricting. I strive for an embodied experience and while I have developed a sense of *cyborg space* and *handless feeling,* in other instances, the immersion can be broken and I become painfully aware of my physical separateness. Further, issues of agency and ableism become conflated as in some ways technical limitations reaffirm and, in some cases, create new forms of disability. As more and more computer science conferences allow this form of 'attendance', we need to consider the social implications for those of us with disabilities. Further, in some instances, I have seen remote participation being used as a way of accommodating disabled persons, instead of ensuring the actual physical space is accessible. Technology, then, can be used to reify these new forms of cyborg disability.

Throughout this experience, I have become a cyborg. Or more accurately accepted that I have become a new type of cyborg. Disability studies scholar, Siebers (2008) theorises disability as a minority identity, and challenges readers to consider embracing it as a positive, writing,

> To reverse the negative connotations of disability… it will be necessary to claim the value and variety of disability in ways that may seem strange to readers who have little experience with disability studies. But it is vital to show to what extent the ideology of ability collapses once we "claim disability" as a positive identity.
>
> (Linton)

He argues doing so improves quality of life for disabled people (Siebers 2008). Thus, by acknowledging, I have become a cyborg, I am making a political statement. It requires a tremendous amount of articulation work to deal with the technology limitations and stigma of disability, both present in everyday life and in the design of the technology itself (which itself create new forms of invisible disability). By embracing the positive aspects of my disability and becoming a cyborg using telepresence, I am afforded a new form of an activist disabled identity. Managing it requires negotiating issues of presence, embodiment and agency, which as I have shown need to be re-theorised to fully consider this new type of hybrid disabled cyborg identity. While this essay has not presented solutions, it provides clear illustration of problems with articulation work to ensure embodiment, agency and prevent ableism. As we move forward with the development of telepresence, the issues of social justice for the disabled need to be carefully considered.

Acknowledgements I would like to thank Ellen Bass, Diane Carr, Paul Dourish, Karen Nakamura, Didem Okzul, Phaedra Shanbaum and my reviewers for feedback on this article.

References

Chalmers M, Galani A (2004) Seamful interweaving: heterogeneity in the theory and design of interactive systems. In: Proceedings of DIS'04, ACM press, NY, pp 243–25
Dourish P (2001) Where the action is: the foundations of embodied interaction. MIT Press, Cambridge
Duncan M (2008) Narrative and its potential contribution to disability studies. In: Smith B, Sparkes AC (eds) Disability & Society, vol 23, no 1, pp 17–28
Ellis C, Adams TE, Bochner AP (2010) Autoethnography: an overview. Forum Qual Soc Res 12(1) (Art 10)
Emerson R, Fretz R, Shaw L (1995) Writing ethnographic fieldwork. Chicago University Press, Chicago
Geertz C (1988) Works and lives: the anthropologist as author. Stanford University Press, Stanford
Gerson EM, Star LS (1986) Analyzing due process in the workplace. ACM Trans OIS 4(3): 257–270

Haraway DJ (1991) A cyborg manifesto: science, technology, and socialist-feminism in the late Twentieth Century. In: Simians, cyborgs and women: the reinvention of nature. Routledge, UK

Herring SC, Fussell SR, Kristoffersson A, Mutlu B, Neustaedter C, Tsui K (2016) The future of robotic telepresence: visions, opportunities and challenges. In: Proceedings of CHI'16 conference extended abstract, ACM, NY, pp 1038–1042

Richards R (2008) Writing the othered self: autoethnography and the problem of objectification in writing about illness and disability. Qual Health Res 18(12):1717–1728

Rode JA (2011) Reflexivity in digital anthropology. In: Proceedings of CHI, ACM, NY, pp 123–132

Siebers TA (2008) Disability theory (corporealities: discourses of disability). Michigian University Press, Ann Arbor

Smith B, Sparkes AC (2008) Narrative and its potential contribution to disability studies. Disabil Soc 23(1):17–28

Thomson RG (1997) Extraordinary bodies: figuring physical disability in American culture and literature. Columbia University Press, NY

Van Maanen J (1988) Tales of the field: on writing ethnography. Chicago University Press Chicago, IL

Vertesi J (2008) Seeing like a rover: embodied experience on the mars exploration rover mission. In: Proceedings of CHI'08 extended abstracts, ACM, NY, pp 2523-25

Breaking Well-Formed Opinions and Mindsets by Designing with People Living with Dementia

Paul A. Rodgers and E. Winton

Abstract This paper presents ongoing research that highlights how design thinking and acting can contribute significantly to breaking down preconceived ideas about what people living with dementia are capable of doing. The research, undertaken in collaboration with Alzheimer Scotland and other dementia organisations across the UK, has adopted a range of disruptive design interventions to break the cycle of well-formed opinions, strategies, mindsets and ways-of-doing that tend to remain unchallenged in the health and social care of people living with dementia. The research has resulted in a number of co-designed interventions that help change the perception of dementia by showing that people living with dementia can offer much to UK society after diagnosis. Moreover, it is envisaged that the co-designed activities and interventions presented here will help reconnect people recently diagnosed with dementia to help build their self-esteem, identity and dignity and help keep the person with dementia connected to their community, thus delaying the need for formal support and avoid the need for crisis responses. The paper reports on three design interventions where the authors have worked collaboratively with nearly 200 people diagnosed with dementia across the UK in co-design and development activities. The paper concludes with a number of innovative recommendations for researchers when co-designing with people living with dementia.

1 Introduction

In the UK, life expectancy over the last few decades has risen steadily. Today, females born in 2015 can expect to live 82.8 years from birth (4 years more than females born in 1991) and males have seen a greater increase in life expectancy of 5.7 years, from 73.4 years for males born in 1991 to 79.1 years for males born in

---

P. A. Rodgers (✉) · E. Winton
Imagination, Lancaster University, Lancaster, UK
e-mail: p.rodgers@lancaster.ac.uk

E. Winton
e-mail: e.winton@lancaster.ac.uk

2015. Life expectancy in the UK is projected to continue increasing; with life expectancy at birth for females projected to be 85.1 years by 2026 and 86.6 years by 2036. Males are also projected to live longer, increasing to 82.1 years by 2026 and 83.7 years by 2036. Improved health care and lifestyles, especially for those aged 65 and over, is the main reason for the increase in life expectancy (Office for National Statistics 2017).

The consequences of these population changes in the UK, however, means the shape of the UK population is transforming with those of a working age shrinking whilst those of a pensionable age is increasing. Whilst a larger population can increase the size and productive capacity of the workforce, it also increases significant pressures and questions the sustainability to provide social services such as education, health and social care and housing. The rise in life expectancy in the UK is a key factor in the forecasted rise of people living with dementia in the UK. The number of people with dementia in the UK is forecast to increase to over 1 million by 2025 and over 2 million by 2051. By the year 2030, over 80% more people aged 65 and over will have some form of dementia compared to 2010.

In the UK, dementia and how we respond to it has reached a crisis point. It is a problem that improved public awareness or a better diagnosis alone will not solve. The management of long-term conditions associated with dementia is the key challenge facing the health and social care system in the UK. The UK Government believes we need to see profound changes to the way we view the person living with dementia as well as the overall system of health and social care (All Party Parliamentary Group on Dementia 2016). With this in mind, the three co-design projects presented in this paper show that people living with dementia can continue to make a significant contribution to society after diagnosis. The approach taken here actively involved a range of stakeholders in the design process such as care workers, people living with dementia and their family and friends to help ensure the three co-design projects met their needs and would be valuable and useful. The three co-design projects were carefully developed to be more appropriate to people living with dementia and their emotional and practical needs. Moreover, the three co-design projects aim to help reconnect people recently diagnosed with dementia to build their self-esteem, identity and dignity and keep the person with dementia connected to their community.

2 The Nature of Dementia

Dementia is a broad umbrella term used to describe a range of progressive neurological disorders. There are many different types of dementia and each person will experience their dementia in their own unique way. Common symptoms of dementia can include problems with short-term memory where new information is difficult to retain. People with dementia can get lost in seemingly familiar places, may experience confusion with names and may also experience confusion in environments which are unfamiliar to them. As a result, people with dementia may lose interest in engaging with others socially, so a person with dementia may become quieter and more introverted, and their self-confidence might become affected. Amongst older people, dementia makes the largest contribution to the need for care, much more so than other types of impairment and chronic disease (Prince et al. 2013). This demand for health and social care services will continue to increase as a result of demographic changes. Responding to this challenge will require innovative ways of supporting people with dementia to live well from the early stages of the illness. Receiving a diagnosis of dementia creates a 'biographical disruption', with the chronically ill 'observing their former self-images crumbling away' (Bury 1982). People need support from the point of diagnosis to come to terms with this life-altering event, remain connected to their community and enable them to live well with this long-term illness. However, people typically do not receive support until the illness is advanced and often at the point of crisis (Alzheimer Scotland 2008). This pattern is becoming more acute as a result of pressure on health and social care budgets.

Philosophical debates on dementia have largely focused around the fundamental nature of being and what constitutes personhood. The failure to recognise personhood and the negative impact of inappropriate caregiving can result in 'malignant social psychology', which includes labelling, disempowerment, infantilisation, invalidation and objectification. One reason behind this malignance is failing to see a person and not showing the respect that properly accords a person (Kitwood 1990). Even when a person seems to have lost a significant part of what made them a unique individual, core elements of their identity will remain. These characteristic gestures and ways-of-doing things are what keep alive the sense of the individual they once were, even if the more sophisticated levels of that individual have been removed. This has important implications for the approach to providing support and what people require in addition to the basics of daily living. A person's sense of self and self-respect can be fostered through 'reinforcing any remaining elements of conscious self-identity'; less conscious elements in a person's identity can be preserved through physical surroundings to retain 'physical links with their past, which help to support a sense of personhood' (Matthews 2006). Whilst mood and behaviour may be profoundly affected, personhood is not; the individual remains the same equally valuable person throughout the course of the illness. Interventions to support the person with dementia should honour their personhood and right to be treated as a unique individual.

3 Designing with People Living with Dementia

The key aim of this ongoing research is to develop a number of disruptive design interventions (e.g. products, systems and services) that break the cycle of well-formed opinions, mindsets and ways-of-doing that tend to remain unchallenged in the health and social care of people living with dementia. Many misconceptions surround people living with dementia, which can result in the perpetuation of stigma, isolation and generally negative reactions. The idea that nothing can be done to help people with dementia often leads to feelings of hopelessness and frustration (Batsch and Mittelman 2012). Many people living with dementia have a sense of inadequacy and low self-esteem. They perceive their status within society has been reduced as a result of their diagnosis (Katsuno 2005). In the main, people living with dementia are not considered capable of designing new products or services. This ongoing work sets out to directly challenge this assumption. The design interventions presented here (i.e. Disrupting Dementia tartan, Designed With Me and 75BC) have all been devised and undertaken from a 'designing with' perspective where the user is not viewed as a 'subject' but rather as an active 'partner' in the project (Sanders and Stappers 2014). The approach taken here encourages the development of richer, more varied solutions to everyday issues by emphasising fun (Bisson and Luckner 1996), 'safe failure', and doing things in ways that those working with people with dementia would not normally do. The three co-design projects presented here adopt a largely interventionist approach, which are based on a number of emerging theories emanating from research in economics, business and design (Christensen and Overdorf 2000; Scharmer 2011; Rodgers and Tennant 2014) that celebrate jumping straight in, doing things in order to learn new things, and valuing failure.

Co-design has been widely used in the commercial sector. However, recent research shows that co-design is increasingly used in the public sector, including the third sector, as a way of engaging citizens in design exploration (Lam et al. 2012). Many co-design techniques and tools, however, assume particular skills, expertise and processes that rely on certain levels of communication, cognitive and creative skills on the part of the participants. As such, many well-established co-design tools and techniques may not be appropriate and need adjustment (Wilson et al. 2015). Indeed when working with people with cognitive and other impairments such as dementia, researchers may have to develop and adopt highly individual co-design approaches and methods (Hendriks et al. 2015). The motivation behind the three projects presented here has been to ensure that everyone involved is engaged fully. As such, great care has been taken to consult with people living with dementia, their family members and care support workers about how they wanted to be involved throughout the projects before they started. In particular, it was vital that the planned co-design projects supported the person living with dementia and that it paid respect to their personhood and their right to be treated as a unique individual (Kinnaird 2012). A co-design approach acknowledges that each individual has their own strengths and weaknesses that they bring to the co-design process. Consequently, the three projects presented here have been carried out with people living with dementia who, it is hoped, will benefit from the experiences. Indeed, the key objective behind this work is to care better for people living with dementia and break down widely held and largely negative preconceived ideas about what people living with dementia are capable of doing.

3.1 Disrupting Dementia Tartan

The first of the three projects presented here is the Disrupting Dementia tartan. This co-design project involved over 130 people living with dementia taking part in co-design workshops held all over Scotland. The project involved in excess of 1900 miles of travel, over 80 h spent travelling and using over half a kilometre of coloured ribbon in the creation of the participants' tartan design prototypes. The main aim of the Disrupting Dementia tartan design project is to help change the perception of dementia by showing that people with dementia can offer much to UK society after diagnosis. Specifically, that people living with dementia are capable of designing a new product that will be sold all over the world. Moreover, this project will help people recently diagnosed with dementia build their self-esteem, identity and dignity and help ensure that every person living with dementia and their families' quality of life and resilience is maximised. In a co-design project such as this one, it is important that the designer does not take an overly dominant role. The instigator of the co-design project should be transparent about the project's objectives and clearly articulate the reasons behind embarking on a co-design project. In other words, the project rationale should always be known from both sides. The goal is to achieve something like a symbiotic collaboration—a mutually beneficial relationship between those involved. Van Klaveren (2012) suggests such an ethical and transparent approach is the foundation for a truly symbiotic co-design relationship.

In this project, each tartan co-design workshop commenced with a short presentation of the basic rules associated with the creation of the Disrupting Dementia tartan. Working closely with Alzheimer Scotland staff and family members, care was taken to ensure that the language used during the workshop was supportive and not offensive to people living with dementia. Also, the researcher supported by care support workers ensured that everyone taking part in the project was kept physically and emotionally safe at all times during the workshop. The creation of each participant's tartan design began with an acetate-based version, followed by a physical prototype constructed using ribbon, and finally the creation of a digital version using a publically available Internet-based tartan design tool (Fig. 1). Each participant was free to determine and shape the tartan design they created during the stages of the design process.

In the example shown in Fig. 1, one can see that the person living with dementia's main colour in their design is purple (Alzheimer Scotland's brand colour), followed by their choice of colours. At this important stage of the co-design process, the researchers adopted an empathic (not sympathetic) manner ensuring they were compassionate, un-patronising, tolerant, understanding and respectful. Many of the workshop participants held a significant position before their diagnosis of dementia including an eye surgeon, an architect and an economist so a respectful attitude was vital to every co-design sessions' success. During the highly iterative stage of co-designing each tartan, the researchers had to consider 'dementia time'. That is, being patient and allowing time and space for each individual and how they might

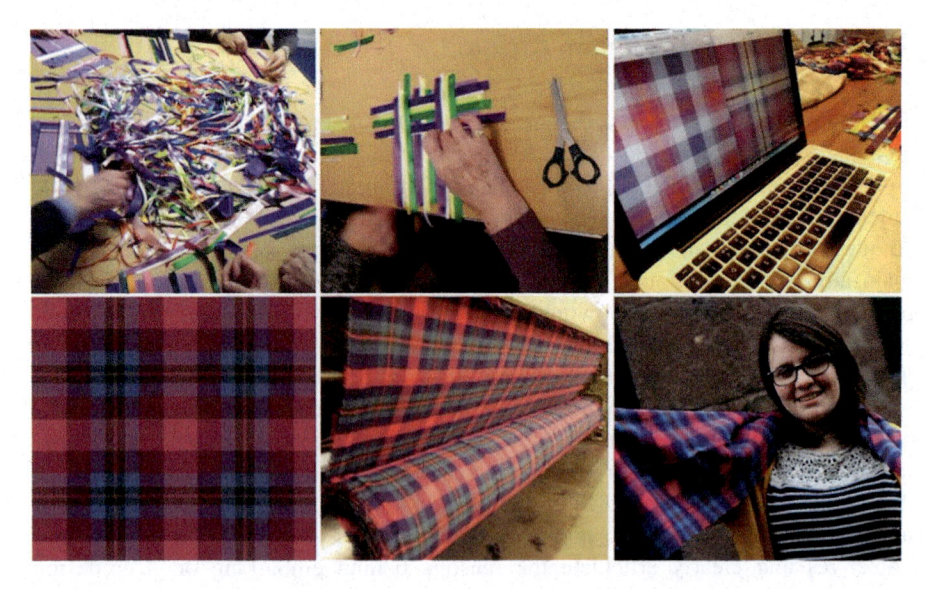

Fig. 1 Tartan design creative process (left to right: acetate, ribbon and digital prototypes)

keep track of their time. Many recent approaches to co-design emphasise the need to rethink and redefine the role of the participants (Van Klaveren 2012). For example, one has to be careful not to imply power relations through the terms we use (Holcombe 2010). In this project, the participants are seen as designers in the process, and their input is valued as much as the co-design facilitator (authors). Like Manzini and Rizzo (2011), this co-design project views the participants as active collaborative co-designers. The participants are creative; they have a range of experiences, skills, knowledge and capabilities and they have enhanced the overall nature of the project by taking part. Several authors have proposed nomenclature such as 'vernacular designers' (Reitan 2006), 'silent designers' (Gorb and Dumas 1987) and 'design amateurs' (Leadbeater 2009; Manzini and Rizzo 2011) to describe the co-design participants. It is worth mentioning that embarking on a co-design project not only changes the role of the participants in the design process, it also changes the role of the designer or researcher (Manzini and Rizzo 2011). Most, if not all, of the co-design literature relates (indeed implies) a collaborative and cooperative effort between two or more equally able agents. Many traditional approaches to involve a person in co-design activities, however, create issues as they assume that the participants are cognitively able, can deal with visual and hands-on techniques and require certain levels of ability. This paper, however, describes co-designing with individuals that are not equal in the sense of their cognitive and communication abilities, which brings new challenges to co-design activities and projects. The remaining sections of the paper report on the significant outcomes of three co-design projects, reflect on the co-designing sessions, and present insights into successful practices when designing together with people living with dementia.

3.2 Designed with Me

Designed With Me is a service design proposition that makes use of the latent creative abilities of an individual's personal knowledge and skills (Kelley and Kelley 2015). Designed With Me adopts a co-design approach where people living with dementia are highly valued and their inputs and collaborations are held in the same esteem as any other participant and collaborator. Designed With Me focusses on the empowerment and inclusion of people living with dementia, along with dementia support workers, carers and the general public, to inform, influence and change local communities. In the process, all participants become co-designers helping to propose possibilities, choose solutions, provide services and 'make things happen'. Co-design is predominately about 'change' (Brown 2009; Heath and Heath 2011), which relates to making a difference in the world around us. Change scenarios develop the collective togetherness in approaching problems and situations. In this scenario, the actions of the designer and the people that they work with are inter-linked by collective responsibility and the desire to make a difference. Work in the Designed With Me project hopes to manifest such change by working with people who have a diagnosis of dementia. The incentive for change and opportunities for co-design do not revolve around resolving the condition of dementia. Rather, this work is interested in the power of the individual, the value of their lived experience, and their continuing inclusion in society. Ultimately, the purpose of this project is to do stuff with people, to try things out and to accept occasional failings as long as the results are evaluated and used to improve the next approach.

Designed With Me started by exploring the attitudes and opinions of people living with dementia to ascertain what is important for them. This initial stage was undertaken to generate a design brief that would be authored by the people living with dementia themselves. The group, all of whom had a diagnosis of dementia, were invited to respond to everyday questions or statements by filling in answers on the back of a set of designed postcards. The questions invited personal and collective opinion utilising the terms 'I' and 'We' the purpose of which was to solicit each participant's opinions and to think and talk about their thoughts, hopes, wishes and desires. The initial sessions stimulated a lot of conversation between the authors and a group of people living with dementia, which resulted in free-flowing collective thinking and views peppered with personal insights. The aim of this workshop was to engender a situation where people living with dementia identified areas of potential where design could make a difference. It was also hoped that the design proposal could ultimately have further value and impact in the local community. With this in mind, the postcards used to prompt the group of people living with dementia were openly ambiguous. The open nature of the postcards invited wider thinking, collective discussion and agreement. Gaining the thoughts and wishes of people living with dementia is essential to the goals of this research. This approach looks to exploit the potential of co-design as a means of raising awareness and developing the voice of people living with dementia. In particular keeping them infused throughout the design process (i.e. formulation of brief, concept generation, development and design delivery). From the first workshop, a number of possible project ideas began to emerge. The considerate and carefully planned approach allowed participants to make explicit their thoughts and considerations. The participants' comments, collected on the postcards, were analysed to identify common themes, thoughts, wants and desires. A number of key themes emerged including:

- Participants wanted more respect and greater communication.
- More appropriate social spaces to meet and mix with others.
- Strong desire to make Sunday special again.

The second co-design workshop focused on the wants, needs and desires expressed by people living with dementia in the first workshop. That is, participants wished to see greater opportunities to make more time and space for social inclusion, understanding, personal esteem and empowerment, and to be nurtured and supported. These key themes were then arranged into a proposition for the second workshop: 'Redesigning Sundays to make them special again, where fun can occur that supports respect and communication'. One particularly powerful piece of feedback from one of the participants that was offered after the first workshop was: '*You made us think more than we are usually asked to do and it is good for us to have to think*'. Also during the lunch that followed the first workshop, the carers or partners of the individuals involved wanted to know more and to understand what had happened during the session. They were interested in the activity offering their own insights as the discussion continued whilst expressing a clear desire to be involved in future events.

The second workshop brought together both carers and people living with dementia to expand upon and propose responses to the brief generated in the first workshop. The larger group (28 participants) assembled in the second workshop allowed for greater involvement, understanding and thinking of all the concerned parties, which supported a sense of togetherness in the discussions and actions. The participants were split into smaller groups of five or six and each group was invited to make marks, scribble details and stick images down in a collage to encourage discussion and communication of the discussion and emerging project ideas. The ideas proposed in the second workshop, from left to right in Fig. 2, are 'Family Day', 'Water/Boats', 'Younger People are a Tonic', 'Local Communities and Big Events', and 'Encourage Interaction'. Currently, the Designed With Me service intervention is considering three concrete proposals with the group of people living with dementia as a response to the brief 'Redesigning Sundays to make them special again, where fun can occur that supports respect and communication'. The three proposed design interventions under consideration are:

- *Our Big Picnic*—allows people of all ages and backgrounds to congregate in an organised event and make the entertainment.
- *Open Street*—will become a local hub for play, talk and local understanding to make the street more like streets from yesteryear.
- *D:Caf*—where people living with dementia deliver a hospitable place for fun, conversation, innovation, play and companionship.

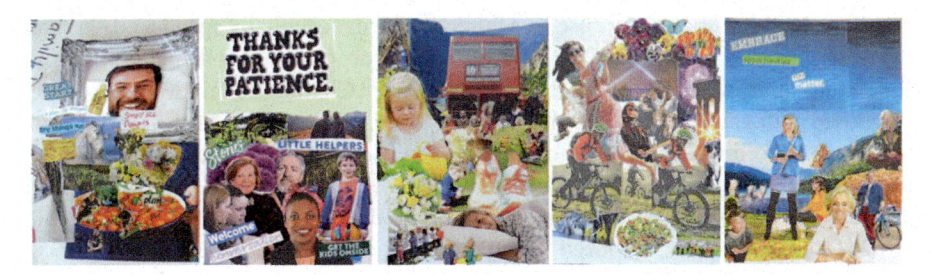

Fig. 2 'Making Sundays special again' initial ideas

3.3 75BC

75BC is a collaborative design project that celebrates the life and work of the Glaswegian comedian Billy Connolly. The co-design project between the authors and a dementia support group based in Bridgeton in the East End of Glasgow has involved a series of recent visits to the 75BC murals in Glasgow and to the American artist Tschabalala Self's exhibition at the Tramway Gallery in Glasgow. During this project, five people living with dementia have produced a range of visual representations of Billy Connolly using collage to create a series of textile designs in the style of Tschabalala Self (Fig. 3). The artworks created by people

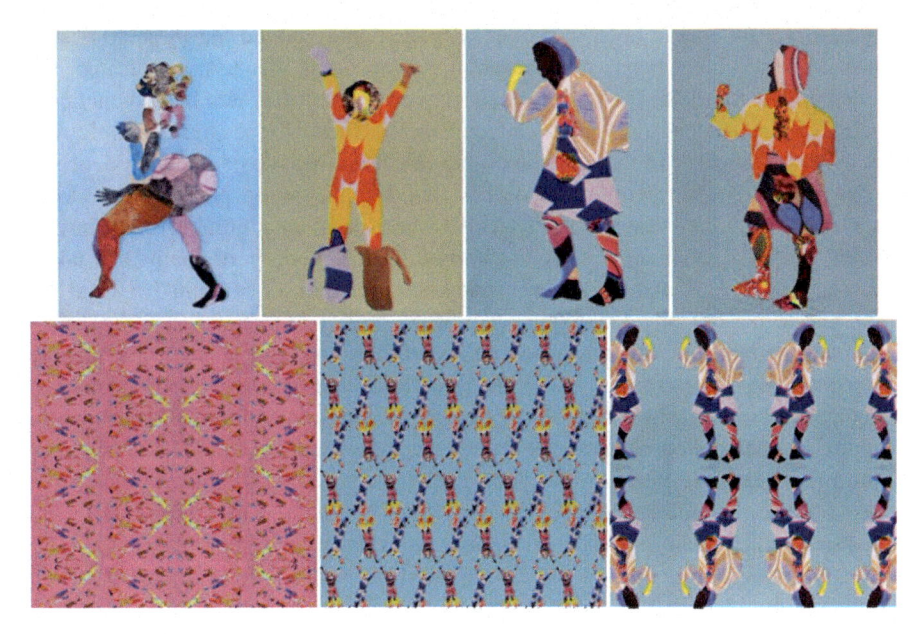

Fig. 3 Tschabalala Self and Billy Connolly collages (top) and new Bridgeton textile fabric design proposals (bottom)

living with dementia make use of fabric patterns originally produced in the Bridgeton area of Glasgow (Turkish Red) alongside patterns from the wider creative community. Works by the legendary designer Charles Rennie Macintosh are composed alongside more contemporary designers Timorous Beasties and Laura Spring. Two forms of Billy Connolly have been used here. One image shows Billy Connolly in his iconic Big Banana Boots from early in his career and the other image shows a more recent picture of Billy Connolly at Dressed to Kilt in 2011. All of the group members composed their patterns and colour schemes in accordance with these two original images. Some followed a clear plan whereas others adopted a much more freeform expression in their representations. The intention of the 75BC co-design project is to use the images created by the five people living with dementia to highlight their inherent creativity and to support the 75BC celebrations. The members of the dementia support group will decide themselves which of these patterns will become a new Bridgeton textile.

4 Conclusions

Reflecting on these three co-design projects, it is abundantly clear that people living with dementia can offer much to society after diagnosis. Working closely with stakeholders including carers, family members and collaborating organisations such as Alzheimer Scotland, the authors have received very positive feedback on the co-design projects. Participants have stated that the co-design experiences had been very positive; they have been interested, engaged and enjoyed the three co-design projects; there had been concentration, focus and discussion during the co-designing activities. Participants felt the three projects had been beneficial. Several of the stakeholders involved considered there to be significant lasting impact for participants in the way the co-design sessions gave people confidence to try new things—some people had been worried about taking part but were very relaxed during the sessions. Impact has also been seen in a number of 'spin-off' projects, discussions, themed activities and outings. Several participants had taken encouragement from the co-design workshops and had since joined a local art group and a number of related spin-off projects have commenced. The three projects presented here show how co-design methods and tools can enable people living with dementia to make a significant contribution to society after diagnosis. Specifically, this work has shown how design thought and action can contribute to changing the perception of dementia and shown that whilst the mood and behaviour of the person may be profoundly affected, their personhood is not. Moreover, the three co-design projects have helped reconnect people recently diagnosed with dementia to build their self-esteem, identity and dignity and keep the person with dementia connected to their local community. The widespread assumption that people living with dementia cannot take part in mainstream activities, and that they have no quality of life or capacity for pleasure and positive involvement has been dismantled by these projects. Whilst the symptoms associated with dementia affect the way a person living with dementia interacts with others, and some activities may be inappropriate as a result, there are many activities such as designing in which they can participate. Moreover, people living with dementia should be encouraged to make decisions or partake in decisions that affect them for as long as possible, to maintain their dignity and self-esteem.

By the year 2030, over 80% more people aged 65 and over will have some form of dementia (a moderate or severe cognitive impairment) compared to 2010. Design, in general, and design research, in particular, needs to embrace these challenges head-on. However, rather than viewing these challenges negatively design has an opportunity to be at the forefront of imagining how we might care and live together better in the future. It is now time, therefore, that design in all its guises grasps this opportunity to envision and realise the future that we will all be proud to share. To envision a future where people living with dementia can make significant contributions to society requires careful consideration and planning. First, researchers should always ask people with dementia how they want to be involved in research, including at what points and in what ways they want to be included. Second, people living with dementia should be involved in setting research priorities. That is, researchers should ask people living with dementia what positive outcomes of the research project might look like for them. Third, researchers must ensure that everyone taking part in the research project is physically and emotionally safe at all times. Fourth, researchers must use language that is supportive of people with dementia whilst avoiding language that may offend. Fifth, researchers need to be 'dementia aware'. They should be compassionate, tolerant, understanding and respectful whilst working with people living with dementia. Lastly, researchers need to consider 'dementia time' in their expectations of research. For instance, finding out the best time to meet and how each individual keeps track of time. Following these guiding principles on how to best conduct co-design projects with people living with dementia will help deliver truly meaningful experiences and outcomes for all involved.

References

All Party Parliamentary Group on Dementia (2016) Dementia rarely travels alone. APPG on Dementia, London, UK
Alzheimer Scotland (2008) Meeting our needs: the level and quality of dementia support services in Scotland. Alzheimer Scotland, Edinburgh, UK
Batsch NL, Mittelman MS (2012) World Alzheimer report 2012: overcoming the stigma of dementia. Alzheimer's Disease International, London, UK
Bisson C, Luckner J (1996) Fun in learning: the pedagogical role of fun in adventure education perspectives. J Exp Educ 19(2):108–112
Brown T (2009) Change by design: how design thinking transforms organisations and inspires innovation. HarperCollins, New York, NY, US
Bury M (1982) Chronic illness as biographical disruption. Sociol Health Illn 4(2):167–182
Christensen C, Overdorf M (2000) Meeting the challenge of disruptive change. Harvard Bus Rev 78(2):66–76

Gorb P, Dumas A (1987) Silent design. Des Stud 8(3):150–156
Heath C, Heath D (2011) Switch: how to change things when change is hard. Random House, London, UK
Hendriks N, Slegers K, Duysburgh P (2015) Codesign with people living with cognitive or sensory impairments: a case for method stories and uniqueness. CoDesign 11(1):70–82
Holcombe S (2010) The arrogance of ethnography: managing anthropological research knowledge. Aust Aboriginal Stud 2:22–32
Katsuno T (2005) Dementia from the inside: how people with early-stage dementia evaluate their quality of life. Ageing Soc 25:197–214
Kelley T, Kelley D (2015) Creative confidence: unleashing the creative potential within us all. William Collins, London, UK
Kinnaird L (2012) Delivering integrated dementia care: the 8 pillars model of community support, September. Alzheimer Scotland, Edinburgh, Scotland, UK
Kitwood T (1990) The dialectics of dementia: with particular reference to Alzheimer's disease. Ageing Soc 10:177–196
Lam B, Dearden A, William-Powlett K, Brodie E (2012) Exploring co-design in the voluntary sector. In: Proceedings of VSSN/NCVO annual conference, University of Birmingham, Birmingham, AL, US
Leadbeater C (2009) We think. Profile Books, London, UK
Manzini E, Rizzo F (2011) Small projects/large changes: participatory design as an open participated process. CoDesign 7(3–4):199–215
Matthews E (2006) Dementia and the identity of the person. In: Hughes JC, Louw SJ, Sabat SR (eds) Dementia: mind, meaning and the person. Oxford University Press, Oxford, UK, pp 163–177
Office for National Statistics (2017) Overview of the UK population: July 2017. ONS, London, UK
Prince M, Prina M, Guerchet M (2013) World Alzheimer report 2013. Journey of caring: an analysis of long-term care for dementia. Alzheimer's Disease International, London, UK
Reitan JB (2006) Inuit vernacular design as a community of practice for learning. CoDesign 2(02):71–80
Rodgers PA, Tennant A (2014) Disrupting health and social care by design. In: Proceedings of the 9th international conference on design & emotion, Bogota, Colombia
Sanders EB-N, Stappers PJ (2014) Probes, toolkits and prototypes: three approaches to making in codesigning. CoDesign 10(1):5–14
Scharmer CO (2011) Leading from the emerging future. In: Minds for change—future of global development ceremony to mark the 50th anniversary of the BMZ Federal Ministry for Economic Cooperation and Development, Berlin, Germany
Van Klaveren R (2012) Artistic participatory practices as a vehicle for togetherness. In: Proceedings of the CUMULUS conference, Helsinki, Finland, pp. 1–11
Wilson S, Roper A, Marshall J, Galliers J, Devane N, Booth T (2015) Codesign for people with aphasia through tangible design languages. CoDesign 11(1):21–34

The Effect of Simulation in Large-Scale Data Collection—An Example of Password Policy Development

J. Chakraborty and N. Nguyen

Abstract Computer networks across the world are increasingly vulnerable to hackers. Network administrators have countered this threat with stronger password policies. However, this has resulted in potential usability challenges for all users. Research has shown that users of these new security requirements would typically do the minimum possible to adhere to these policies. End users have become wary of the potential security risks posed by hackers. Privacy laws and the need to protect user data have further added to the difficulties that researchers must overcome in order to better understand user needs. As a result, large sets of data containing password patterns are very difficult to collect and analyse. In this article, we present a possible solution to this data collection challenge by using simulation. This offers us the ability to generate large amounts of user data that can be used to illustrate different trends of password use. Our simulations of a scenario in an academic setting consist of four types of users—undergraduate and graduate students, faculty and staff. By making conservative assumptions of user behaviours based on literature, our findings show that while users of different education and technical backgrounds face different levels of challenges in setting up passwords, nearly all users displayed similar characteristics when updating passwords. These findings from our simulation illustrate the ability to overcome data collection challenges in this field and could potentially allow us to design more inclusive password policies.

1 Introduction

The increasing number of business and government agencies that rely on a web-based presence to conduct business places an emphasis on the need for strong password policies. Allied with a growing threat from Internet-based hackers,

J. Chakraborty (✉) · N. Nguyen
Towson University, Towson, MD, USA
e-mail: jchakraborty@towson.edu

N. Nguyen
e-mail: npnguyen@towson.edu

© Springer International Publishing AG, part of Springer Nature 2018
P. Langdon et al. (eds.), *Breaking Down Barriers*,
https://doi.org/10.1007/978-3-319-75028-6_23

network administrators are increasingly reliant on ever more complex security password requirements to protect their client's networks. Examples of typical policies can range from having passwords with 10 or more characters to changing passwords every 3–6 months. However, while these types of policies are manageable for the modern day, tech-savvy digital native, they have proven to be an obstacle to those who are not as familiar with the demands of these technology policies (Besnard and Arief 2004). These stringent policies place an increased cognitive burden on users who may not be accustomed to the robust password policy needs. As a result, research has shown that these users typically set up passwords that might compromise security (Keith et al. 2007; Anderson and Agarwal 2010; Richards 2017).

The complexity of establishing and managing the password requirements of most web-based tools requires special care and attention (Keates et al. 2000). The security policies in these websites typically require users to set up and maintain passwords following very strict guidelines that are often difficult to comply with and remember. The multistep guidelines required to set up passwords of sufficient complexity or strength makes heavy demands of the cognitive load that end users must overcome. Research has shown that users tend to gravitate towards passwords with personal connections, such as parts of their names, birthdays of loved ones, or favourite television characters. This practice is usually borne out of frustrations with the complex security policies that have been set up. Such practices make password-enabled accounts more vulnerable to hackers who may be able to guess the user's account details (Duggan et al. 2012; Gulenko 2014).

The need to secure systems with stronger password requirements and the typical users desire to create memorable passwords has resulted in a need for usable security (Persad et al. 2007). The literature in this field reports significant efforts towards bridging this gap by trying to understand the end user needs using traditional methods of data collection and analysis (Mohamed et al. 2017). However, navigating through the ethical constraints of data collection related to passwords has proven to be a major challenge to researchers. The human–computer interaction (HCI) literature indicates that most password behaviours from end users are gathered through surveys, questionnaires or interviews (Brown et al. 2004). These methods of data collection are typically slower and face rigorous challenges from ethics boards regarding privacy concerns. As a result, these datasets are typically smaller and offer limited scope of generalisable findings.

In this paper, we examine a potential solution to this problem of data collection by conducting a simulation in a controlled environment applying data gathered from the literature. The use of simulation in the computing field is not new. Indeed, it is often used in automated manufacturing or supply chain management analysis as a way to predict outcomes. However, simulation is rarely used in HCI to study human behaviours, as it is very difficult to predict. The usable security literature has identified password behaviours as one of the few user outcomes that are predictable (Brown et al. 2004). Therefore, we sought to apply these known password behavioural outcomes to illustrate the effect of simulation using a sample password policy in the scenario of a public university. The aim of this paper is to analyse the findings of this large-scale simulation with four classes of end users: undergraduate and graduate students, faculty and staff. It is envisioned that the findings of this study of these four groups of users will serve to highlight the broader need to design more inclusive password security policies. Specifically, the contributions of this paper are:

- A simulation of user behaviours based on four types of users: undergraduate students, graduate students, faculty and staff.
- Analysis of simulation and recommendations for policy changes.

This work is an extension of the body of literature towards usable and inclusive security in the HCI domain. The remainder of this paper is as follows. Section 2 provides a brief summary of the literature on usable security and the need for a flexible data collection methodology. Section 3 outlines the details of the simulation exercise that was carried out. Section 4 offers some explanation of the results derived from our simulation exercise. Section 5 summarises the implication of the results and, finally, Sect. 6 outlines the limitations of our study and offers suggestions for future password policy designers.

2 Background

Designing password policy that ensures security and is also usable remains a challenge. This entails making the system easy and efficient for the users to accomplish their tasks, while at the same time making it difficult for the intruders to compromise the system; above all, the system must be inclusive of all users. The body of work on the interaction between usability and security has only recently started gaining attention, as reported by (Schultz et al. 2001; Flechais et al. 2007; González et al. 2009). Indeed, the importance of usability in security rests in the fact that most of security functionalities and controls are embedded in the user interface (UI) and good interface design results in more effective security functionalities (Mohamed et al. 2017).

Existing literature in this body of work addresses several aspects of usable security such as security policy and standards of authentication (Mohamed et al. 2017). Studies of user behaviours report that users typically compromise security when they feel overwhelmed (Besnard and Arief 2004). Other user behaviour studies related to password security support a variety of emotional, psychological and cognitive explanations in response to challenges faced with maintaining password security (Anderson and Agarwal 2010; Gulenko 2014; Richards 2017). The literature also reports that users typically rely upon personal information in password creation. Personal data can be in the form of birth date or home address. The literature suggests that the volume of information available through social computing has increased this problem of achieving usable security (Brown et al. 2004).

Gathering data about the end user requirements to design usable security policies pose significant challenges such as privacy and logistics. Typically, users are cautious about sharing their personal data. Protecting the privacy of the user's password data is paramount and must satisfy all ethical provisions. As a result, it is difficult to conduct any type of password behaviour analysis on large datasets (Brown et al. 2004). The majority of research studies in usable security have been carried out using known data gathering and analysis techniques in HCI such as surveys, interviews and focus groups. The findings of these methods are quite revealing and have helped to further the field. However, the data collection process using these methods can slow down the data gathering process significantly, and the typical sample sizes are also smaller (Mohamed et al. 2017; Richards 2017).

The need exists for a different data collection technique that can generate a larger sample size of user behaviour data fairly quickly that would not violate the stringent ethics or privacy concerns. This scientifically validated method should be fairly easy to set up and have the ability to produce large datasets in a short time that can be analysed using various statistical methods. Inspired by these needs and a scientific curiosity to try a cross-disciplinary approach to analyse usable security, we propose the use of a simulation methodology. The use of simulation by the scientific community is not new. It is primarily used in fields where there is very little variation in the development process such as supply chains or automated manufacturing. However, it can be argued that in a controlled environment with known upper and lower limits of variations, the use of simulation techniques can be useful in the generation of large amounts of data for analysis. We developed our study using this reasoning and known values of human behavioural characteristics that have been identified in the literature. These include user preferences for the following personal details in their passwords: name or parts of name, date of birth, the numbers 1 through 0 from a qwerty keyboard and the following special characters ! @#$%^&*() (Brown et al. 2004; Duggan et al. 2012; Richards 2017).

3 Simulation Design

We designed a simulation using a very specific scenario of four types of users in a public university—undergraduate (U) and graduate (G) students, faculty (F) and staff (S). Our study extends the work of (Duggan et al. 2012) who analysed data collected from computer scientists, administrative staff and students in an academic environment also using interviews and diaries of password used to create models of password behaviour. We extended their study by using a simulation of a carefully controlled similar academic institution. For our design, we first gathered an example of existing password policies from the website of a typical public university in the USA. Table 1 shows this example of a typical set of policies that are designed by public institutions to restrict access to networks. For our experiment, we used this policy.

Table 1 Password policy from public university

Each password must: (A) Be at least 8 characters in length (B) Use at least 3 of the following 4 different types of characters: (B1) uppercase letters (B2) lowercase letters (B3) numbers (B4) symbols: !#$%&*+,-/:;()<=>?_ (C) Not contain any part of your name (D) Not be one of your last 10 passwords

We then designed our simulation programme for two scenarios with the following assumptions: all users were neurotypical; users could come from four types of education backgrounds—Undergraduate students (U), graduate students (G), faculty (F) and staff (S); all our users had some degrees of computer literacy; all users had managed their respective passwords at least once. We chose these four user types to closely emulate the Duggan et al. (2012) study who carried out their experiments using three user groups. The two scenarios were (1) to create a new password and (2) updating or changing an existing password. In both cases, the chosen password has to satisfy the institution policy towards passwords found in Table 1. We assigned known password design behaviours, such as using a name or a date of birth, as a part of a password (Brown et al. 2004; Duggan et al. 2012). We wanted to understand the following factors in scenario (1).

1.1 The success rate of users with different education levels in *creating* a new password.
1.2 The distribution of core components (using characteristics A through D from Table 1) in a successful password.
We also analysed the following user behaviours in scenario (2)
2.1 The success rate of users with different technical levels in *changing* their password.
2.2 The similarity of the user's new password to their last two passwords.

3.1 Simulation Design

To conduct the experiment, we divided the simulation into two phases according to the two aforementioned scenarios. Each participant belongs to one of the four groups U, G, S and F. Each group is assigned a probability corresponding to their educational levels. We assumed the following order of increasing education proficiency from the users—U, S, G and F. In each test, we simulated four groups

Table 2 Probability distribution of group policy adherence

Group	A	B1	B2	B3	B4	C	D
U	0.70	0.70	0.90	0.70	0.50	0.60	0.50
S	0.60	0.50	0.90	0.50	0.40	0.40	0.40
G	0.85	0.80	0.90	0.85	0.75	0.75	0.70
F	0.92	0.85	0.95	0.90	0.85	0.80	0.75

simultaneously with N participants each, with the maximum number of trials of each participant K allowed was set to 10, i.e. each participant could try to create or change their password up to 10 times. Finally, for the sake of consistency, each test was repeated 1000 times. The results for each group of users were then averaged out for analysis.

In the second phase, we set the probabilities that a user in a group can successfully create a new password that satisfies all policy conditions A–D. Table 2 describes those probabilities.

Using a combination of the literature (Brown et al. 2004; Duggan et al. 2012) and experiences in higher education, we made the following assumptions: U has a 70% chance of being successful in understanding and setting up a password using policy A (from Table 2), 70% chance of success with policy B1 (from Table 2), 90% chance of success with policy B2 (from Table 2), 70% chance of success with policy B3 (from Table 2), 50% chance of success with policy B4 (from Table 2), 60% chance of success with policy C (from Table 2) and 50% chance of success with policy D (from Table 2). Table 2 outlines the assumptions for groups U, S, G and F. We also make the assumption that each user group will tend to recreate a new password closely similar to the previous edition as a convenience and to improve memorability, as found in the literature (Brown et al. 2004).

3.2 Simulation Execution—Scenario 1: Setting up Password

A test in any group was executed using the following steps:

1. Randomise a probability that represents the chance that a user in that group could successfully complete a requirement from (A) to (D) (from Table 1).
2. The user could try again (up to 10 times) if they did not meet the most recent requirement. In requirement (B) (from Table 1), if the user failed to meet more than one sub-requirements (B1–B4) (from Table 1), they would have to try again.
3. The number of successful users together with their number of trials and passwords were recorded for each test in any group. The successful password of each user would be used in the second procedure in the simulation. We only recorded successful users because any unsuccessful user must have made more than 10 attempts to create a password.

4. For each successful password, we also recorded the distributions of essential elements (i.e. name, date of birth and other factors).
5. For consistency, the test was repeated 1000 times and the results were averaged.

3.3 Experiment Execution—Scenario 2: Changing Password

A test in any group was executed using the following steps:

1. For each successful password P developed, we compared P to the new password P' generated by adding one or two numbers to P. This simulated the regular habit of a user when creating a new password based on the old one, as identified in the literature (Brown et al. 2004).
2. We simulated the user behaviour through a permutation of parts of a password before adding one or two numbers. For instance, if P was 'Br@ndonSm1th', then a new password P' could be 'Sm1thbr@ndon12' where the two parts were permutated.
3. To compare the similarity between the old and new password, we utilised the Sorensen–Dice index which was commonly used in string similarity comparison (Dice 1945).
4. Finally, we repeated each test over 1000 executions for consistency and the results were averaged.

4 Results and Discussions

The purpose of our study was to demonstrate the potential value of simulation as a methodology to generate large amounts of data related to user behaviours in setting up and updating passwords using complex password policies in a short time. Based on the literature, we assumed that all users would create passwords that were meaningful to them personally. We also assumed that given the complexity requirements for updating or changing passwords setup by organisations, most users would change passwords with slight modifications (one or two characters). Figures 1, 2 and 3 show the results of our simulations of 3000 users per category—U, G, S and F.

As seen in Table 1, the password policy in a public university is complex and has multiple variables that have to be taken into consideration. In Fig. 1, the coloured shapes in the graphs represent the averaged data points from the simulation for each set of users (U, G, F and S). Trials (in Y-axis) represents the average number of attempts each group of users makes in order to set up passwords for the first time in order to meet the password policy requirements. While number of

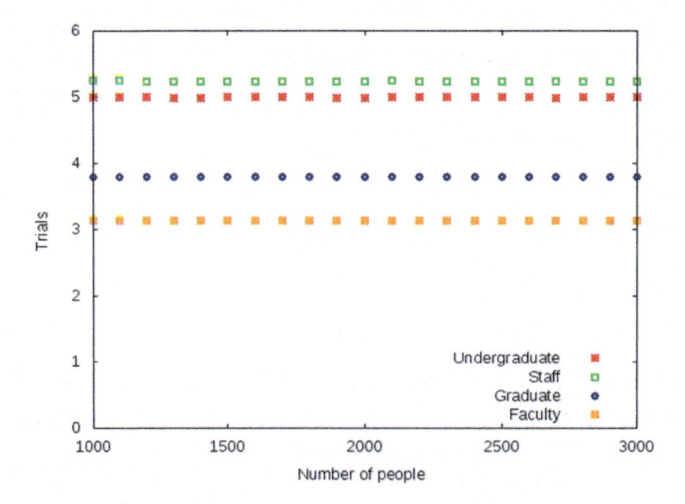

Fig. 1 Results of simulation showing number of trials needed to successfully set up password

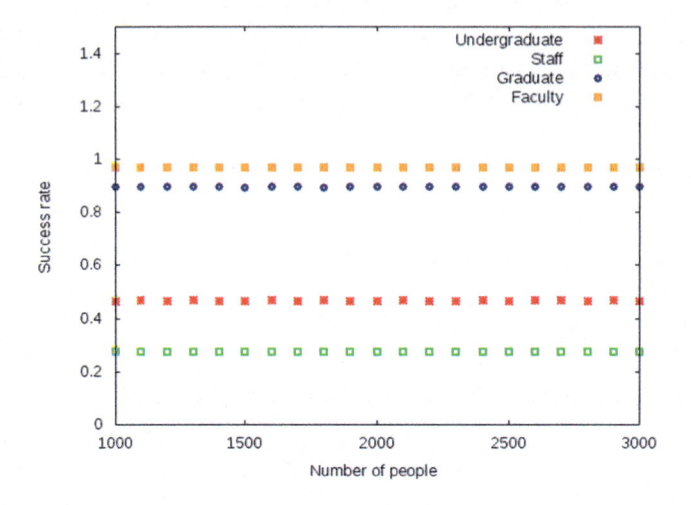

Fig. 2 Results of simulation showing success rate of password creation

people (in X-axis) shows the variation in data as our experiment progressed. Our simulation of 3000 users in the categories of U and S was based on the probability assumptions in Table 2 and showed that both these sets of users would require five or more attempts to set up a password. Similarly, the simulation shows that G would require almost four attempts and F are usually successful at just over three attempts.

The simulation findings in Fig. 2 closely follow the pattern in Fig. 1 in that S had the lowest rates of success in setting up passwords (about 27%), followed by U (46%). G and F fared much better (89% and 96%, respectively). The analysis of this

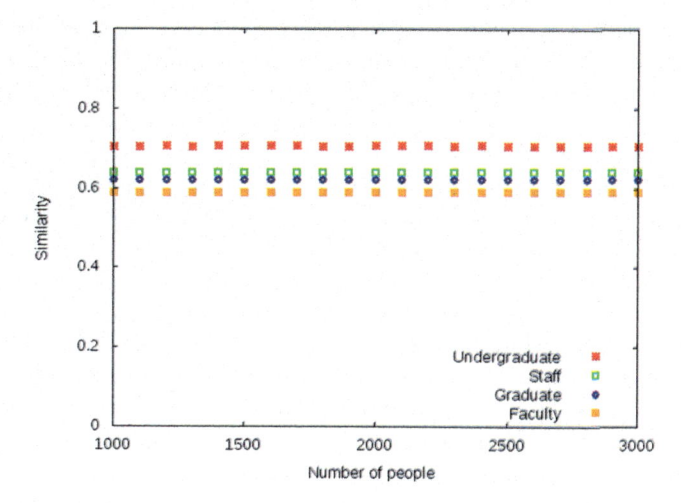

Fig. 3 Results of simulation showing similarities of password and recently changed password

larger dataset produced some interesting results. Based on our findings, it could be suggested that education levels could be the factor that leads to these outcomes. This could suggest that the more familiar one is with technology, the easier it becomes to set up complex passwords. Inversely, our simulation suggests that users who are digital immigrants might find it difficult to set up similarly complex passwords.

Although Fig. 2 suggests that G and F are better at setting up passwords for the first time, our simulation analysis in Fig. 3 suggests all users display similar behaviours when updating passwords. With the slight exception of U, all other users recreated passwords with minimal changes to the original password. From our simulation, it could be argued that educational background does not alter poor password behaviours when faced with a complex security policy.

5 Conclusions

The aim of this paper was to demonstrate the viability of simulation as a rapid data collection tool in the analysis of user behaviour related to password policies. We conducted our experiments using conservative assumptions of known behavioural patterns exhibited by users based on the literature (Brown et al. 2004; Duggan et al. 2012). Our findings were consistent with the literature and validate the work of Duggan et al. (2012). Our study demonstrated the potential of using simulation to generate large datasets of user preferences under a controlled environment. Our simulation was not affected by the complexities arising from protecting user privacy and small sample sizes that traditional HCI methods (such as surveys, interviews and questionnaires) must overcome. Our simulation of behaviours of four types of users (U, G, F and S) managing complex password policies in a controlled scenario illustrates the increasing difficulties that all users might face. The findings suggest that while education may have some bearing on the success rates of setting up passwords for the first time, they do not appear to be significant in updating passwords using complex policy requirements. This suggests the influence of other factors, such as memorability, may influence how users update passwords. These findings shed light on the challenges that all users would have to overcome to comply with complex password policies.

In designing security policy, administrators have to pay attention to user requirements as well as the network security. The consequences of implementing security policies that are too complex for users are well documented. Our simulation suggests that users will seek the easiest route to circumvent password policy that might cause memorability and retention challenges. This illustrates the importance of gathering information about user requirements in the design of any security policy. We demonstrated the value of using simulations towards this goal. This methodology has the potential to generate large volumes of user data that can be used to test out a policy before implementation. By understanding the potential effects on the users of any security policy, it is possible to design more usable security.

6 Limitations and Future Direction

The potential limitations of our study might arise from some of the assumptions of human behaviour that we have made in Table 2. It could be argued that users would change more than one or two characters in their passwords to be fully compliant with a security policy. It could also be argued that memorability is an important factor in password creation, an idea which is supported by the technology acceptance model (TAM) (Mohamed et al. 2017). Given the increasing body of scientific literature on cybersecurity, it is clear that we need to expand our knowledge of user behaviours while designing password policies. The use of simulation can potentially help identify different trends and limitations of policies before they are implemented.

As a continuation of this study, we hope to emulate our simulation using inclusive policies designed with the help of domain experts in usability and security. We hope to further the usable security literature by conducting more simulations using different controlled scenarios. It is envisioned that such findings could be presented to security policymakers to help to create more inclusive security policies.

References

Anderson CL, Agarwal R (2010) Practicing safe computing: a multimedia empirical examination of home computer user security behavioral intentions. MIS Q 34:613–643

Besnard D, Arief B (2004) Computer security impaired by legitimate users. Comput Secur 23:253–264

Brown AS, Bracken E, Zoccoli S, Douglas K (2004) Generating and remembering passwords. Appl Cogn Psychol 18:641–651

Dice LR (1945) Measures of the amount of ecologic association between species. Ecology 26:297–302

Duggan GB, Johnson H, Grawemeyer B (2012) Rational security: modelling everyday password use. Int J Hum Comput Stud 70:415–431

Flechais I, Mascolo C, Sasse MA (2007) Integrating security and usability into the requirements and design process. Int J Electron Secur Digit Forensics 1:12–26

González RM, Martin MV, Arteaga JM, Rodríguez FÁ, Zezzatti CAOO (2009) Web service-security specification based on usability criteria and pattern approach. JCP 4:705–712

Gulenko I (2014) Improving passwords: influence of emotions on security behaviour information. Manag Comput Secur 22:167–178

Keates S, Clarkson PJ, Harrison L-A, Robinson P (2000) Towards a practical inclusive design approach. In: Proceedings on the 2000 conference on universal usability, ACM, pp 45–52

Keith M, Shao B, Steinbart PJ (2007) The usability of passphrases for authentication: an empirical field study. Int J Hum Comput Stud 65:17–28

Mohamed MA, Chakraborty J, Dehlinger J (2017) Trading off usability and security in user interface design through mental models. Behav Inf Technol 36:493–516

Persad U, Langdon P, Clarkson J (2007) Characterising user capabilities to support inclusive design evaluation. Univ Access Inf Soc 6:119–135

Richards KE (2017) Risk analysis of the discoverability of personal data used for primary and secondary authentication. University of Maryland Baltimore County, MD, US

Schultz EE, Proctor RW, Lien M-C, Salvendy G (2001) Usability and security an appraisal of usability issues in information security methods. Comput Secur 20:620–634

Education and Existing Knowledge of Architects in Germany About Accessibility and Building for the Older Generation

E. Rudolph and S. Kreiser

Abstract A prerequisite for the development of architecture's potential to support a safe and independent living of all people is the planning of demographically sustainable buildings. In practice, however, there are currently great obstacles realising buildings for the older generation. An essential starting point for overcoming these difficulties is to improve the education and further training of architects. This interdisciplinary research project *MATI: Mensch—Architektur—Technik—Interaktion für demografische Nachhaltigkeit* aimed at finding out whether, and where, there are obstacles for architects to implement more demographically sustainable buildings. To evaluate the role of accessibility in the work of the architects the education at the nine leading technical universities in Germany (TU9) was analysed. In addition, architects in practice were asked via an online survey to assess their knowledge of building for older adults and people with disability. Planning of accessible buildings is often underrepresented in the education at the faculties of architecture of the TU9. Although the offered courses, which are dealing with this issue, are very well accepted and attended by students, the universities only partially recognised the importance and potential of the topic. The majority of the architects who participated in the online survey stated that they have a good knowledge about accessible planning. However, accessibility often has a negative connotation for these architects. In summary, it can be stated that the education on the accessibility and design of demographically sustainable buildings needs improvements and should be an integral part of architectural education.

E. Rudolph (✉) · S. Kreiser
Faculty of Architecture, TU Dresden, Dresden, Germany
e-mail: elisa.rudolph@tu-dresden.de

S. Kreiser
e-mail: stefanie.kreiser@tu-dresden.de

© Springer International Publishing AG, part of Springer Nature 2018
P. Langdon et al. (eds.), *Breaking Down Barriers*,
https://doi.org/10.1007/978-3-319-75028-6_24

1 Introduction

A prerequisite for the development of architecture's potential to support a safe and independent living of all people is the planning of demographically sustainable buildings. This includes age-appropriate, accessible architecture and the use of ambient assisted living systems. In practice, however, there are currently great obstacles realising buildings for the older generation. An essential starting point for overcoming these difficulties is to improve the education and further training of architects.

The interdisciplinary research project *MATI: Mensch—Architektur—Technik—Interaktion für demografische Nachhaltigkeit (human—architecture—technology—interaction for demographic sustainability) (MATI)* was aimed at finding out whether and where the obstacles for architects to implement more demographically sustainable buildings are. In order to support diversity and to avoid exclusion, every architect should have expertise in planning accessible buildings suitable for all generations.

2 Education, Further Training and Existing Knowledge of Architects

Our study took a closer look at education, further training and existing knowledge of architects in Germany. Therefore, we subdivided it into three main parts. First, we examined the official websites of the faculties of architecture (at TU9) which introduced their study guides, lesson plans and module contents. A keyword search was used to help to identify the lectures dealing with accessibility. Additional semi-structured questionnaire-based interviews with the responsible teachers completed our data.

Second, we asked 65 architects to participate in our online survey to evaluate their existing knowledge about accessibility and ambient assisted living systems (AAL). The study was completed in the third step by an evaluation of the further trainings about accessibility that took place in the last 3 years.

2.1 Education of Architecture Students at the Nine Leading Technical Universities in Germany

At first, the research was carried out at the faculties of architecture of TU9 to determine the importance of accessible and age-appropriate buildings in their curriculums during the summer semester 2012 until winter semester 2014.

TU9 is the alliance of leading Institutes of Technology in Germany, which includes RWTH Aachen University, TU Berlin, TU Braunschweig, TU Darmstadt, TU Dresden, Leibniz Universität Hannover, Karlsruhe Institute of Technology (KIT), TU Munich and University of Stuttgart. The study took a closer look at the official websites of the faculties of architecture which introduced their study guides, lesson plans and module contents. A keyword search, including the terms accessibility, inclusive design, housing, older adults, intergenerational equity and multi-generation, was used to help to identify the lectures dealing with these topics. Moreover, the attendance figures gave assumptions about the lectures' attractiveness.

Additional information (study guides, lesson plans and module contents) about the last semesters was handed in inter alia by the study course coordinators. Questionnaire-based interviews with the responsible teachers achieved the comparability of the statements. Furthermore, each basic questionnaire was complemented by specific questions about the particular university and the personal view on accessibility of the teachers.

At faculty level: The evaluation of the analysis showed that only two of the TU9 have a chair for healthcare buildings and design:

1. TU Berlin, Chair of Architecture for Health.
2. TU Dresden, Chair for Social and Healthcare Buildings and Design.

Although the University of Stuttgart has no specific chair for healthcare buildings and design, it has a close link with the social studies and architecture department at the Institute Housing and Design (IWE). Therefore, the accessibility and inclusive design are principles in teaching and design tasks at the IWE.

At other universities, minor elective modules or individual seminars are devoted to the subject (Table 1). Specialised courses often refer to other topics such as energy-efficient construction. In many cases, the chairs of building construction and design anchor the specialties of accessible construction in their teaching, as it is the case at the RWTH Aachen University, TU Berlin or TU Munich. Until 2013, the *Competence Centre for accessible planning and design* existed in addition to the regular education programme at TU Berlin.

Courses teaching the basics of accessibility and inclusive design are only mandatory for the students at the TU Dresden and the University of Stuttgart.

At student level: At every university, there are a few students who work intensively with the issue during their basic studies. Although the courses relating to the issue are very well attended and accepted by the students, not all of the TU9 seem to have recognised the importance and potential of the subject.

The results of the research point out an underrepresented role of accessible architecture in the teaching agenda of architecture faculties at the TU9. It seems to be an unattractive topic for the teaching architects. The interviews suggested that the following issues might be the reasons for such a situation:

1. Whether semester design projects focus on accessibility, therefore, depends on the interests and skills of the academic mentors. The lectures dealing with inclusive design and accessibility often arise out of personal interests of academic staff (RWTH Aachen University, TU Munich and University of Stuttgart) or from a personal contact between professors and research associate and lecturers

Table 1 Survey about education of architecture students at TU9 in Germany

	TU Dresden	TU Berlin	TU Braunschweig	TU Munich	RWTH Aachen University	Karlsruhe Institute of Technology	University of Stuttgart	TU Darmstadt	Leibniz Universität Hannover
Chair for healthcare buildings and design	X	X							
Outstanding offers							X		
Courses offered by lecturers or honorary professors			X	X				X	
Minor elective modules		X	X		X	X			
Mandatory courses (basics)	X						X		
Mandatory courses (design course related)		X						X	

(TU Darmstadt and TU Munich), so that after retirement (TU Darmstadt), staff turnover or completing a teaching assignment (TU Munich, TU Berlin: *Competence Centre for accessible planning and design*) the courses are not continued.
2. Due to the shortened education as one part of the Bologna Process, there is less space for lectures focusing on accessibility. This raises the question how the fundamental knowledge of accessible construction and design for older adults can be integrated into the shortened bachelor studies.
3. Teaching assignments that address accessibility in small modules or seminars can barely cover basic education and do not reach all of the students since they are often optional.
4. Interdisciplinary cooperation projects rarely take place in education due to the lack of communication during the scheduling process. However, during the research at some universities of the TU9 (i.e. RWTH Aachen University, TU Berlin, TU Braunschweig, TU Dresden and KIT), the interdisciplinary teams emerge. The University of Stuttgart takes a special position in this case by linking the teaching of housing and design with the department of sociology of architecture and housing.
5. There is a lack of outstanding architectural projects considering this topic that could be shown in lectures as best practice examples. Scientific journals intensely used by teachers and students also lack articles focusing on best practice examples dealing with accessibility.

The participants of the interviews emphasise the importance of the general education of architects where inclusive design has no special position, but should be taught by all teachers. So far, however, this is not the case at any university of TU9.

2.2 Existing Knowledge of Architects

The online survey examined whether and how architects consider specific user requirements such as the ones of older adults in their practical work. This survey should serve as a guide to assess the skills of practicing architects in the field of accessibility, building for older adults and ambient assisted living systems (AAL). The online survey was sent to the Architectural Associations of the federal states of Germany with the request for publication and subsequent distribution. Participants were invited by e-mail and informed about the study's goal.

The survey was subdivided into four parts:

1. general data,
2. knowledge and expertise on accessibility and inclusive design,
3. accessibility in planning and practice and
4. accessibility—aims and visions.

In total, 65 architects completed the survey, including 28 office leaders, 31 employees (14 as registered members at the Architectural Association), five self-employed architects and one participant who made no reference to his/her professional status. 46% of the participants acquired many years of experience (more than 16 years), no special qualifications and also never attended a further training on accessible architecture.

Only 17% of the 65 participating architects stated that they had 'excellent' expertise in the field of accessibility and building for older adults. The majority (52%) described their knowledge as 'good'. Almost a third gave 'fair' and a small group (3%) 'poor' or 'very poor' as an answer (Fig. 1).

When asked whether accessibility is attractive for architects, 80% answered 'no'. The arguments range from the high-cost factors to the need of additional construction requirements and the restrictive planning regulations to aesthetic design issues. The result is comparable to the result of the research in Flanders (Belgium) where they interviewed one group of participants from 10 different architecture firms (Van der Linden et al. 2016).

According to the survey, DIN standards (German industry norm) and other regulations were greatly used as the resources of information on accessible construction. Other resources included the relevant literature, the Internet and the best practice projects. Only very few architects would call planning specialists on inclusive design, as they, according to their answers, already owned the adequate skills themselves (Fig. 2).

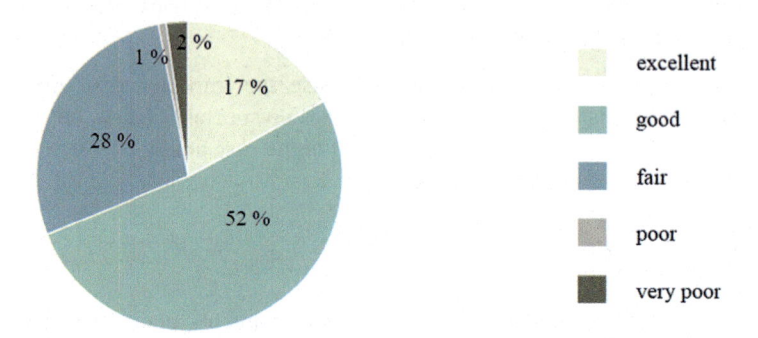

Fig. 1 Evaluation of answers to the question, 'How do you evaluate your knowledge of building for older adults and disabled people?'

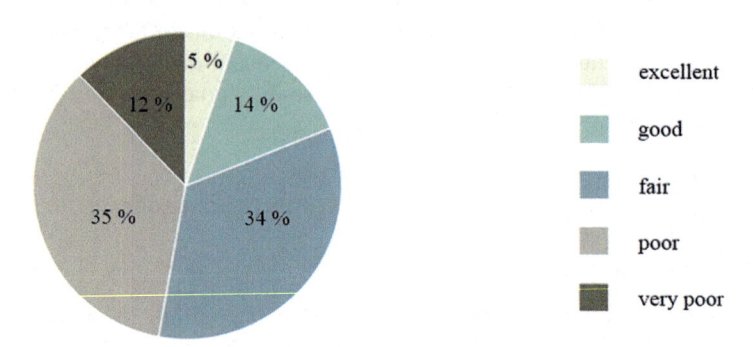

Fig. 2 Evaluation of answers to the question: 'How do you evaluate your knowledge of AAL systems?'

Raising awareness of the clients was regarded by 56% of the participants as the most important reason towards the planning of demographically sustainable buildings. It is stated that these clients have a negative attitude to accessibility due to the fear of additional costs and disinterest.

The knowledge of AAL is to be regarded as insufficient among architects. Only 19% stated that they have 'excellent' or 'good' knowledge about it. The majority (84%) has used none of these technical systems in construction projects yet. According to the survey results, this was mainly due to the lack of project tasks emphasising on the needs of older adults (56%), the lack of knowledge about planning with AAL systems (27%) and their high construction costs (19%). In particular, the access to expertise and information about AAL are desired more than the training, the best practice projects or the literature. Furthermore, the interview results suggest that architects want to be informed via newsletters or online information.

Overall, the survey confirmed the assumption that architects dislike dealing with the issues of accessibility. It is perceived as a negative connotation associated with illness, old age and disability, but also as a restrain to aesthetic design possibilities. Therefore, it is important to break down prejudices among architects and change their views towards a holistic, inclusive understanding of design that takes the needs of every generation into account. One way to achieve this goal is to invite people with disabilities to the teaching course so that they can attract attention to their requirements for a better understanding and consideration during the planning process for further architects (Vermeersch and Heylighen 2015), Fig. (3).

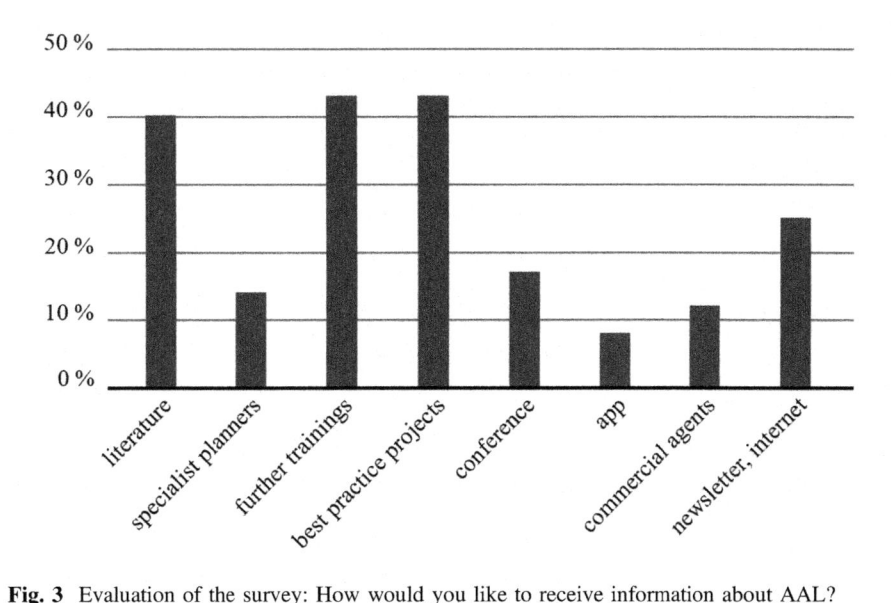

Fig. 3 Evaluation of the survey: How would you like to receive information about AAL?

2.3 Further Training of Architects

In practice, architects have to realise the accessibility in private and public building projects due to its anchoring in building regulations of the federal states of Germany (e.g. MBO § 50). In recent years, an amendment to the relevant DIN standards (DIN 18040 parts 1, 2 and 3) for accessibility took place, so that Architectural Associations offered further trainings.

At the Architectural Associations of the federal states of Germany, the following data were surveyed:

- date,
- title,
- brief description,
- organiser,
- speakers,
- type and
- number of participants of the events offered on the subject of accessibility from 2012 to 2014.

Even though a lot of courses were very well attended and sometimes overbooked; some others were cancelled due to a lack of interest. This lack of interest is assumed to be linked to the relevance of the content, the cost factors and the time. In order to make a statement about the proportion of the architects, which are developing their knowledge of accessibility, the latest numbers of architects registered at the Architectural Associations was requested from the Association of German Architects. Considering the number of members of all federal states of Germany (excluding Baden-Wuerttemberg, Hamburg, Saxony-Anhalt and Thuringia), only 1.5%—1149 out of 78,778 registered architects—continued their education in this topic. The percentage would possibly be higher since not all of the listed members of the Architectural Association are actually working as architects in the construction industry.

3 Conclusions

In sum, it can be stated that the accessibility and demographically sustainable planning should be a part of the general education in architecture. At the same time, architecture teachers, who are dealing with this topic long-term, are needed. In such a way the latest developments, trends, as well as the research, can be integrated into the teaching process.

Although the Validation Organization for Study Programmes Architecture and Planning (ASAP) demands: 'By the end of their studies students should have acquired skills in designing, planning and construction as well as knowledge and skills that enable them to fulfil their role as generalists and coordinate interdisciplinary program aims. Because this competence distinguishes architects from other providers of services in the field of built environment [...]' (ASAP 2013). The Association of German Architects also supports this request (BDA 2014). In the accreditation guidelines and content requirements of the leading agencies (ASAP, ASIN, ACQUIN and ZEVA) for the development of specialised criteria and assuring the quality of architectural education, a concrete anchoring of the competence to plan accessible buildings suitable for all generations is still missing.

An important step towards a self-evident integration of accessibility in the German architecture education would be its specific mention in the accreditation catalogue for courses in architecture. Future architects should develop an understanding of demography that includes not only '[an] understanding of the live cycle of materials, issues of ecological sustainability [or] the impact on the environment [...].' (ASAP 2013) but also the changes in requirements and needs of the occupants.

Formulations for learning skills such as '[an] understanding of the social context in which building projects originate, in relation to ergonomic and space requirements and issues of equality and access' (ASAP 2013) should be clarified. They should include the basics of an accessible environment. At international level, in the 'UNESCO-UIA Charter on architectural education', it has also clearly defined statements about accessibility do not exist (UIA 2011, 2014).

Attractive training offers for demographically sustainable planning, which also deal with the latest and aesthetically best examples from practice, are useful in any case. The content has mostly not been taught during the studies. It is yet to investigate how the contents of further trainings should be designed to attract and achieve a large number of participating architects. However, the basic knowledge should be taught during the studies and then supplemented and deepened by further education and training in practice.

Further research influenced by international research is needed on how knowledge transfer of accessibility should take place in Germany. Data about how Universities of applied science and arts (Fachhochschulen) deal with the topic of accessibility in teaching do not exist.

According to the German HOAI (Fee Structure for Architects and Engineers), German architects have to inform and consult their customers about the importance of accessibility. As a consequence, German architects should integrate the topic as a natural part into their planning process and attribute it a higher priority. If during the later use of the building structural barriers are constituted as insurmountable, the costs of necessary restructuring measures will be even higher—especially in relation to the costs that would have occurred during the new construction.

Architects should contribute to their social responsibility to convey the importance of the topic to their respective clients. Another important measure lies in the sensitisation of authorities, who often refuse inclusive design, according to the statements of the survey participants.

There is also a lack of knowledge during the architecture education in Germany, which is, how to transfer the best practice, including their design concepts and aesthetic standards. This also requires more cooperation from journals and other publications. Specialist standard reference, journals and other publications should give more space to this subject and publish it regularly rather than as a special topic. International research should also be taken into account.

The technical planners or the producers should present information on new ambient assisted living systems in a well-prepared and understandable way.

Acknowledgements The interdisciplinary research project MATI: Mensch—Architektur—Technik—Interaktion für demografische Nachhaltigkeit (human—architecture—technology—interaction for demographic sustainability) (MATI) was funded by the Federal Ministry of Education and Research (BMBF). The authors thank the participating universities, professors, teachers and architects for sharing their time and insights and the TU Dresden for supporting the research.

References

ASAP (2013) Fachliche Kriterien für die Akkreditierung von Studiengängen der Architektur. 5. Auflage. Berlin: ASAP. http://www.asap-akkreditierung.de/dateien/dokumente/de/fachliche_kriterien_architekur_5._ueberarbeitete_auflage_2013.pdf. Accessed 28 Aug 2017

BDA (ed) (2014) Zur Ausbildung der Architekten. Thesen des 1. BDA Hochschultags der Architektur. BDA, Berlin, Germany

UIA (2011) UNESCO/UIA Charta für die Ausbildung von Architekten. Überarbeitete Fassung 2011. UIA Architects, Paris, France. http://www.uia-architectes.org/sites/default/files/GERMAN_CHAR_2011_0.pdf. Accessed 28 Aug 2017

UIA (2014) UIA accord on recommended international standards of professionalism in architectural practice. Amended August 2014 at the XXVI general assembly (Durban, South Africa). http://www.uia-architectes.org/sites/default/files/UIAAccordEN.pdf. Accessed 28 Aug 2017

Van der Linden V, Dong H, Heylighen A (2016) From accessibility to experience: opportunities for inclusive design in architectural practice. Nord J Architectural Res 28(2):33–58

Vermeersch P, Heylighen A (2015) Mobilizing disability experience to inform architectural practice. Lessons learned from a field study. J Res Pract 11(2):1–27

Author Index

A
Alwani, R., 3
Alyami, R., 227
Amanatidis, T., 207
Annemans, M., 215

B
Bichard, J., 3
Bradley, M., 65
Bradley, O., 65
Bridge, C., 101
Bueter, K., 125

C
Carmien, S., 89
Chakraborty, J., 263
Choi, Y. M., 29
Clarkson, P. J., 17, 41, 65, 195, 207

D
Danschutter, S., 159
Darzentas, J. S., 89
Deroisy, B., 159
Dickerson, T., 195

F
Ferati, M., 135

G
Giannoumis, G. A., 135
Goodman-Deane, J., 41, 65

H
Heitor, T. V., 77
Heylighen, A., 77, 215

J
Jellema, P., 215

K
Karam, M., 51
Kevdzija, M., 147
Kirch, J., 125
Kreiser, S., 275
Krivonos, D., 135

L
Langdon, P. M., 17, 41, 51, 181, 207
Lazar, J., 171
Liu, Y., 195

M
Marquardt, G., 125, 147
Moody, W., 51
Morris, J., 113
Mouzakitis, A., 17

N
Nguyen, N., 263

P
Pandya, U., 135
Pereira, C. M., 77
Persad, U., 41
Petrie, H., 89
Pey, T., 135

R
Raby, E., 3
Rode, J. A., 239
Rodgers, P. A., 251
Rudolph, E., 275

S
Skrypchuk, L., 17
Spencer, J., 3
Strickfaden, M., 181

W
Waddingham, P., 195
Wallace, T., 113
Waller, S. D., 65, 195

Wei, H., 227
West, J., 3
Winton, E., 251